Fetal Heart Rate Monitoring

FIFTH EDITION

AF704626

EDITORS

Alison G. Cahill, MD, MSCI

Associate Dean of Translational Research
Professor, Department of Women's Health
Director, Dell Medical School Health Transformation Research Institute
University of Texas at Austin, Dell Medical School
Austin, Texas

Nandini Raghuraman, MD, MSCI

Assistant Professor, Division of Maternal-Fetal Medicine
MFM Fellowship Program Director
Chief, Division of Clinical Research
Department of Obstetrics and Gynecology
Washington University, St. Louis

Wolters Kluwer

Philadelphia • Baltimore • New York • London
Buenos Aires • Hong Kong • Sydney • Tokyo

Acquisitions Editor: Chris Teja, Nicole Dernoski
Development Editor: Cindy Yoo
Editorial Coordinator: Anju Radhakrishnan
Marketing Manager: Kirsten Watrud
Production Project Manager: Frances Gunning
Manager, Graphic Arts & Design: Stephen Druding
Art Director, Illustration: Jennifer Clements
Manufacturing Coordinator: Lisa Bowling
Prepress Vendor: Lumina Datamatics Ltd.

Fifth Edition

9 8 7 6 5 4 3 2 1

Printed in Mexico

Library of Congress Cataloging-in-Publication Data

ISBN-13: 978-1-9752-1618-4

Cataloging in Publication data available on request from publisher.

shop.lww.com

QUADM1124

The authors dedicate this book in the hope that an in-depth, physiologically oriented understanding of electronic fetal heart rate monitoring (EFM) will result not only in the best possible outcome for babies and mothers but also in an understanding of the limits of this technology. Fetal heart rate (FHR) monitoring is after all a diagnostic, not a therapeutic, device, and no thermometer, EKG, or other diagnostic tool can do more than give us better information and help us make better decisions. It cannot in and of itself improve outcomes. The unrealistic expectations that EFM has created and the frequency of abnormal FHR patterns have together led to a labor and delivery environment that is one of high anxiety, for both patients and their caregivers. Clearly, EFM very accurately identifies the fetus that is well oxygenated (category I patterns) and the fetus with hypoxia sufficient to result in death or damage (category III patterns), but the challenge continues to identify those patterns that will deteriorate and without timely intervention may lead to category III patterns. We hope that with a better understanding of EFM, we are not only able to optimize outcomes and understand the limits of this technology but also to react more appropriately—minimizing interventions and making the labor and delivery unit the happy, fulfilling environment it should be.

Contributors

Katherine H. Campbell, MD, MPH
Associate Professor
Obstetrics, Gynecology, & Reproductive Sciences
Yale School of Medicine
New Haven, Connecticut

Aaron Caughey, MD, MPP, MPH, PhD
Professor and Chair
Obstetrics and Gynecology
Oregon Health & Science University
Portland, Oregon

Suneet Chauhan, MD
Professor and Director, Maternal-Fetal Medicine Division Principal Investigator, Eunice Kennedy Shriver NICHD Maternal-Fetal Medicine Units Network
Department of Obstetrics, Gynecology, & Reproductive Sciences
McGovern Medical School-UTHealth
Houston, Texas

Ngina K. Connors, MD, MBA
Chair, Department of Obstetrics and Gynecology
Obstetrics and Gynecology
Atrium Health
Charlotte, North Carolina

Heather Frey, MD, MSCI
Associate Professor
Obstetrics and Gynecology
The Ohio State University College of Medicine
Columbus, Ohio

Antonina Frolova, MD, PhD
Assistant Professor
Obstetrics and Gynecology
Washington University in St. Louis
Saint Louis, Missouri

Christy Gandhi, BA, MD
Maternal Fetal Medicine Clinical Fellow
Department of Obstetrics & Gynecology
Columbia University
New York, New York

Anna Graseck, MD, MSCI
Assistant Professor
Obstetrics and Gynecology
University of Pennsylvania
Philadelphia, Pennsylvania

Josiah Hawkins, MD, MBA
Assistant Professor
Department of Obstetrics & Gynecology
UT Southwestern Medical Center
Dallas, Texas

Scott Infusino, MD
Fellow
Maternal Fetal Medicine
University of Wisconsin Hospitals and Clinics
Madison, Wisconsin

Christian M. Pettker, MD
Professor
Obstetrics, Gynecology, & Reproductive Sciences
Yale School of Medicine
New Haven, Connecticut

Patrick S. Ramsey, MD, MSPH
Professor and Chief, Division of Maternal-Fetal Medicine
Obstetrics & Gynecology
University of Texas Health Science Center at San Antonio
San Antonio, Texas

Uma M. Reddy, MD, MPH
Professor and Vice Chair of Research
Obstetrics and Gynecology
Columbia University
New York, New York

Janine Rhoades, MD
Assistant Professor
Obstetrics and Gynecology
University of Wisconsin School of Medicine and Public Health
Madison, Wisconsin

Joshua I. Rosenbloom, MD, MPH
Attending Physician
Obstetrics and Gynecology
Hadassah Hebrew University Medical Center
Jerusalem, Israel

Catherine Spong, MD
Tenured Professor and Chair
Obstetrics and Gynecology
University of Texas Southwestern Medical Center
Dallas, Texas

Lorene Atkins Temming, MD, MSCI
Assistant Professor
Obstetrics and Gynecology
Atrium Health Wake Forest University School of Medicine
Charlotte, North Carolina

Lauren Theilen, MD, MSCI
Assistant Professor
Obstetrics and Gynecology
University of Utah
Salt Lake City, Utah

Xiao-Yu Wang, MD
Fellow
Maternal Fetal Medicine
Ohio State University
Columbus, Ohio

Rachel Wiley, MD, MPH
Maternal Fetal Medicine Fellow
Department of Obstetrics and Gynecology
University of California San Diego
San Diego, California

Oxana Zarudskaya, MD, PhD
Physician
Obstetrics and gynecology
University of Texas Health Science Center at San Antonio
San Antonio, Texas

Preface

With inspiration, scholarly commitment, background, and experience in the scientific basis and technology of fetal heart rate (FHR) monitoring, Dr. Roger K. Freeman revered and recognized expert in the field, along with his first partner, Dr. Thomas J. Garite, embarked on the creation of the first and foremost textbook in FHR monitoring in 1981. They dedicated this first edition to the founding fathers of FHR monitoring, Dr. Edward Hon and Dr. Edward Qulligan. After the publication of this first edition, Dr. Michael P. Nageotte joined as the third author. This second edition and subsequently the third and fourth became the well-known and leading textbook on the subject. In the fourth and last edition published in 2003, Lisa A. Miller, CNM, JD, was added as the fourth and final author. This book is also unique as it originally included only the primary authors. The textbook also became the backbone of many teaching conferences that Dr. Freeman, Dr. Garite, Dr. Nageotte, and Ms. Miller conducted around the country.

FHR monitoring is a complex and inexact science with the goal of detecting the absence of fetal hypoxia and acidosis. We emphasize the ABSENCE, as this is where the technology is most accurate and irrefutable. Knowing the fetus is not suffering from intrapartum hypoxia allows the attendant to be reassured and not interfere with the normal process of labor and delivery. Unfortunately, the FHR often exhibits changes that make the determination of the presence and severity of hypoxia, its evolution to acidosis, and the need to intervene a complex and difficult process. This is exactly where the need for this textbook became evident and provided the reader with the most thorough and scientifically based knowledge to process and understand this more difficult aspect of evaluating the nuances of FHR patterns.

Now we are grateful that the most prominent expert in FHR monitoring and the effects of hypoxia on the fetus before and during labor, Dr. Alison G. Cahill and her colleague, Dr. Nandini Raghuraman, have taken on the process of continuing the publication of our textbook. Dr. Cahill's studies on the many aspects of the determination of hypoxia and acidosis using FHR monitoring as well as the understanding the effects of hypoxia and acidosis and its severity and duration have added substantially to our understanding of and ability to continue to use this technology in everyday Obstetrics. We are so very pleased that she, Dr. Raghuraman and the contributing authors, all well-recognized experts in this field, have agreed to lead the effort of sustaining this important series of this textbook that lasted over 22 years. The format of the chapters has largely been retained.

We are extremely thankful that this updated, expert revision will now be available for physicians, nurses, midwives, and other related healthcare professionals to enable them to provide the best care possible to insure the health of our mothers and babies through pregnancy, labor, and delivery, the newborn period, and beyond.

Roger K. Freeman, MD
Retired
Long Beach, California

Thomas J. Garite, MD
Professor and Chairman Emeritus
Obstetrics and Gynecology
University of California
Irvine, California

Michael P. Nageotte
Medical Degree
Associate Chief Medical Officer, Miller Children and Women's Hospital, Long Beach
Maternal-Fetal Medicine
Miller Children's and Women's Hospital
Long Beach, California

Lisa A. Miller, RN, BSN, CNM, JD
Nurse Educator
Self-employed
Perinatal Risk Management & Education Services
Vancouver, Washington

Contents

CHAPTER 1

History of Fetal Monitoring

Oxana Zarudskaya and Patrick S. Ramsey

The ability to hear the fetal heart was not described until the 17th century when Phillipe LeGaust first depicted fetal heart tones in his poetry in an ancient French dialect. LeGaust was a colleague of Marsac, a physician of the province of Limousin, who is credited with first having heard the fetal heart. Marsac's observation, however, went unnoticed until 1818, when Swiss surgeon Francois Mayor reported the presence of fetal heart sounds when he placed his ear on the maternal abdomen in an attempt to hear the fetus splash about in the liquor amnii. Three years later, the French nobleman Lejumeau Kergaradec, apparently unaware of Mayor's report, described both the fetal heart tones and the uterine souffle. He suggested auscultation to be of value in the diagnosis in singleton and twin pregnancy and in determining fetal lie and presentation.

As with many discoveries, the obstetricians of the time were slow to respond to Kergaradec's observations and recommendations. To convince clinicians of the value of Kergaradec's findings, Evory Kennedy of Dublin published an extensive book in 1833, *Observations on Obstetric Auscultation*.[1] The text contains many anecdotal examples of cases in which auscultation was clearly beneficial. In addition, Kennedy described the funic souffle for the first time.

THE FETOSCOPE

Before the development of the fetoscope, much attention was paid to whether mediate (stethoscopic) auscultation, using Laennec's instrument, or immediate auscultation, with direct application of the ear to the gravid maternal abdomen, was the more appropriate choice. Rauth, quoted in Hirst,[2] suggested vaginal stethoscopy as more valuable in the early detection of fetal life. The development of the head stethoscope (fetoscope) is a story of controversy and professional jealousy. It was first reported, in 1917, in *The Journal of the American Medical Association* (Fig. 1.1), by David Hillis,[3] an obstetrician then working in Chicago Lying-In Hospital. In 1922, J. B. DeLee,[4] who was chief of staff at the same institution and who became a legend in American obstetrics for many contributions, published his report of a similar instrument. Although

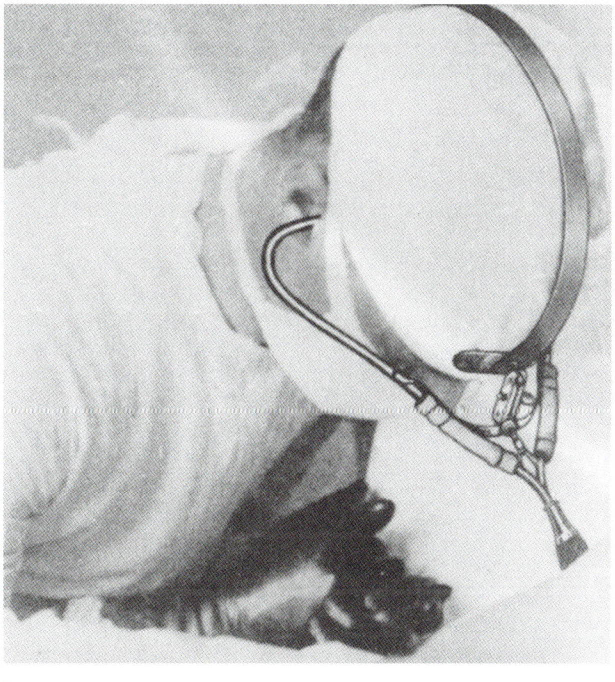

Figure 1.1. The original illustration of the head stethoscope or fetoscope. (From Hillis DS. Attachment for the stethoscope. *JAMA*. 1917;68(12):910.)

the order of publications was clear, DeLee claimed that he openly talked of this idea for many years preceding the Hillis publication. The instrument, which subsequently came to be known as the DeLee-Hillis stethoscope, has changed little since its early development.

DIAGNOSIS OF FETAL DISTRESS

Thirty years after Mayor first described heart sounds, Kilian, quoted in Goodlin,[5] first proposed that changes in the fetal heart rate (FHR) might be used to diagnose fetal distress and to indicate when the clinician should intervene on behalf of the fetus. He formulated what is sometimes called "the stethoscopal indication for forceps delivery" and suggested that heart rates below 100 or above 180 beats per minute (bpm) and those with loss of purity of tone or distinct intermission, or in which only one tone could be heard, were indications for forceps application without delay. In 1893, Von Winckel[6] described the criteria of fetal distress, which were to remain essentially unchanged until the arrival of fetal scalp sampling and electronic heart rate monitoring: tachycardia (heart rate >160 bpm), bradycardia (heart rate <100 bpm), irregular heart rate, passage of meconium, and gross alteration of fetal movement. Few studies either challenged or supported the validity of these auscultative and clinical criteria for fetal distress. It was not until 1968, when Benson et al[7] published the results of the Collaborative Project, commissioned by the National Institute of Neurologic Diseases and Blindness, bringing these criteria under serious scrutiny. The Benson study reviewed the benefits of FHR auscultation in the management of intrapartum fetal distress in 24,863 deliveries. Benson concluded that there was "no reliable indicator of fetal distress in terms of fetal heart rate save in extreme degree." Ten years earlier, Hon[8] asked 15 obstetricians to count several rates from audiotape. He found a wide divergence in counting and pointed out the unreliability of human computation of the FHR (Fig. 1.2).

As new information has emerged, the term fetal distress has been determined as an inappropriate term to describe FHR patterns that may be associated with decreases in fetal oxygenation. Because a large proportion of such patterns do not result in neonates with signs of fetal hypoxia and/or acidosis, the term "nonreassuring FHR pattern" has been adopted to refer to such tracings. In addition, the original recommendations for intervention based on periodic FHR patterns alone are undergoing an evolution in which the presence of spontaneous or evoked accelerations, FHR variability, fetal pH, and

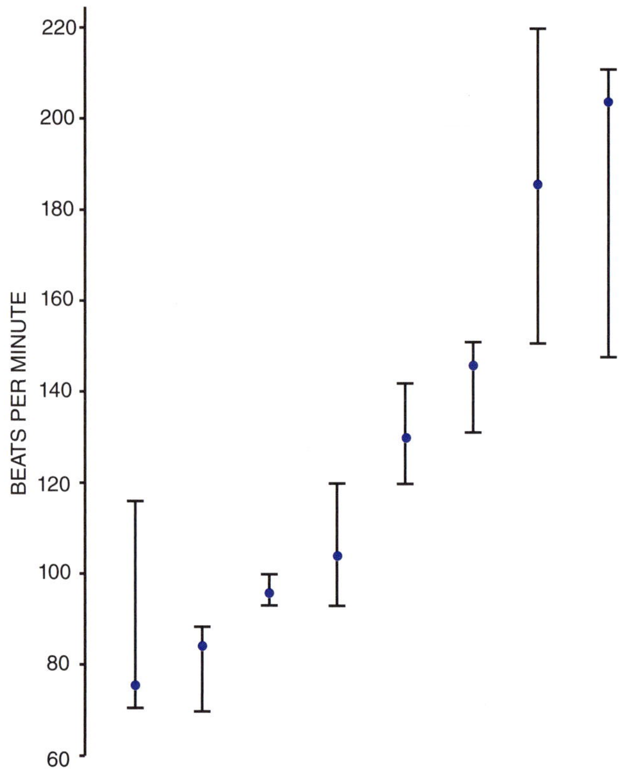

Figure 1.2. Range of error in auscultative counting of fetal heart rate (FHR) by 15 obstetricians asked to count from recorded FHR. Count as reported by obstetrician on vertical scale versus actual count on horizontal scale. (From Hon EH. The electronic evaluation of the FHR. *Am J Obstet Gynecol.* 1958;75(6):1215–1230.)

fetal pulse oximetry allow the clinician to sometimes avoid intervention for nonreassuring patterns. These approaches will be discussed in Chapter 8.

With these serious doubts, and with the age of electronic technology fast making its impact on modern medicine, it was inevitable that obstetric research would turn to more sophisticated methods of fetal evaluation.

THE FETAL ELECTROCARDIOGRAPH

Cremer[9] recorded the FHR electronically for the first time in 1906, by means of abdominal and intravaginal leads. For the first half of the century, the application of fetal electrocardiography was used primarily for the diagnosis of fetal life. It was Southern[10] who, in 1957, suggested that certain changes in fetal electrocardiograph (ECG) might correlate with fetal hypoxia. Shortly thereafter, Hon and Hess[11] reviewed all the applications of fetal electrocardiography, including fetal presentation, diagnosis of twins, antenatal diagnosis of

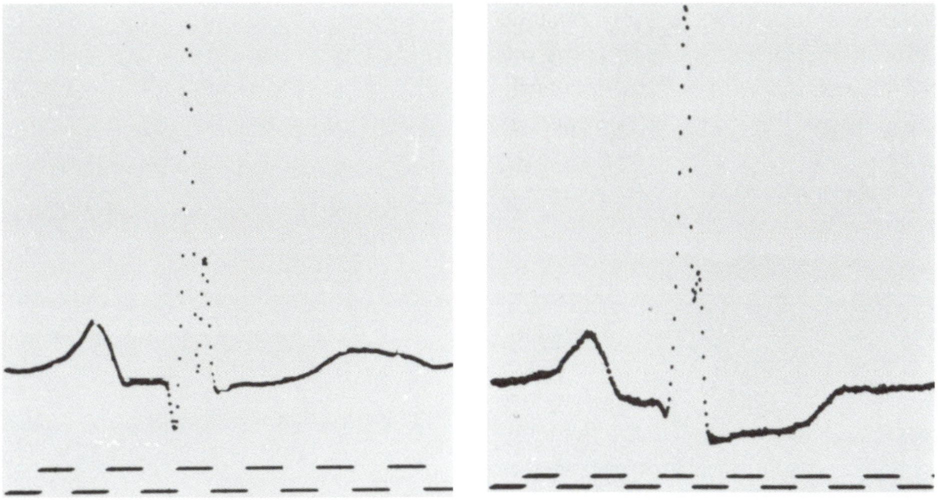

Figure 1.3. **Left:** An average of 25 electrocardiograph (ECG) complexes performed before the onset of a contraction: baseline 160 beats per minute. **Right:** Average of 25 ECG complexes performed immediately after the end of the same contraction, during a late deceleration. Notice the depression of the ST segment. Scalp capillary blood pH 7.34, Apgar score 4/9, umbilical artery pH 7.25. (From Crosignani PG, Pardi G. *Fetal Evaluation during Pregnancy and Labor*. Academic Press; 1971:235.)

congenital heart disease, diagnosis of fetal maturity, and fetal distress. They concluded that the ECG waveform was not of consistent value in any of these situations and, specifically, that in 75 cases of fetal distress, "no consistent fetal ECG changes could be detected." Subsequently, Pardi et al[12] used group-averaging techniques to demonstrate ST segment depression with fetal hypoxia (Fig. 1.3). Unfortunately, this technique has not been developed to the point where it has become clinically applicable.

The history of the development of electronic FHR monitoring, or cardiotachometry, is a complex merger of technologic development with empirical observations of those heart rate patterns associated with various causes of fetal distress.

The earliest preliminary report of FHR monitoring came in 1958 from Edward Hon,[8] then at the Yale University School of Medicine. He reported on the continuous instantaneous recording of FHR via fetal ECG monitor on the maternal abdomen. He began to elucidate the causes of fetal bradycardia and, more specifically, defined when bradycardia was indicative of fetal distress. In the years that followed, Hon, Caldeyro-Barcia in Uruguay, Hammacher in Germany, and their coworkers reported their observations on the various heart rate patterns associated with fetal distress. Bradycardia and tachycardia were well-known signs of fetal compromise. In 1959, Hon[13] defined the type of variable deceleration associated with umbilical cord compression and proposed a mechanism for the hypoxic uteroplacental causes of delayed decelerations. In 1963, Caldeyro-Barcia et al[14] reported their observations on the "prognostic significance" of similar heart rate decelerations, which they called Types II and III. In addition, short- and long-term FHR variability was defined for the first time. Hammacher[15] subsequently described this parameter's significance in terms of loss of heart rate variability in association with fetal distress.

With many investigators throughout the world making similar observations, FHR terminology became extremely confusing. Hon, Caldeyro-Barcia, and many of their colleagues met at an international conference on monitoring of the fetal heart in December 1971 in New Jersey and in March 1972 in Amsterdam to discuss nomenclature and develop standards for FHR monitoring. They developed and agreed upon a common nomenclature. Efforts were made to agree upon universal scales and paper speed for fetal monitors, but these remained variable. Much of the subsequent history has been one technological development for the clinical application of electronic FHR monitoring. The first practical commercially available fetal monitor to be of clinical use was produced by Hammacher and Hewlett-Packard in 1968 using external tocography and phonocardiography (Fig. 1.4). Before this, monitors were bulky and generally limited to research, although attempts were made to market some equipment for

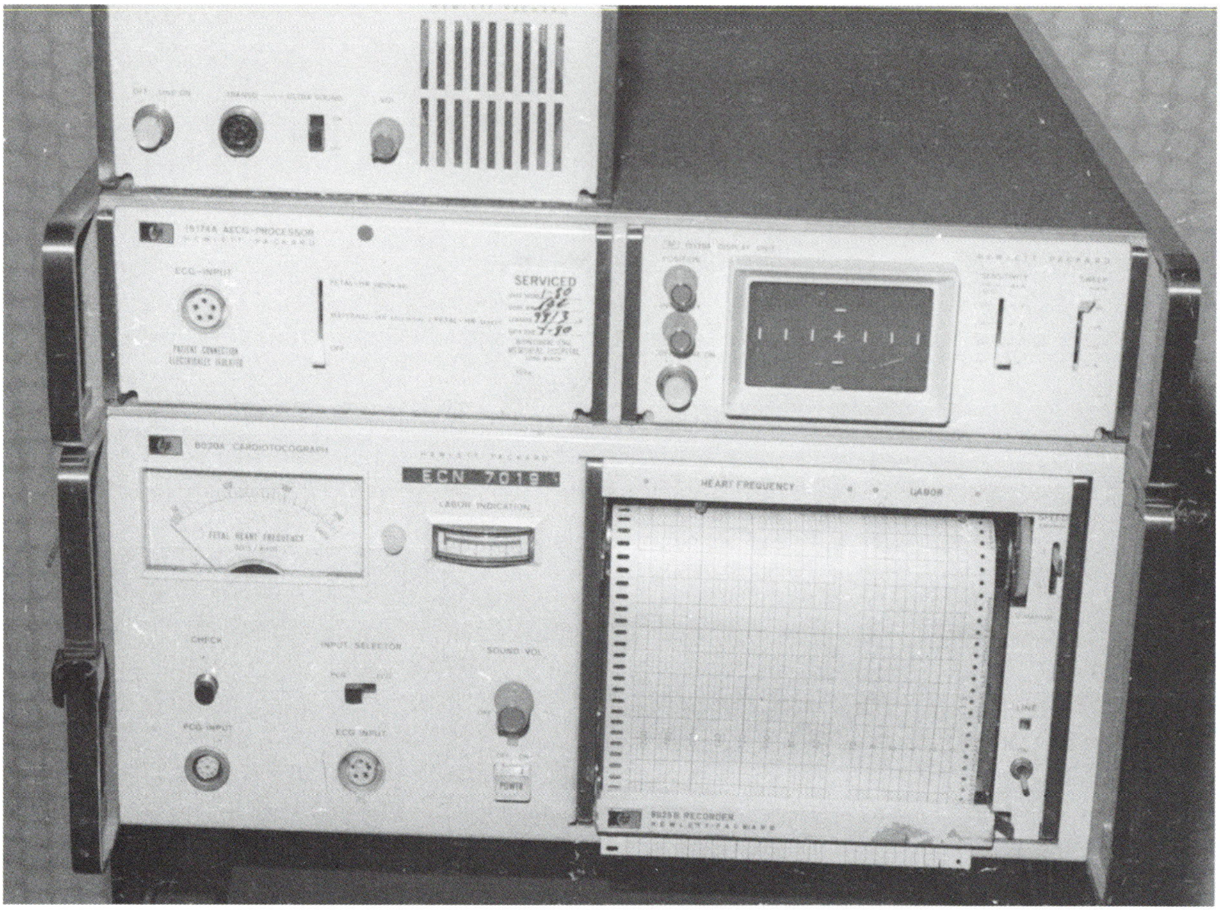

Figure 1.4. The first generation of practical commercially available fetal monitors. The original model used external monitoring with phonocardiography only. The upper two modules were subsequently added, allowing the addition of external ultrasound and internal fetal electrocardiographic monitoring (Hewlett-Packard Model 8020A).

general use (Fig. 1.5). Technological advances since that first generation of fetal monitors have allowed further and more accurate definition of FHR patterns and have provided the clinician with a practical tool.

Direct ECG monitoring was realized with Hon's introduction of an electrode that could be applied directly to the fetal scalp.[16] This was originally a modification of a surgical skin clip (Fig. 1.6). This technique was most famously used in STAN monitors. STAN monitors (Neoventa Medical, Mölndal, Sweden) with an invasive scalp electrode have the capability to measure FHR as well as a derivative for the ST segment of fetal QRS complex. Studies of the sheep fetus showed depression in the ST segment with hypoxia, which became the basis for these monitors. Additional studies demonstrated that the combination of the ST metric with FHR monitoring was better than FHR monitoring alone to reduce the incidence of hypoxic-ischemic encephalopathy and even reduce the incidence of cesarean delivery. However, the main disadvantage with these monitors is the invasive technique.[17] Subsequently, Hon developed a more convenient disposable spiral electrode (Fig. 1.7) that is widely used in the United States. A new device under research and development is the MindChild MERIDIAN monitor. ECG waveforms collected using this noninvasive monitor are being compared with invasive monitoring systems, and initial results are promising.[17] MindChild monitor was approved for clinical use by the FDA in September 2012. Doppler ultrasound and external ECG and logic systems that provide adequate approximations of the real beat-to-beat heart rate have been more recent developments.

Challenges with noninvasive voltage technologies are associated with the need to improve the filtering of noise charges from the mother. Despite the fact that voltage-based technologies are the most active in the fetal monitoring market, developers are working on

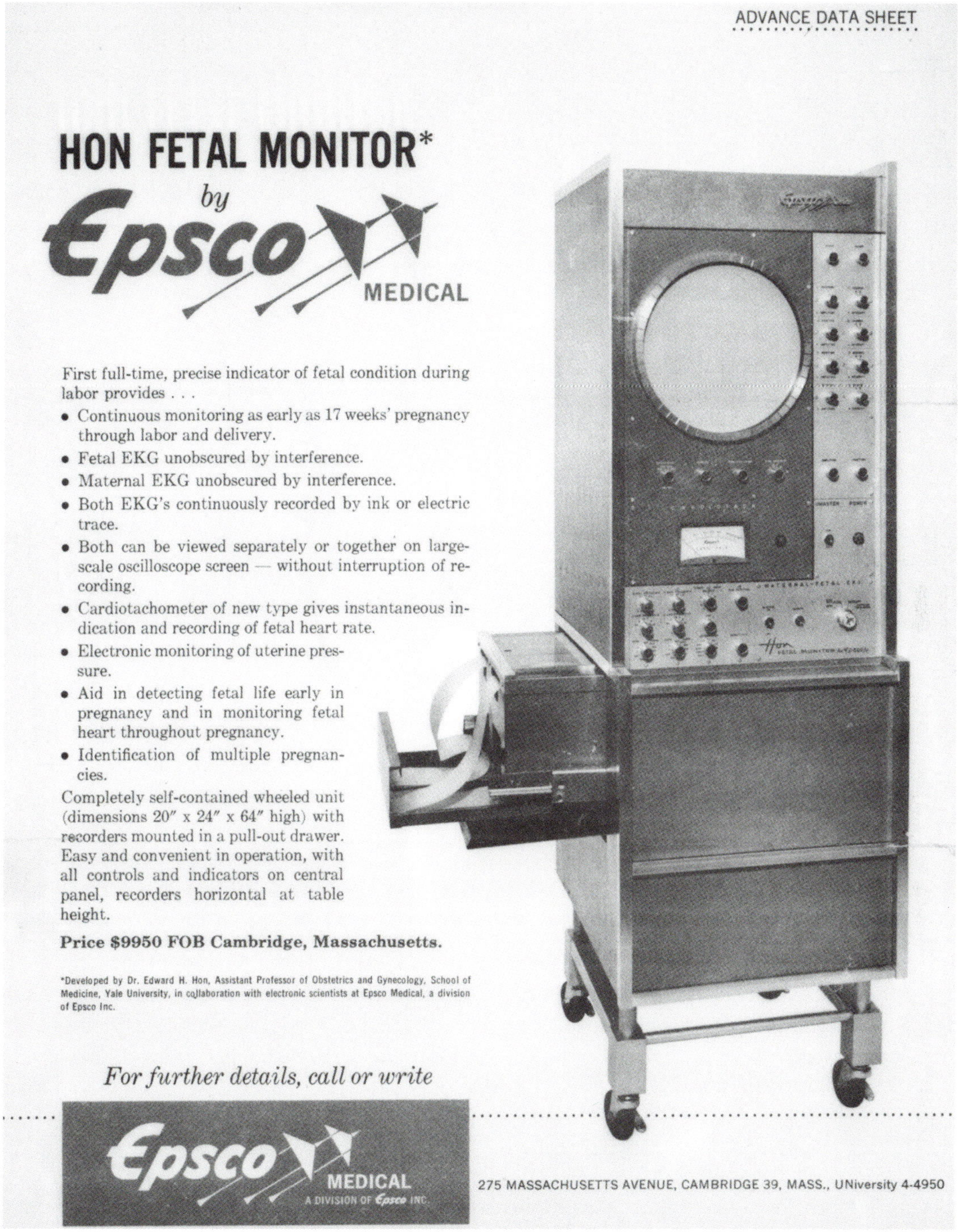

Figure 1.5. This bulky machine was the first attempt at making a commercially available fetal monitor. (Courtesy of Epsco, Inc.)

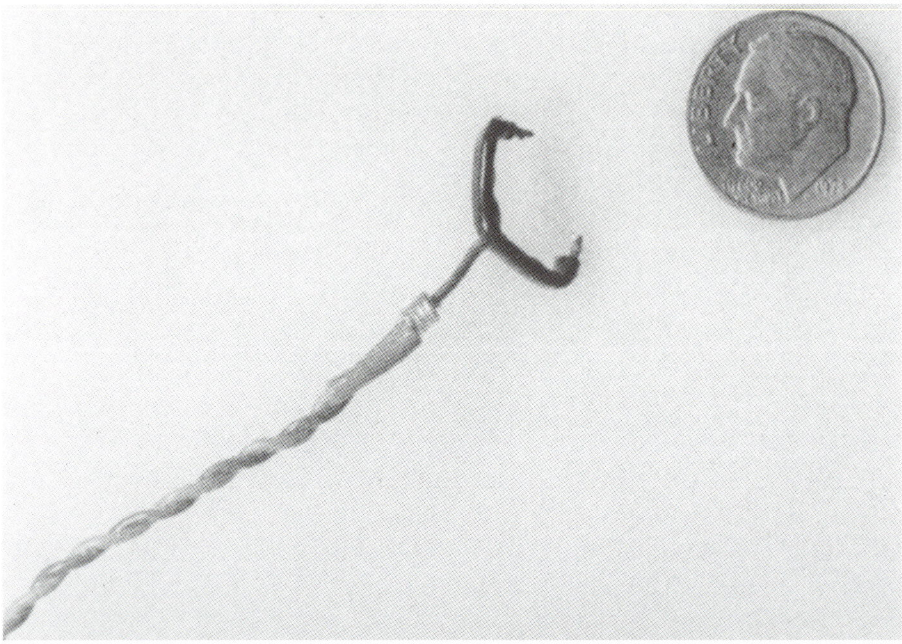

Figure 1.6. Vaginal fetal scalp electrode as described by Dr. Edward Hon.[16] This is a modification of a Michelle surgical skin clip. A specially made long forceps and a vaginal speculum are necessary for application.

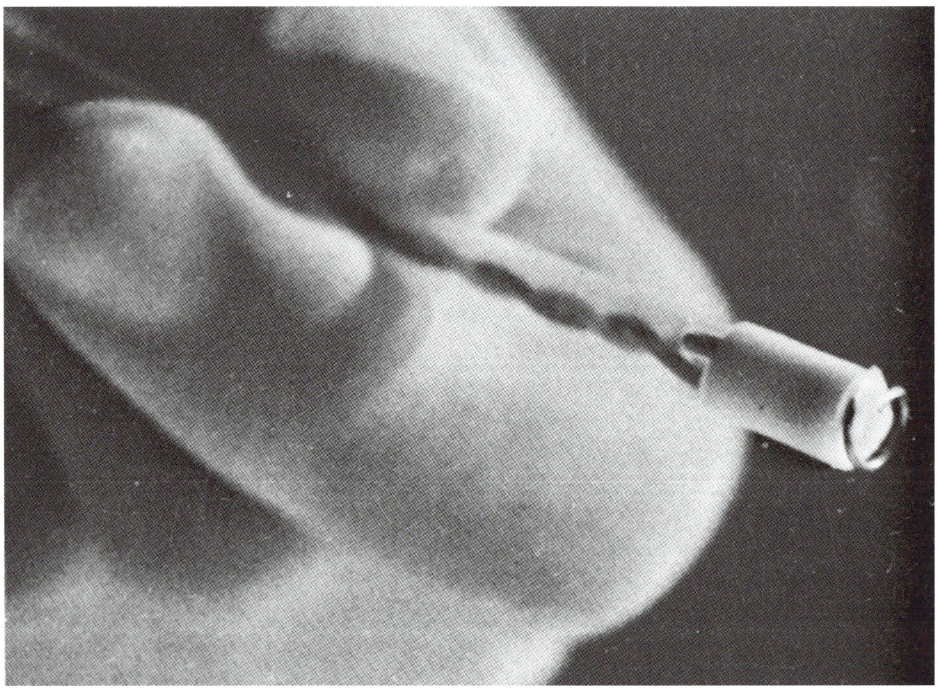

Figure 1.7. A spiral silver–silver chloride fetal scalp electrode described by Hon[17] in 1972. This is packaged within a plastic sheath, which allows direct application without the aid of a speculum.

other technologies as well. Lifewave, Inc. (Los Altos, CA) is building a technology for measuring fetal heart using radar technology (emits a low-energy electromagnetic signal and analyzes the return waveform that has bounced off moving fetal structures to calculate the FHR). This device will potentially be portable and small but is yet to be approved by the FDA. Magnetocardiography and fetal magnetic resonance imaging are also being evaluated to assess fetal cardiac activity, but their role in active labor is questionable owing to the fixed nature of these instruments.[17]

FETAL PULSE OXIMETRY

Another potential adjunct for fetal monitoring during labor is fetal pulse oximetry. This technique uses a probe that sits on the baby's head while in the uterus or in the vagina during labor, and it measures the amount of oxygen being carried by the baby's blood. This tool can act as an adjunct to differentiate the cases that require further investigations like fetal scalp sampling from those that don't[18]; however, initial trials did not demonstrate that knowledge of the fetal oxygen saturation reduces the need for cesarean delivery or improved neonatal outcomes.[19]

ERA OF QUESTIONING

Benson's report on the data collected by the Collaborative Project set the stage for rejection of auscultation and the boom in electronic cardiotachometry. By 1978, it was estimated that fetal monitoring was in routine use in over half of labors.[18] Enthusiasm for its use, however, came without clear documentation of its efficacy and safety. There were many retrospective analyses of fetal monitoring and nearly all agreed to a beneficial effect, including reduction of intrapartum stillbirth rate and perinatal mortality as well as improved Apgar scores.[20-22] Randomized controlled trials have now been reported.[23-26] While mixed, they do not uniformly show electronic monitoring as beneficial and, indeed, suggest that such monitoring may substantially increase the rate of cesarean sections. Details of all these studies and an analysis of the risks and benefits of fetal monitoring are reviewed in Chapter 3. The era of consumer demand in obstetrics, in particular, coupled with a period of heightened government intervention into cost, risks, and benefits of medical care, has provided further impetus for questioning electronic fetal monitoring.

Electronic fetal monitoring has become a common practice for patients during labor. However, further applications will depend on continuing evaluation and adjustment of current methodologies, as well as on the development of new technology. It is clear, however, that the assessment of the human fetus for hypoxia is one end result of the development of electronic FHR monitoring.

REFERENCES

1. Kennedy E. *Observations on Obstetric Auscultation*. Hodges and Smith; 1833.
2. Hirst BC. *An American System of Obstetrics*. Lea Brothers Co.; 1888.
3. Hillis DS. Attachment for the stethoscope. *JAMA*. 1917;68(12):910.
4. DeLee JB. Ein neues Stethoskop, für die Geburtshilfe besonders geeignet. *Zentralbl Gynaekol*. 1922;46:1688.
5. Goodlin RC. History of fetal monitoring. *Am J Obstet Gynecol*. 1979;133(3):325.
6. Von Winckel F. *Lehrbuch der Geburtshilfe*. Wiesbaden; 1893:634.
7. Benson RC, Shubeck F, Deutschberger J, Weiss W, Berendes H. Fetal heart rate as a predictor of fetal distress: a report from the collaborative project. *Obstet Gynecol*. 1968;32(2):529-566.
8. Hon EH. The electronic evaluation of the fetal heart rate. *Am J Obstet Gynecol*. 1958;75(6):1215-1230.
9. Cremer M. *Munch Med Wochenschr*. 1906;53:811.
10. Southern EM. Fetal anoxia and its possible relation to changes in the prenatal fetal electrocardiogram. *Am J Obstet Gynecol*. 1957;73(2):233-247.
11. Hon EH, Hess OW. The clinical value of fetal electrocardiography. *Am J Obstet Gynecol*. 1960;79:1012-1023.
12. Pardi G, Brambati B, Dubini S, Luchetti D, Polvani F, Candiani GB. Analysis of the fetal electrocardiogram by the group-averaging technique. In: *Proceedings of the 2nd European Congress of Perinatal Medicine*. London; 1970.
13. Hon EH. Observations on "pathologic" fetal bradycardia. *Am J Obstet Gynecol*. 1959;77(5):1084-1089.
14. Caldeyro-Barcia R, Mendez-Bauer C, Poseiro JJ, et al. Control of human fetal heart rate during labor. In: Cassels D, ed. *The Heart and Circulation in the Newborn Infant*. Grune & Stratton, Inc.; 1966.
15. Hammacher K. Die kontinuierliche elektronische Überwachung der fetalen Herztätigkeit vor und während der Geburt. In: Kaser O, Friedberg V, Oberk KG, Thomsen K, Zander J, eds. *Gynakologie v Gerburtshilfe BD II*. Georg Thieme, Stuttgart; 1967, p. 793.
16. Hon EH. Instrumental on of fetal heart rate and electrocardiography. II. A vaginal electrode. *Am J Obstet Gynecol*. 1963;86: 772-784.
17. Adam J. The future of fetal monitoring. *Rev Obstet Gynecol*. 2012;5(3-4):e132-e136.
18. Luttkus AK, Dudenhausen JW. Fetal pulse oximetry. *Baillieres Clin Obstet Gynaecol*. 1996;10(2):295-306. doi: 10.1016/s0950-3552(96)80039-3.

19. Bloom SL, Spong CY, Thom E, et al.; National Institute of Child Health and Human Development Maternal-Fetal Medicine Units Network. Fetal pulse oximetry and cesarean delivery. *N Engl J Med.* 2006;355(21):2195-2202.
20. Hon EH, Paul RH, Hon RW. Electronic evaluation of fetal heart rate. XI. Description of a spiral electrode. *Obstet Gynecol.* 1972;40(3):362-365.
21. Williams RL, Hawes WE. Cesarean section, fetal monitoring, and perinatal mortality in California. *Am J Public Health.* 1979; 69(9):864-870.
22. Task Force on Predictors of Fetal Distress, NICHD Consensus Development Committee on Antenatal Diagnosis, NIH Publication 79-1973, 1979.
23. Haverkamp AD, Thompson HE, McFee JG, Cetrulo C. The evaluation of continuous fetal heart rate monitoring in high-risk pregnancy. *Am J Obstet Gynecol.* 1976;125(3):310-320.
24. Renou P, Chang A, Anderson I, Wood C. Controlled trial of fetal intensive care. *Am J Obstet Gynecol.* 1976;126(4):470-476.
25. Kelso IM, Parsons RJ, Lawrence GF, Arora SS, Edmonds DK, Cooke ID. An assessment of continuous fetal heart rate monitoring in labor: a randomized trial. *Am J Obstet Gynecol.* 1978;131(5):526-532.
26. Haverkamp AD, Orleans M, Langendoerfer S, McFee J, Murphy J, Thompson HE. A controlled trial of the differential effects of intrapartum fetal monitoring. *Am J Obstet Gynecol.* 1979; 134(4):399-412.

CHAPTER 2

Physiologic Basis of Fetal Monitoring

Catherine Spong and Josiah Hawkins

INTRODUCTION

The intent of fetal heart rate (FHR) monitoring is surveillance of heart rate patterns with a goal of detecting potential fetal compromise. An understanding of fetal physiology is key to the interpretation of the FHR pattern. This chapter will describe the variables that contribute to normal and abnormal fetal physiology and how these changes are reflected in the FHR pattern.

CELLULAR RESPIRATION

A discussion of the physiology behind electronic fetal monitoring would be incomplete without a discussion of cellular respiration, as clinicians employ fetal monitoring to guard against the development of "acidemia" and related diagnoses such as "hypoxic ischemic encephalopathy."

Normal cellular respiration includes an anaerobic phase and an aerobic phase. Glycolysis, the metabolism of glucose to pyruvic acid, is anaerobic and generates eight molecules of ATP (four ATP directly and two NADH which equate to four ATP). If the pyruvic acid subsequently enters the aerobic phase, an additional 30 molecules of ATP are generated, for a net total of 38 molecules of ATP, in exchange for one molecule of glucose under conditions of aerobic metabolism.

However, when there is oxygen deprivation, continued anaerobic metabolism ensues. The pyruvic acid, which would otherwise be shuttled into the aerobic phase under aerobic conditions, is converted to lactic acid under anaerobic metabolism. This continued anaerobic metabolism is costly: glycolysis generates eight molecules of ATP, of which the metabolism of pyruvic acid to lactic acid uses six molecules of ATP, for a net gain of only two molecules of ATP. Aerobic metabolism is thus favored by the cell, but under adverse conditions, anaerobic metabolism will proceed, in order to produce at least some energy. Anaerobic metabolism is inefficient and carries another potential cost, the buildup of lactic acid by-products, which can contribute to metabolic acidemia and cellular dysfunction.[1]

Metabolic acidemia is not the only mechanism for acidemia: an organism requires exhalation of CO_2 to maintain a normal pH. For the fetus "breathing" through the placenta, this exhalation of CO_2 will be impeded with cord occlusion, and any buildup in CO_2 that is associated with cord occlusion can generate a respiratory acidosis, which when detected at delivery is generally rapidly cleared.

In the absence of maternal diseases that compromise respiratory function, the mother is usually normally oxygenated. How then can a fetus become "hypoxic"? This requires an understanding of blood flow within the maternal and fetal units, as well as adaptations that protect the fetus during intrauterine life.

BLOOD FLOW AT THE MATERNAL-FETAL INTERFACE

Uterus and Placenta

The bilateral uterine arteries primarily perfuse the uterus, with the ovarian arteries providing another 17% of estimated blood flow near term, for a total of 841 mL/minute.[2] These uterine arteries continue as arcuate arteries that span the surface of the uterus longitudinally, with basal arteries branching at 90 degrees and continuing as spiral arteries that traverse the thickness of the myometrium. Brosens and Dixon[3] reported that approximately 120 spiral arteries enter the intervillous space (Fig. 2.1).

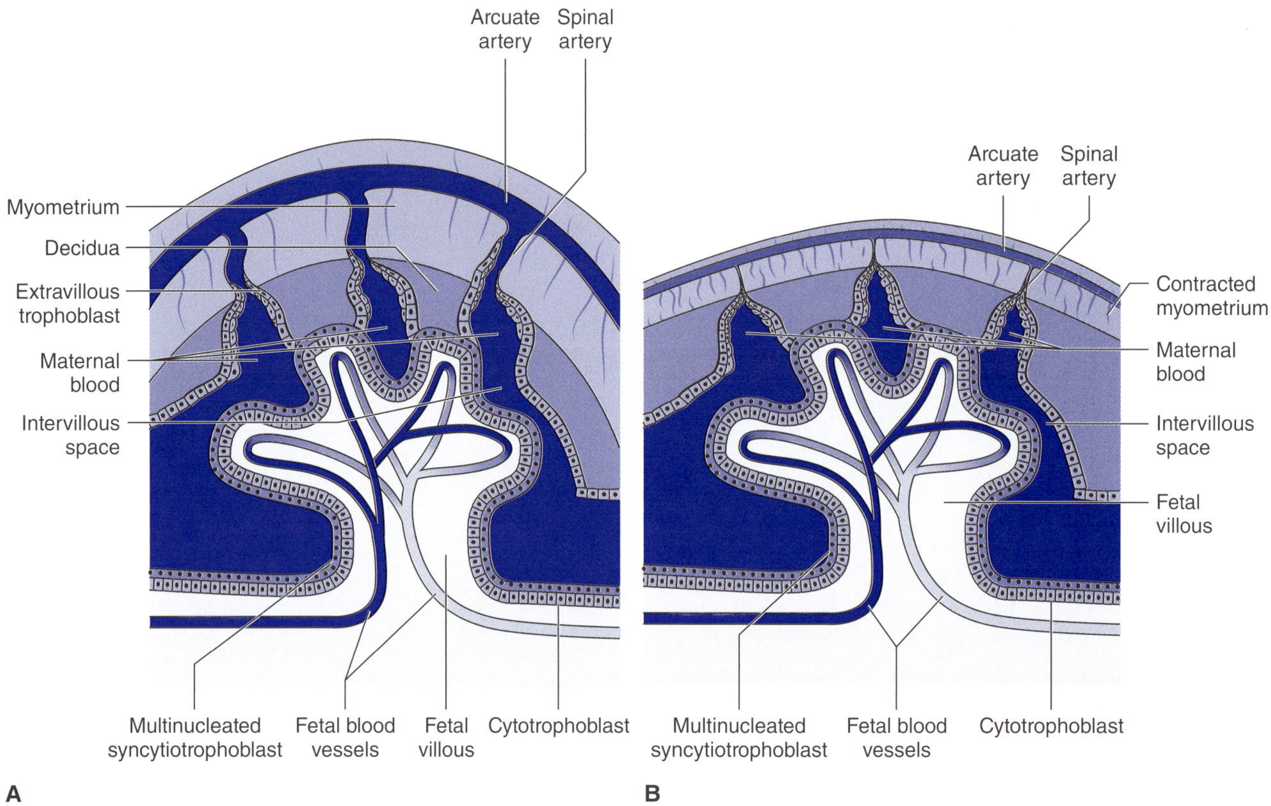

Figure 2.1. Maternal-fetal interface illustrating the fetal villi containing fetal vessels with overlying cytotrophoblast and multinucleated syncytiotrophoblast with extravillous trophoblast having remodeled the maternal spinal arteries to larger-caliber vessels carrying a high volume of blood at low pressure. **A.** Before contraction, mean arterial pressure of spinal arteries 85 mm Hg, relaxed intramyometrial pressure 10 mm Hg, amniotic fluid pressure 10 mm Hg. **B.** During contraction, mean arterial pressure of spinal arteries 90 mm Hg, but spinal arteries collapsed because of intramyometrial pressure being 120 mm Hg, and amniotic fluid pressure 60 mm Hg. Circulatory stasis within the intervillous space prone to hypoxemia, hypercapnia, acidemia. (Source: Data from Poseiro et al, 1969.[4])

The intervillous space is a critical component of the maternal and fetal interface, and derangements in its development are hypothesized to lead to reduced blood flow at term as well as obstetrical syndromes, such as preeclampsia and fetal growth restriction.[5,6] Normally, the blastocyst implants in the decidualized endometrium, where extravillous trophoblasts contact maternal spiral arterioles and remodel these muscular vessels into larger-caliber, thin-walled canals carrying a high volume of blood at low pressure. This low-pressure blood flow bathes the fetal villi within the intervillous space, providing nutrients and oxygen while removing waste. Thus, the placenta functions as an extra-corporeal organ with pulmonary, renal, and other roles, in addition to producing steroid hormones that are important to pregnancy physiology.

The placental unit is described as hemochorial because the maternal blood directly contacts the fetal villi, a characteristic of primate and rodent placentas.[7] This contrasts with the epitheliochorial placenta of ruminants including the sheep (a species frequently studied in fetal physiology experiments), in which the maternal and fetal vessels are separated by a layer of trophectoderm and a layer of endometrium. The fetal villus from a hemochorial placenta is composed of an outer multinucleated syncytiotrophoblast layer and an inner cytotrophoblast layer that surround the fetal vessels. The fetal villi within the intervillous space have numerous twists adding to the high surface area to volume ratio that facilitates gas exchange.

Fetal Circulation

The fetal vessels within this placental system are in continuity with the thin-walled umbilical vein carrying blood to the fetus and the umbilical arteries that

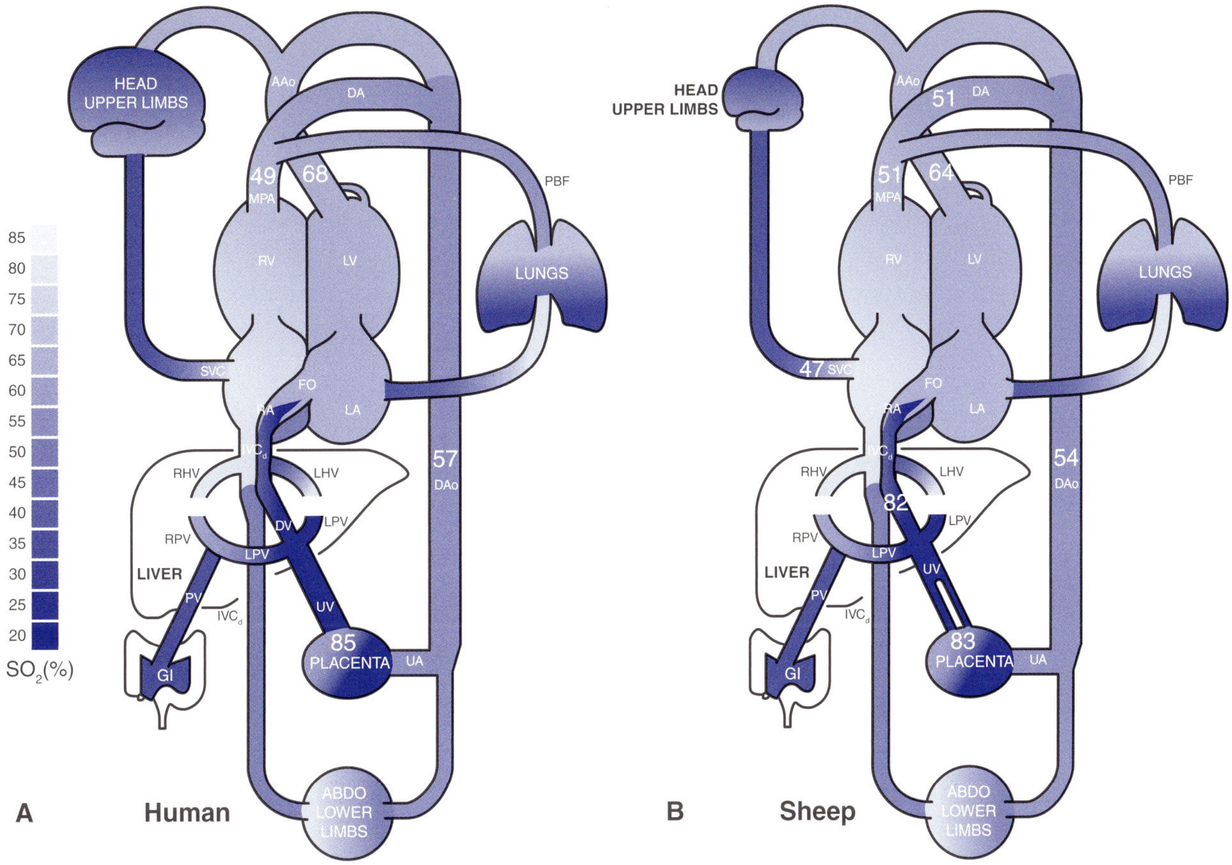

Figure 2.2. T2-weighted MRI in human pregnancies to confirm previous observations from the sheep[9] that the oxygen saturation of blood entering the fetus is 85%. This figure compares the human **(A)** and sheep **(B)** fetal circulations, showing the great similarity. Importantly, much of the research in fetal physiology has used the sheep model. (Reproduced with permission from Saini BS, Darby JRT, Portnoy S, et al. Normal human and sheep fetal vessel oxygen saturations by T2 magnetic resonance imaging. *J Physiol.* 2020;598(15):3259-3281.)

branch from the hypogastric arteries and curve around the fetal bladder as they exit into the umbilical cord. Saini et al[8] used T2-weighted MRI in human pregnancies to confirm previous observations from the sheep[9] that the oxygen saturation of blood entering the fetus is 85% (Fig. 2.2).

This oxygenated blood returning to the fetus through the umbilical vein is preferentially diverted via the ductus venosus into the inferior vena cava and into the right side of the fetal heart, and most of this blood flow is then preferentially shuttled through the atrial septum into the left-sided circulation where oxygen saturation is 68%. This left-sided circulation preferentially perfuses the heart and brain, with blood in the right ventricle showing a lower oxygen saturation of 49%. Most of the right heart output is preferentially directed via the ductus arteriosus toward the lower body, approximately one-third of combined fetal cardiac output directed back to the placenta in the second trimester and one-fifth at term.[10]

Nicolaides et al[11] used cordocentesis to measure pO_2, SaO_2, and hemoglobin in 208 normally grown pregnancies advancing from 18 to 38 weeks. They reported that venous and arterial pO_2 decreased from 45.8 to 35.4 mm Hg and from 37.6 to 32.6 mm Hg, respectively. This is compensated by a rise in hemoglobin concentration from 10.8 to 14.5 g/dL from 18 to 38 weeks.

How Is the Fetus Able to Survive at a Lower Oxygen Saturation While Intrauterine?

It is notable that the oxygenated venous blood entering the fetus has a pO_2 of only 35.4 mm Hg at term, which would be incompatible with survival for an adult. The adaptions that facilitate fetal survival include:

1. A higher fetal hemoglobin concentration which allows for more oxygen carrying capacity.

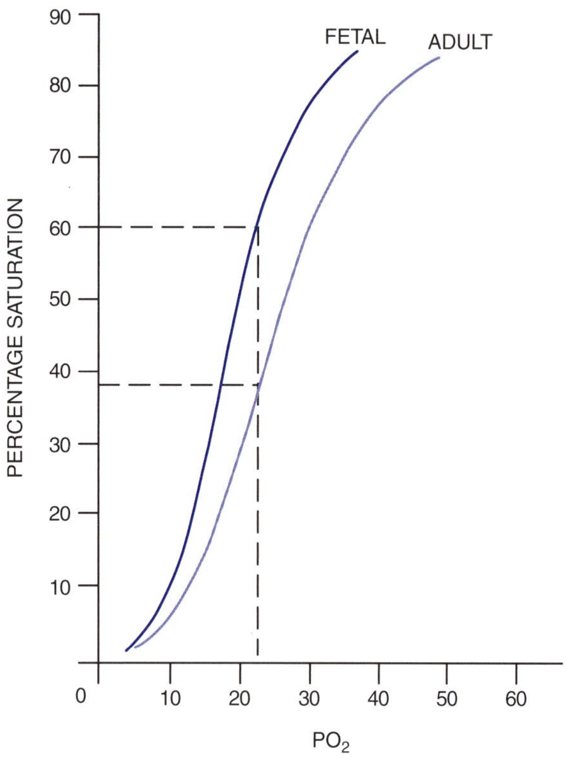

Figure 2.3. Adult and fetal hemoglobin dissociation curves.

2. A steeper fetal hemoglobin dissociation curve, such that a pO_2 of 35 mm Hg corresponds to an oxygen saturation of approximately 85% (Fig. 2.3), whereas in the adult it would correspond to approximately 65%.
3. High levels of 2,3-disphosphoglycerate during pregnancy lowers maternal affinity for oxygen, thereby increasing delivery of oxygen to the fetus.
4. The fetal cardiac output exceeds adult cardiac output on a volume per unit of weight basis, such that a greater amount of oxygen can be moved more quickly to the tissues.

Historically, oxygen has been administered to laboring individuals when FHR abnormalities have been encountered. This practice has been questioned with respect to effectiveness, as well as that hyperoxygenation may be associated with toxicity from lipid peroxidation. A large meta-analysis reported that for laboring individuals, the addition of oxygen as part of intrauterine resuscitation was not effective.[12] A randomized controlled trial to assess efficacy as well as potential toxicity is currently underway (ClinicalTrials.gov Identifier: NCT03581214).

Whether maternal hyperoxygenation during labor is beneficial or not, most cases of fetal hypoxia are attributable to reduced blood flow on either side of the placenta. Thus, the addition of oxygen to a normally-oxygenated laboring individual is unlikely to be as helpful as restoring blood flow. This leads to the importance of understanding the mechanisms of reduced blood flow on the maternal and fetal sides of the placenta.

FACTORS THAT DECREASE UTERINE BLOOD FLOW

Maternal Position

When supine, the enhanced lumbar lordosis of pregnancy may cause hypotension from compression of the inferior vena cava by the gravid uterus. This hypotension results from reduced blood flow back to the heart, with consequent reduced preload and cardiac output. Depending on the amount of compression, blood flow through the aorta may also be reduced, further reducing blood flow to the uterus. The effect of aortocaval compression has long been recognized.[13] Abitol[14] studied 902 laboring individuals and noted 126 (14%) had late decelerations, and in 24, the late decelerations occurred only in the supine position. Changing to the lateral position resolved the decelerations and associated abnormalities, including reduced femoral blood pressure and a lower fetal scalp pH. Simpson and James used pulse oximetry to randomize 142 individuals into different groups to compare interventions for intrauterine resuscitation.[15] They reported that a lateral recumbent position significantly increased oxygen saturation (left mean 48.3%, right mean 47.7%) compared to a supine position (mean supine 37.5%, P = .03). More recently, Walker et al[16] performed a Cochrane meta-analysis of studies of maternal position in the second stage of labor and found no increase in the primary endpoint of operative delivery, but noted that all studies used the left or right lateral or semi-recumbent positions and that positions "flat on the back or lithotomy are not generally used due to the possibility of aortocaval compression."

Uterine Contractions

Myometrial contractions can collapse the spiral arterioles if intra-myometrial pressure exceeds arterial pressure (Fig. 2.1). This reduces perfusion at the placenta by ~60%[17] and appears to be a consequence of even normal labor, as the pre-labor umbilical artery mean pH decreases from 7.38 to 7.25 at delivery.[18] When uterine blood flow is already pathologically diminished owing to other conditions that result in poor placentation, the fetus may not be able to tolerate normal labor. Pathologic contractile activity, such as with tachysystole or tetanic contractions, including from the use of oxytocin or prostaglandins, may result in contractions that effectively cause intervillous perfusion to cease until the uterus is relaxed. Placental abruption can also result in tetanic contractions,[19] but the mechanism for reduced perfusion with abruption is also significantly mediated by a reduced placental surface area for exchange.

Surface Area

As mentioned earlier, the reduced placenta surface area associated with placental abruption is an important pathologic entity, but there are numerous potential causes for reduced effective surface area. The placenta itself may be pathologically small owing to an intrinsic genetic abnormality such as confined placental aneuploidy triploidy or a chromosomally abnormal pregnancy. In monochorionic twin pregnancies, there can be unequal sharing of the placenta, such that one twin suffers because of reduced blood flow. Placental insufficiency can develop later in pregnancy in association with hypertensive disorders, as well as from maternal floor infarction/massive perivillous fibrin deposition, which can occur with maternal autoimmune disease, antiphospholipid antibody syndrome, and possibly certain viral infections.[20] Infarcts of the placenta caused by either maternal or fetal vascular malperfusion can also reduce placental perfusion.[21]

Maternal Hypotension

Anything that reduces maternal cardiac output to the placenta can reduce placental perfusion. A common example is conduction anesthesia causing sympathetic blockade and maternal hypotension, which generally responds to positional changes, intravenous fluid administration, and the use of a combined alpha- and beta-adrenergic agent such as ephedrine. Lappen et al[22] reported that evidence of maternal hypovolemia/dehydration on admission was more likely associated with FHR decelerations during labor compared to euvolemic individuals. The use of anti-hypertensive agents, including dihydropyridine-based (such as nifedipine) drugs for tocolytic therapy, has been reported to cause severe maternal hypotension and FHR abnormalities.[23] Important considerations in the face of maternal hypotension include maternal sepsis, acute coronary events, concealed hemorrhage, and other life-threatening maternal conditions.

Diffusion Distance and Other Abnormalities

Placental edema can increase the thickness of the distance from the villous membrane to the fetal capillary, impeding gas exchange. Conditions associated with marked placental edema include the various causes of hydrops fetalis, although the underlying etiology of the hydrops can itself cause poor placental perfusion and gas exchange (eg, erythroblastosis fetalis causing severe fetal anemia, with villous edema as an associated finding). Avagliano et al[24] described villous edema in 38.2% of cases of fetal pH less than 7.0 versus controls (pH > 7.0), but a significantly greater number of syncytial knots (38.2% vs 13.7%), choriangiosis (8.8% vs 2.9%), and villous branching abnormalities (35.3% vs 14.7%), suggesting placental developmental abnormalities predating labor may also predispose to acidemia.

Other Factors that Decrease Fetal Uterine Blood Flow

Fetal hemodynamic compromise can occur in response to fetal sepsis, fetal heart failure, and fetal anemia. Placental infarcts caused by fetal vascular malperfusion can also compromise blood flow.[21,25]

FETAL CIRCULATORY RESPONSE TO INSUFFICIENT PLACENTAL PERFUSION

The consequence of insufficient placental perfusion is a reduction in the partial pressure of oxygen. The subsequent response by the fetus, and the adaptive mechanisms that can protect it, has been summarized by Turner et al.[17] Briefly, the reduction in the partial pressure of oxygen will activate fetal chemoreceptors that stimulate the sympathetic and parasympathetic systems. Activation of the sympathetic system increases peripheral vascular resistance and centralizes blood flow to the brain, heart, and adrenals, whereas activation of the parasympathetic system slows the FHR and decreases myocardial oxygen demand. Both sympathetic and parasympathetic activations increase end-diastolic volume and cardiac output, which may increase mean arterial pressure and cerebral blood flow. Decompensation can result from worsening hypoxemia, academia, and depletion of myocardial glycogen stores.

Electronic fetal monitoring is used to evaluate fetal well-being with a goal to identify fetal compromise; its use in low-risk pregnancies has been questioned, owing to such monitoring being associated with more interventions (operative and cesarean delivery) without reducing the rate of cerebral palsy. The American College of Obstetricians and Gynecologists[26] has recommended (Level C evidence) that individuals with high-risk conditions have continuous fetal monitoring in labor.

CONTROL OF THE FETAL HEART RATE

The following describes the physiology behind the control of the FHR, as well as the physiology behind FHR changes. Much of this understanding involves studies by legendary investigators.

Experimental Evidence

Mathematically, the FHR is equal to the reciprocal of the interval between two successive beats. This can be calculated using a fetal electrode attached to the fetal scalp to measure the peak of the fetal electrocardiogram, the R wave, to signify the timing of the fetal heartbeat. This internal electrode is more precise than an external Doppler wave that averages between beats.

The FHR decreases with advancing gestational age,[27] by about 10 beats per minute (bpm) from approximately 160 bpm at 15 weeks. Preterm fetuses may have a slightly increased baseline heart rate compared to more mature fetuses, but any baseline FHR over 160 bpm should be investigated for potential fetal compromise. The gradual decrease in the FHR is likely because of maturation of the parasympathetic nervous system and increased vagal tone, as atropine administered to the fetus results in a greater magnitude increase in FHR with increasing gestational age (summarized in Schifferli and Caldeyro-Barcia).[27]

Renou et al[28] showed that direct administration of atropine to the human fetus has three effects. First, the previous increase in the baseline heart rate described by Schifferli and Caldeyro-Barcia[27] was confirmed. Second, atropine administered directly to the fetus decreased the variability of the FHR, suggesting the balance of the parasympathetic and sympathetic systems was altered. Last, the atropine accentuated FHR accelerations, suggesting that suppression of the parasympathetic system unmasked sympathetic impulses causing accelerations. When Renou and colleagues administered a beta-adrenergic blocker (propranolol) to the fetuses that had received atropine, the accelerations were abolished and the FHR decreased, illustrating the effect of sequential abolishment of the parasympathetic and sympathetic nervous impulses.

Variability: Converging Effects of the Intact Sympathetic and Parasympathetic Nervous Impulses

The normal FHR baseline in the third trimester ranges between 110 and 160 bpm.[29] This baseline and its associated variability are determined by the atrial pacemaker, with converging regulatory effects of intact sympathetic and parasympathetic nervous impulses. This sympathetic and parasympathetic controls originate in the medulla at the rostroventrolateral medulla and nucleus ambiguous, respectively.[30] The parasympathetic activity to the heart is mediated directly by the vagal nerve, whereas the sympathetic activity is a combination of direct innervation from the bilateral thoracolumbar sympathetic chains, as well as from adrenal catecholamines circulating in the blood. An abnormal or absent cortex in the presence of an intact brainstem, as in some cases of fetal anencephaly, can be associated with FHR variability.[31,32] Notably, Pereg and Goldman[33] reported that the presence of good short-term variability was correlated with a more conserved midbrain at autopsy.

FHR variability increases with increasing central nervous system (CNS) maturation, particularly after 32 weeks.[29] Reactivity is the association between fetal movement and episodes of FHR acceleration. Fetal accelerations are often associated with fetal movement, although fetal movements can occur without accelerations.[34] Accelerations are less common during periods of fetal sleep. Before 23 weeks, reactivity is infrequent, but increases during the third trimester in association with CNS maturation.[35,36] Periods of reactivity may last 20 to 40 minutes or more, and normal fetuses rarely go more than 80 minutes without reactivity.[37,38] Both maternal heart rate and a fetal circadian rhythm have been correlated with reactivity.[37,39]

According to the 2008 NICHD criteria,[29] baseline FHR variability is determined over a 10-minute interval, while excluding accelerations and deceleration. Baseline variability is defined as fluctuations in the baseline heart rate that are irregular in frequency and amplitude, quantified as the amplitude from peak to trough in bpm. The classifications of variability include absent, minimal (0-5 bpm), moderate (6-25 bpm), and marked (>25 bpm).

Moderate variability is generally viewed as reassuring, whereas marked variability has been associated with hypoxemia in both fetal sheep and humans.[40,41] This increased variability in response to acute hypoxemia may be mediated by peripheral chemoreceptors that increase parasympathetic and sympathetic neural activity. The balance of the neural inputs, with the parasympathetic system decreasing the FHR and the sympathetic system stimulating broad vasoconstriction to maintain perfusion, is affected by vasoactive mediators (including catecholamines) after at least 1 minute,[42] consistent with the generally transient nature of the marked variability of acute hypoxemia.

Chronic hypoxia affects FHR variability, with reduced sympathetic contribution after 72 hours in sheep.[43] Similarly, in labor characterized by repeated umbilical cord compression, parasympathetic neural activity dominates and can be associated with decreased fetal heart variability.[42] The impact of either chronic hypoxia or an acute antepartum asphyxia event on subsequent FHR variability in sheep is complex and may reflect the timing from an event.[44] Tan cautions that inappropriate reliance on fetal tracing may lead to inappropriate decisions about the timing of antepartum insults to the CNS.[45]

Drugs may also affect the FHR and its variability, ostensibly through effects on the CNS. For example, Ramirez-Cacho et al[46] reported that a median maintenance dose of 70 mg of methadone (range: 20-130 mg) was associated with a reduction in the variability, baseline, and frequency of accelerations in the first stage of labor. Hatjis and Meis[47] reported that butorphanol was strongly associated with a sinusoidal fetal heart pattern.

This sinusoidal fetal heart pattern is unusual and characterized by a relatively smooth, sine-like wave pattern. The sinusoidal pattern has long been associated with fetal anemia, including erythroblastosis fetalis[48] and fetal-to-maternal hemorrhage[49]; a successful fetal transfusion for Rh disease has been associated with the resolution of the sinusoidal pattern.[50,51] A sinusoidal pattern is uncommonly seen acutely in labor and is generally considered to be alarming; the 2008 consensus guidelines[29] specify that at least 20 minutes of sinusoidal activity is consistent with a nonreassuring or category III tracing. There is some evidence that arginine vasopressin is correlated with this pattern. Indeed, Murata et al[52] reported that anemic fetal sheep had high levels of arginine vasopressin, but the infusion of arginine vasopressin did not induce a sinusoidal tracing except in the cases of high-dose atropine or in vagotomized fetal sheep. It is possible that altered parasympathetic activity caused by cerebral ischemia, in the presence of high levels of arginine vasopressin induced by stress, mediates this sinusoidal character.[53]

In summary, the CNS, mediated by the balance of sympathetic and parasympathetic effects, plays an important role in the regulation of the FHR and its variability. Moderate variability and the presence of accelerations are generally associated with reassuring fetal status, but the absence of accelerations does not necessarily imply fetal danger nor does reduced variability in all situations; context is important. In the next section, we will discuss the effect of uterine contractions on the FHR under various conditions.

UTERINE CONTRACTIONS AND FETAL HEART RATE

Early Decelerations

The 2008 consensus classification for fetal heart monitoring[29] defines early decelerations as visually apparent decelerations that are usually symmetric, with a decrease to the nadir of at least 30 seconds and a gradual return that is associated with a uterine contraction. In most cases, the nadir occurs at the same time as the peak of the contraction, and the onset and recovery correspond to the beginning and ending of the contraction, respectively.

These early decelerations are not associated with hypoxia or acidemia,[54] and administration of atropine with pressure on the fetal head diminished or abolished the decelerations, consistent with a vagally mediated action.[55] Paul et al[56] later associated early FHR decelerations with fetal head compression mediated via vagal nerve activity.

As described in the fourth edition,

> Hon (personal communication, 1974, Los Angeles) studied neonates, using different-sized donut pessaries, and found that placing the circular pessary over the fetal vertex, when the inside diameter of the pessary was 4 to 6 cm in diameter, usually result in post pressure from the edge of the pessary over the anterior fontanelle.

And this was associated with a heart rate deceleration. These experiments ostensibly simulated FHR decelerations that typically occur between 4 and 6 cm in labor.

Variable Decelerations

Before variable decelerations were termed such, Sir Joseph Barcroft, during his time as Chair of the

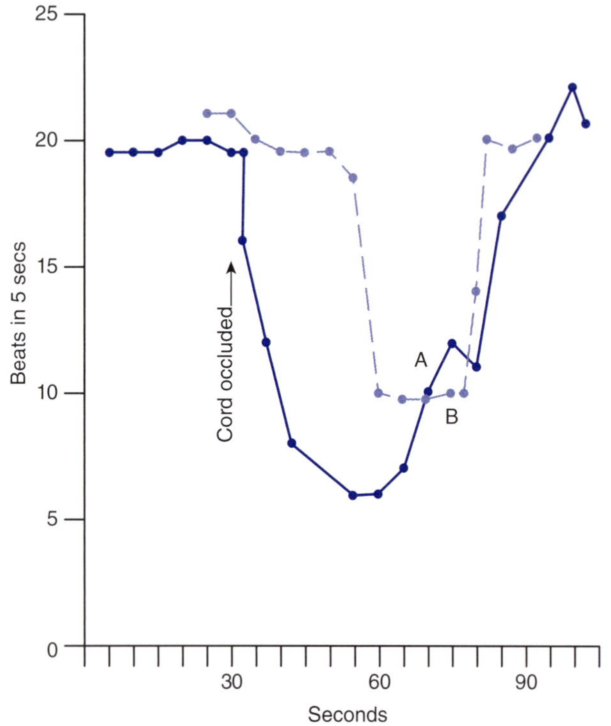

Figure 2.4. Umbilical cord occlusion of the fetal goat (solid line, intact vagus nerve; broken line, with vagotomy). (Reproduced with permission from Marshall FHA. Researches on Pre-Natal Life.)

Department of Physiology at Cambridge University in 1937, worked with Dr. DJ Bauer to study the effect of umbilical cord occlusion in the goat. As seen in Figure 2.4, from Barcroft's seminal monograph Researches on Pre-Natal Life,[57] umbilical cord occlusion of the exteriorized fetal goat produced a rapid and profound drop in the FHR. However, after bilateral vagotomy of the exteriorized fetal goat, umbilical cord occlusion produced a drop in the FHR, but it was significantly delayed. This suggested that the instantaneous decrease in the heart rate of the intact exteriorized goat was mediated by the vagus nerve, but the delayed decrease in heart rate of the exteriorized goats with bilateral vagotomy was mediated by another mechanism. Later, Hon et al[55] showed that atropine administered to human fetuses with cord compression significantly reduced or abolished the rapid deceleration associated with umbilical cord compression, supporting part of Barcroft's findings.

Hemodynamically, total cord occlusion is associated with increased afterload and fetal hypertension that is sensed by baroreceptors, which communicate with the central vagal nuclei and mediate a parasympathetic-driven slowing of the FHR.[58] The shape, duration, depth, and timing of the deceleration varies with the location of the cord and degree of compression, such that these decelerations are described as Variable. In a seminal experiment by Lee et al,[59] a hysterotomy was made without delivery of the fetus. The cord was identified and the BP and heart rate of the fetus were measured during progressive compression of the cord. Partial occlusion of the cord, with only the thin-walled umbilical vein compressed, reduced afferent blood flow to the fetus, which reduced blood pressure and stimulated baroreceptors to increase the FHR. Total compression reproduced the findings of Barcroft and Hon, and decompression of the cord reversed this sequence. This is depicted in Figure 2.5, from Lee et al.[59] It is notable that accelerations, sometimes termed "shoulders" bordering the deceleration, can frequently accompany variables.

Several studies involving amnioinfusion support the idea of cord compression as an etiology for variable

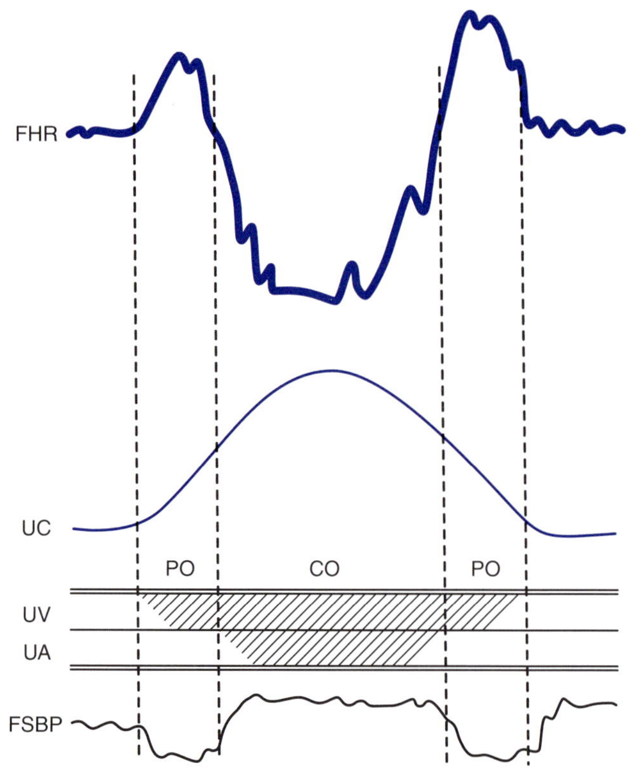

Figure 2.5. Physiologic mechanism of fetal heart rate changes by degree of umbilical cord compression. PO, partial occlusion; CO, complete occlusion; UC, uterine contraction; UV, umbilical vein; UA, umbilical artery; FSBP, fetal systemic blood pressure. (Reproduced with permission from Lee CY, Di Loreto PC, O'Lane JM. Study of fetal heart rate acceleration patterns. *Obstet Gynecol.* 1975; 45(2):142-146.)

decelerations when amniotic fluid is low. Gabbe et al[60] was one of the first to demonstrate this after amniotomy in the laboratory, and a prospective randomized study of saline amnioinfusion via a transcervical catheter was reported to improve repetitive variable decelerations.[61] Spong et al[62] correlated the success of amnioinfusion with a lower amniotic fluid index at the outset, and failure of amnioinfusion to resolve the variable decelerations was associated with increased prevalence of true knots in the cord and nuchal cords. Amnioinfusion for meconium-stained amniotic fluid, in the absence of variable decelerations, did not improve outcomes and was associated with more chorioamnionitis/endometritis.[63]

At some point, intermittent cord occlusion will sufficiently interrupt blood flow to reduce perfusion, resulting in lower oxygen tension, increased CO_2 levels, and acidemia from metabolic (lactic acid production) and respiratory (reduced removal of pCO_2) causes. Significant acidemia may depress myocardial action sufficiently to reduce function and the heart rate, which may be the cause of the delayed fall in the heart rate of vagotomized fetal goats with total cord compression in Barcroft's experiments above. There is a potential role for the action of chemoreceptors with progressive umbilical cord occlusion. For example, Siassi et al[64] studied the effect of 60 seconds of complete cord occlusion at progressively higher oxygen tension (20-220 mm Hg) and found the normally brisk reduction in the FHR is markedly less at higher oxygen tension, suggesting that chemoreceptor activity is complementary to baroreceptor function.

Late Decelerations

As noted earlier in this chapter, intervillous blood flow can be reduced by numerous causes. When this intervillous blood flow is reduced, then there is a decrease in perfusion of the fetal villi. This state is frequently termed "uteroplacental insufficiency." Like inadequate perfusion from frequent or prolonged cord compression, decreased perfusion caused by uteroplacental insufficiency can result in lower oxygen tension, increased CO_2 levels, and acidemia. When this occurs chronically, the result can be fetal growth restriction and stillbirth; however, acutely during labor, uteroplacental insufficiency may manifest as acidemia and fetal injury.

The FHR change associated with uteroplacental insufficiency was termed a late deceleration by Hon[65] and a Type II deceleration by Caldeyro-Barcia et al.[66] In a series of comprehensive experiments, Itskovitz et al[67] studied fetal sheep that were normal and chronically hypoxemic. In normal fetal sheep, reduced uterine blood flow that was prolonged resulted in chemoreceptor-mediated reflex bradycardia when carotid arterial pO_2 fell below 20 mm Hg. This was associated with a substantial decrease in left ventricular output measured using an electromagnetic flowmeter. Both the bradycardia and decrease in left ventricular output were abolished with atropine. In chronically hypoxemic fetal sheep, reduced uterine blood flow resulted in a delayed heart rate deceleration caused by reflex bradycardia (mediated by both chemoreceptors and baroreceptors), as well as a non-reflex bradycardia attributed to secondary hypoxic myocardial depression. This bradycardia was related to baseline fetal oxygenation: With a lower carotid artery pO_2, the sooner the bradycardia occurred and with a deeper and more prolonged deceleration.

CONCLUSION

Normal cellular respiration utilizes aerobic metabolism for maximum energy production. Under conditions of oxygen deprivation and anaerobic metabolism, the cell will produce less energy with the buildup of lactic acid as a by-product. Robust uterine blood flow as well as several fetal adaptations are protective and help to ensure optimal oxygen delivery and clearance of waste such as CO_2 and acid. When uterine blood flow is reduced, either through reduced uteroplacental perfusion or through umbilical cord occlusion, evidence can manifest in the FHR tracing. Variability is a key indicator of fetal status and is a result of the converging effects of the parasympathetic and sympathetic nervous impulses. In labor, the parasympathetic system predominates and may be associated with reduced variability, particularly under conditions of repetitive umbilical cord occlusion or placental insufficiency. The addition of decelerations can be informative. Early decelerations are associated with fetal head compression and are generally considered benign, whereas variable decelerations reflect the physiology of cord occlusion which can become pathologic with prolonged or frequent compression, and late decelerations indicate reflex (chemoreceptor and baroreceptor), as well as non-reflex (direct myocardial depression), responses to hypoxemia.

REFERENCES

1. Naifeh J, Dimri M, Varacallo M. Biochemistry: aerobic glycolysis. In: *StatPearls* [Internet]. StatPearls Publishing; 2022.

2. Moore LG, Wesolowski SR, Lorca RA, Murray AJ, Julian CG. Why is the human uterine artery blood flow during pregnancy so high? *Am J Physiol Regul Integr Comp Physiol.* 2022;323(5):R694-R699.
3. Brosens I, Dixon HG. The anatomy of the maternal side of the placenta. *J Obstet Gynaecol Br Commonw.* 1966;73(3):357-363.
4. Poseiro JJ, Mendez-Bauer C, Pose SV, et al. Perinatal factors affecting human development. Pan American World Health Organization, Scientific Publication No 185, Washington, DC; 1969:161-171.
5. Brosens I, Pijnenborg R, Vercruysse L, Romero R. The "Great Obstetrical Syndromes" are associated with disorders of deep placentation. *Am J Obstet Gynecol.* 2011;204(3):193-201.
6. Miller D, Garcia-Flores V, Romero R, Galaz J, Pique-Regi R, Gomez-Lopez N. Single-cell immunobiology of the maternal-fetal interface. *J Immunol.* 2022;209(9):1450-1464.
7. Furukawa S, Kuroda Y, Sugiyama A. A comparison of the histological structure of the placenta in experimental animals. *J Toxicol Pathol.* 2014;27(1):11-18.
8. Saini BS, Darby JRT, Portnoy S, et al. Normal human and sheep fetal vessel oxygen saturations by T2 magnetic resonance imaging. *J Physiol.* 2020;598(15):3259-3281.
9. Rudolf AM. Distribution and regulation of blood flow in the fetal and neonatal lamb. *Circ Res.* 1985;57(6):811-821.
10. Kiserud T, Ebbing C, Kessler J, Rasmussen S. Fetal cardiac output, distribution of the placenta and impact of fetal compromise. *Ultrasound Obstet Gynecol.* 2006;28(2):125-136.
11. Nicolaides KH, Economides DL, Soothill PW. Blood gases, pH, and lactate in appropriate and small-for-gestational-age fetuses. *Am J Obstet Gynecol.* 1989;161(4):996-1001.
12. Raghuraman N, Temming LA, Doering MM, et al. Maternal oxygen supplementation compared with room air for intrauterine resuscitation: a systematic review and meta-analysis. *JAMA Pediatr.* 2021;175(4):368-376.
13. Howard BK, Goodson JM, Mengert WIT. Supine hypotensive syndrome in late pregnancy. *Obstet Gynecol.* 1951;1(4):371-377.
14. Abitol MM. Supine position in labor and associated fetal heart rate changes. *Obstet Gynecol.* 1985;65(4):481-486.
15. Simpson KR, James DC. Efficacy of intrauterine resuscitation techniques in improving fetal oxygen status during labor. *Obstet Gynecol.* 2005;105(6):1362-1368.
16. Walker KF, Kibuka M, Thornton JG, Jones NW. Maternal position in the second stage of labour for women with epidural anaesthesia. *Cochrane Database Syst Rev.* 2018;11(11):CD008070.
17. Turner JM, Mitchell MD, Kumar, SS. The physiology of intrapartum fetal compromise at term. *Am J Obstet Gynecol.* 2020;222(1):17-26.
18. Arikan GM, Scholz HS, Petru E, Haeusler MC, Haas J, Weiss PA. Cord blood oxygen saturation in vigorous infants at birth: what is normal? *BJOG.* 2000;107(8):987-994.
19. Ananth CV, Lavery JA, Vintzileos AM, et al. Severe placental abruption: clinical definition and associations with maternal complications. *Am J Obstet Gynecol.* 2016;214(2):272.e1-272.e9.
20. Redline RW. Extending the spectrum of massive perivillous fibrin deposition (maternal floor infarction). *Pediatr Dev Pathol.* 2021;24(1):10-11.
21. Kulkarni VG, Sunilkumar KB, Nagaraj TS, et al. Maternal and fetal vascular lesions of malperfusion in the placentas associated with fetal and neonatal death: results of a prospective observational study. *Am J Obstet Gynecol.* 2021;225(6):660.e1-660.e12.
22. Lappen JR, Chien EK, Mercer BM. Contraction-associated maternal heart rate decelerations: a pragmatic marker of intrapartum volume status. *Obstet Gynecol.* 2018;132(4):1011-1017.
23. Oei SG. Calcium channel blockers for tocolysis: a review of their role and safety following reports of serious adverse events. *Eur J Obstet Gynecol Reprod Biol.* 2006;126(2):137-145.
24. Avagliano L, Locatelli A, Danti L, Felis S, Mecacci F, Bulfamante GP. Placental histology in clinically unexpected severe fetal acidemia at term. *Early Hum Dev.* 2015;91(5):339-343.
25. Leon RL, Sharma K, Mir IN, et al. Placental vascular malperfusion lesions in fetal congenital heart disease. *Am J Obstet Gynecol.* 2022;227(4):620.e1-620.e8.
26. American College of Obstetricians and Gynecologists. Intrapartum fetal heart rate monitoring: nomenclature, interpretation, and general management principles. Practice Bulletin 106, reaffirmed 2021.
27. Schifferli P, Caldeyro-Barcia R. Effects of atropine and beta adrenergic drugs on the heart rate of the human fetus. In: Boreus L, ed. *Fetal Pharmacology.* Raven Press; 1973:259-279.
28. Renou P, Warwick N, Wood C. Autonomic control of fetal heart rate. *Am J Obstet Gynecol.* 1969;105(6):949.
29. Macones GA, Hankins GD, Spong CY, Hauth J, Moore T. The 2008 National Institute of Child Health and Human Development workshop report on electronic fetal monitoring: update on definitions, interpretation, and research guidelines. *Obstet Gynecol.* 2008;112(3):661-666.
30. Coote JH, Spyer KM. Central control of autonomic function. *Brain Neurosci Adv.* 2018;2:2398212818812012.
31. Park YJ, Kim YJ, Hoh JK, Park MI. Fetal heart rate parameters of anencephalic fetuses according to gestational age. *J Reprod Med.* 2011;56(5-6):241-246.
32. Terao T, Kawashima, Y, Noto H, et al. Neurological control of fetal heart rate in 20 cases of anencephalic fetuses. *Am J Obstet Gynecol.* 1984;149(2):201-208.
33. Pereg D, Goldman JA. Fetal heart rate patterns: a study of the anencephalic fetus. *Obstet Gynecol.* 1979;53(4):530-533.
34. Navot D, Yaffe H, Sadovsky E. The ratio of fetal heart rate accelerations to fetal movements according to gestational age. *Am J Obstet Gynecol.* 1984;149(1):92-94.
35. Smith CV, Phelan JP, Paul RH. A prospective analysis of the influence of gestational age on the baseline fetal heart rate and reactivity in a low-risk population. *Am J Obstet Gynecol.* 1985;153(7):780-782.
36. Druzin ML, Fox A, Kogut E, Carlson C. The relationship of the non-stress test to gestational age. *Am J Obstet Gynecol.* 1985;153(4):386-389.
37. Patrick J, Campbell K, Carmichael L, Probert C. Influence of maternal heart rate and gross fetal body movements on the daily pattern of fetal heart rate near term. *Am J Obstet Gynecol.* 1982;144(5):533-538.
38. Brown R, Patrick J. The nonstress test: how long is enough? *Am J Obstet Gynecol.* 1981;141(6):646-651.

39. Patrick J, Campbell K, Carmichael L, Natale R, Richardson B. Patterns of gross fetal body movements over 24-hour observation intervals during the last 10 weeks of pregnancy. *Am J Obstet Gynecol.* 1982;142(4):363-371.
40. Parer JT, Dijkstra HR, Vredebregt PP, Harris JL, Krueger TR, Reuss ML. Increased fetal heart rate variability with acute hypoxia in chronically instrumented sheep. *Eur J Obstet Gynecol Reprod Biol.* 1980;10(6):393-399.
41. Thaler I, Timor-Tritsch IE, Blumenfeld Z. Effect of acute hypoxia on human fetal heart rate: the significance of increased heart rate variability. *Acta Obstet Gynecol Scand.* 1985;64(1):47-50.
42. Tournier A, Beacom M, Westgate JA, et al. Physiological control of fetal heart rate variability during labour: implications and controversies. *J Physiol.* 2022;600(3):431-450.
43. Shaw CJ, Allison BJ, Itani N, et al. Altered autonomic control of heart rate variability in the chronically hypoxic fetus. *J Physiol.* 2018;596(23):6105-6119.
44. Yamaguchi K, Lear CA, Beacom MJ, Ikeda T, Gunn AJ, Bennet L. Evolving changes in fetal heart rate variability and brain injury after hypoxia-ischaemia in preterm fetal sheep. *J Physiol.* 2018;596(23):6093-6104.
45. Tan S. Fault and blame, insults to the perinatal brain may be remote from time of birth. *Clin Perinatol.* 2014;41(1):105-117.
46. Ramirez-Cacho WA, Flores S, Schrader RM, McKay J, Rayburn WF. Effect of chronic maternal methadone therapy on intrapartum fetal heart rate patterns. *J Soc Gynecol Investig.* 2006;13(2):108-111.
47. Hatjis CG, Meis PJ. Sinusoidal fetal heart rate pattern associated with butorphanol administration. *Obstet Gynecol.* 1986;67(3):377-380.
48. Manseau P, Vaquier J, Chavinié J, Sureau C. Sinusoidal fetal cardiac rhythm: an aspect evocative of fetal distress during pregnancy. *J Gynecol Obstet Biol Reprod (Paris).* 1972;1(4):343-352.
49. Modanlou HD, Freeman RK, Ortiz O, Hinkes P, Pillsbury G Jr. Sinusoidal fetal heart rate pattern and severe fetal anemia. *Obstet Gynecol.* 1977;49(5):537-541.
50. Lowe TW, Leveno KJ, Quirk JG, Santos-Ramos R, Williams ML. Sinusoidal fetal heart rate pattern after intrauterine transfusion. *Obstet Gynecol.* 1984;64(3 Suppl):21S-25S.
51. Hatjis CG, Mennuti MT, Sacks LM, Schwarz RH. Resolution of a sinusoidal fetal heart rate pattern following intrauterine transfusion. *Am J Obstet Gynecol.* 1978;132(1):109-111.
52. Murata Y, Miyake Y, Yamamoto T, et al. Experimentally produced sinusoidal fetal heart rate pattern in the chronically instrumented fetal lamb. *Am J Obstet Gynecol.* 1985;153(6):693-702.
53. Lear CA, Kasai M, Drury PP, et al. Plasma vasopressin levels are closely associated with fetal hypotension and neuronal injury after hypoxia-ischemia in near-term fetal sheep. *Pediatr Res.* 2020;88(6):857-864.
54. Kubli FW, Hon EH, Khazin AF, Takemura H. Observations on heart rate and pH in the human fetus during labor. *Am J Obstet Gynecol.* 1969;104(8):1190-1206.
55. Hon EH, Bradfield AH, Hess OW. The electronic evaluation of the fetal heart rate. V. The vagal factor in fetal bradycardia. *Am J Obstet Gynecol.* 1961;82:291-300.
56. Paul WM, Quilligan EJ, MacLachlan T. Cardiovascular phenomenon associated with fetal head compression. *Am J Obstet Gynecol.* 1964;90(6):824-826.
57. Barcroft J. *Researches on Pre-Natal Life.* Blackwell Scientific Publications; 1946.
58. Lee ST, Hon EH. Fetal hemodynamic response to umbilical cord compression. *Obstet Gynecol.* 1963;22:553-562.
59. Lee CY, Di Loreto PC, O'Lane JM. Study of fetal heart rate acceleration patterns. *Obstet Gynecol.* 1975;45(2):142-146.
60. Gabbe SG, Ettinger BB, Freeman RK, Martin CB. Umbilical cord compression associated with amniotomy: laboratory observations. *Am J Obstet Gynecol.* 1976;126(3):353-355.
61. Miyazaki FS, Nevarez F. Saline amnioinfusion for relief of repetitive variable decelerations: a prospective randomized study. *Am J Obstet Gynecol.* 1985;153(3):301-306.
62. Spong CY, McKindsey F, Ross MG. Amniotic fluid index predicts the relief of variable decelerations after amnioinfusion bolus. *Am J Obstet Gynecol.* 1996;175(4 Pt 1):1066-1067.
63. Spong CY, Ogundipe OA, Ross MG. Prophylactic amnioinfusion for meconium-stained amniotic fluid. *Am J Obstet Gynecol.* 1994;171(4):931-935.
64. Siassi B, Wu PY, Blanco C, Martin CB. Baroreceptor and chemoreceptor responses to umbilical cord occlusion in fetal lambs. *Biol Neonate.* 1979;35(1-2):66-73.
65. Hon EH. Observations on pathologic fetal bradycardia. *Am J Obstet Gynecol.* 1959;77(5):1084-1099.
66. Caldeyro-Barcia R, Casacuberta C, Bustos R, et al. Correlation of intrapartum changes in fetal heart rate with fetal blood oxygen and acid base state. In: Adamson K, ed. *Diagnosis and Treatment of Fetal Disorders.* Springer-Verlag; 1968:205-225.
67. Itskovitz J, Goetzman BW, Rudolph AM. The mechanism of late deceleration of the heart rate and its relationship to oxygenation in normoxemic and chronically hypoxemic fetal lambs. *Am J Obstet Gynecol.* 1982;142(1):66-73.

CHAPTER 3

Intrauterine Hypoxia and Other Causes of Neonatal Encephalopathy and Cerebral Palsy

Aaron Caughey

The basic assumption that the predominant cause of cerebral palsy (CP) is intrauterine hypoxia is false. Although intrauterine hypoxia and its causal predecessors of cord compression, placental abruption, cord prolapse, uterine rupture, and others may lead to severe intrauterine hypoxia, neonatal acidosis, hypoxic-ischemic encephalopathy, and ultimately, neurodevelopmental delay and injury, they are probably only the causal etiology for a third or fewer of cases.

Electronic fetal heart rate (FHR) monitoring has been studied with respect to the effects of hypoxemia on the FHR. The relationship between uteroplacental insufficiency, umbilical cord compression, and FHR changes is useful in studying the mechanism of FHR change with respect to intrauterine fetal oxygenation. FHR changes also occur when the fetal central nervous system (CNS) control of FHR is impaired. This impairment may or may not have a hypoxic cause. The concept of CNS damage caused by intrauterine fetal conditions is no longer believed to be limited to hypoxia and trauma. Myriad associations have been described, even though a substantial percentage of children with neurologic problems never have a precise etiology assigned. Recent research has pointed to mechanisms other than hypoxia, including infection, hypercoagulable states, maternal thyroid disease, genetic abnormalities, and a family history of neurologic abnormalities. It is generally agreed that intrauterine hypoxia that progresses to metabolic acidosis in a term fetus, proximate to birth, sufficient to result in later CNS damage, will always be associated with neonatal encephalopathy.[1] Recent studies have also pointed to the fact that a substantial portion of cases of neonatal encephalopathy are not caused by intrauterine global fetal hypoxia. Furthermore, localized ischemia caused by cerebral infarcts without global hypoxia may cause neonatal encephalopathy and later neurologic damage. Finally, prematurity has the largest association with later CP and the patterns of neurologic deficits differ from those of children who sustained intrauterine damage at or near term.

INTRAUTERINE FETAL HYPOXIA

There can be intrauterine fetal hypoxia from a variety of factors. Oxygen comes to the fetus from the placenta, so if the fetal-placental circulation is disrupted, most commonly through compression of the umbilical cord, this will lead to fetal hypoxia. Gas exchange at the level of the placenta may also be suboptimal owing to placental pathology and during contractions. Upstream, if the mother is hypoxic, hypovolemic, or hypotensive, placental perfusion and/or placental oxygenation may be impacted. When the fetus is exposed to insufficient oxygen to allow the complete metabolism of glucose, lactic acid accumulates and results in metabolic acidosis. Acute impairment of the umbilical circulation will result in hypercarbia and respiratory acidosis caused by decreased exchange of CO_2, but uteroplacental insufficiency may or may not be associated with hypercarbia because the exchange of CO_2 at the placenta is more efficient than is exchange of oxygen. The term fetal asphyxia is overused and vague. More appropriately, terminology should refer to fetal hypoxia with or without metabolic acidosis. Additionally, although it is a popular legal theory, there remains no scientific basis for the notion that cerebral ischemia caused by the pressures of labor on the fetal skull and in the absence of fetal hypoxia with metabolic acidosis is a cause of CP.

Fetal circulatory responses to hypoxia include redistribution of blood flow to the more vital organs resulting in preservation of circulation to the brain, myocardium, and adrenal glands. There is a resulting decrease in blood flow to the kidneys, gastrointestinal tract, and muscles. This is why there is commonly acute kidney and liver damage in cases of hypoxic-ischemic encephalopathy. Another consequence of hypoxia is a loss of cerebral vascular autoregulation resulting in pressure-passive circulation. When the level of hypoxemia is near lethal, there is a decrease in fetal cardiac output resulting in hypotension and decreased cerebral blood flow.[2-4] It appears that when fetal cardiac output declines, resulting in a decrease in cerebral blood flow below a critical level, neuronal necrosis results. Subsequent development of cerebral edema in the neonate further compromises cerebral blood flow, aggravating the degree of neuronal necrosis.

When fetal hypoxia occurs at sublethal levels, permanent damage to the fetus may result; however, the frequency with which this occurs in the intrapartum period and the ability of the clinician to use fetal monitoring to prevent it are a subject of intense debate. References to perinatal brain damage can be found earlier, but the English orthopedic surgeon, Little,[5] is credited with the first specific hypothesis suggesting adverse perinatal events as the main etiologic factors in infantile spastic palsies. He reviewed the histories of more than 200 cases of spasticity of congenital origin and presented his paper entitled "On the influence of abnormal parturition, difficult labors, premature birth and asphyxia neonatorum, on the mental and physical condition of the child, especially in relation to deformities" to the Obstetrical Society of London. He concluded that these 200 cases had one thing in common, that is, some abnormal characteristics of parturition. The form of CP that he described has often been called "Little's disease." Little later went so far as to conclude that virtually nothing other than abnormalities of birth could cause the clinical picture he described.[5] Subsequently, other neurologic problems including mental retardation, epilepsy, and behavioral and learning disorders have been attributed to various intrapartum problems.

Animal data corroborating the concept that perinatal asphyxia may cause profound sublethal neurologic damage can be found in the classic papers of Windle and Becker.[6] Between 1943 and 1963, Windle[7] performed experimental asphyxiation of rhesus monkeys and evaluated the immediate, long-term, and neuropathologic effects. The monkeys were asphyxiated in one of two ways, both involving hysterotomy. Either the placenta and membranes were delivered with the fetus within the intact amniotic sac or the fetal head was covered by a fluid-filled sac and the umbilical cord was completely occluded. The fetal oxygen supply was completely interrupted for 5 to 20 minutes. Monkeys allowed to breathe in 6 minutes or less showed no neurologic deficits and no pathologic brain changes. Asphyxiation for more than 7 minutes produced at least transient motor and behavioral changes and relatively consistent brain pathology, along with necrosis of brain stem cells in the inferior colliculi and ventrolateral thalamic nuclei with secondary glial proliferative scarring. The most profound changes were found in monkeys left anoxic for 12 to 17 minutes. Resuscitation was invariably necessary. More severe brain stem lesions were created. Initially, the monkeys were hypoactive and hypotonic. Seizures, ataxia, and athetosis were often seen. The monkeys were observed for eight years and, as they matured, most deficits gradually improved, leaving residual hypoactivity and clumsiness. Although this model indeed supported the hypothesis that perinatal asphyxia is associated with permanent neurologic damage, the pattern of damage did not seem to correspond with the mental retardation and spasticity seen most commonly in humans. In later experiments, Windle[7] subjected monkeys to prolonged labor with oxytocin, and the asphyxiated neonates did not show the midbrain and brain stem lesions of acute total asphyxia but rather primarily cortical damage.

Myers[8] suggested that total asphyxia may not be the usual case in humans and that prolonged partial asphyxia is more likely. Myers was able to produce partial asphyxia in the rhesus monkey by various techniques including oxytocin-induced tachysystole, compression of the maternal abdominal aorta, maternal infusion of catecholamines, and inspiration by the pregnant monkey of reduced oxygen concentrations. These were controlled by maintaining fetal pO_2 at 5 to 9 mm Hg. Myers et al[9] later demonstrated that late decelerations of the FHR were caused by this fetal hypoxemia. Fetuses were maintained in these partially asphyctic states for at least 1 hour, then delivered and resuscitated. The immediate effect on the newborn was flaccidity, which evolved after several hours into generalized hypertonus and decerebrate posturing, at which time the newborns began to have periodic generalized seizures. Many fetuses developed ileus and cardiogenic shock and then died. A minority of fetuses survived. Extensive histopathologic examination of the brain led Myers to conclude that such prolonged partial hypoxia led to a vicious cycle of brain swelling, which caused decreased cerebral blood flow that further aggravated the brain swelling. In extreme degrees, such diminished blood flow led to total hemispheric cortical necrosis. In lesser degrees, cortical damage was seen in the middle third of the paracentral cerebral cortex and in the basal ganglia. Such lesions correspond closely with the intellectual deficits and spastic motor defects seen in humans in whom prolonged intermittent asphyxia is more common than acute total asphyxia as described by Windle.

ETIOLOGIC FACTORS IN CEREBRAL PALSY

Many authors have reviewed obstetric histories of children with congenital neurologic damage. Early in his career, Freud became interested in the etiology of CP. In his 1897 monograph, *Die Infantile Cerebrallahmung*,[10] Freud concluded that one-third of the cases were the result of traumatic birth, one-sixth were consequent to prematurity, one-sixth were of prenatal or postnatal cause, and one-third were unknown. Interestingly, Freud questioned whether the real etiology of the damage was the birth process or if abnormalities seen at birth were a reflection of a previously existing abnormality. For example, one study[11] found that a third of breech deliveries had major malformations, hence a conclusion that abnormal development was caused by breech delivery rather than the reality that existing fetal abnormalities contribute to the incidence of breech presentation. Another study[12] found a 3.8-fold increase in CP for breech-delivered children compared to those presenting as a vertex. In a study of 561 congenitally spastic children, upon review of their birth certificates, the authors found a very high incidence of abruptio placentae and placenta previa.[13] In an analysis of 96 obstetric records of infants in whom CP developed, only 18 of these births were uncomplicated, 34 babies were premature, and of the 96 infants, 30% had apnea of more than 30 seconds at birth.[14] Compared with controls, there was a doubling of third-trimester hemorrhage, a 3-fold increase in breech delivery, a 4-fold increase in both anesthetic complications and fetal distress by auscultation, and a 10-fold increase in shoulder dystocia among affected infants. In a subsequent, more extensive review[15] of 753 cases are summarized in Table 3.1.

A study in 1962 reviewed 317 patients with CP and concluded that 5% were a result of kernicterus, 8% were caused by congenital defects and neurologic infections, and 87% were cases "with possible obstetric causes."[16] Thus, for many years, it has been the impression that CP

TABLE 3.1 Obstetric background of 753 cases of CP[16]

Background	CP (%)	Control (%)
Postnatally acquired	8.5	
Premature (<2500 g)	29.0	8.0
Twins (rate twin A = rate twin B)	7.0	1.0
Mid/high forceps	8.0	5.0
Breech	9.0	3.5
Resuscitated at birth	27.0	3.0
Hypoxia	11.0	4.0
Cord prolapse	3.0	.3
Abruptio placentae	4.0	1.3
Toxemia	5.0	2.0
Prolonged labor	2.4	1.6
Hemolytic disease	6.0	.3
Congenital anomalies	5.0	1.3

CP, cerebral palsy.

was primarily caused by perinatal events. Fetal monitoring was developed with the hope that, by identifying fetal hypoxia early enough and with prompt and appropriate intervention, death and damage could be prevented.[17]

Contrary to the classic theory of intrapartum hypoxia as the major cause of CP, epidemiologic studies have shown that only a minority of CP cases are attributable solely to intrapartum events and that most cases of CP with intrapartum factors also have antepartum risk factors. In a 1998 case-controlled study that compared 164 term infants with moderate or severe neonatal encephalopathy to 400 term control infants without neonatal encephalopathy, antepartum and intrapartum risk factors for the development of CP were categorized. When adjusting for antepartum risk factors, they concluded that only maternal pyrexia during labor, occipital posterior position, an acute intrapartum event, instrumental vaginal delivery, emergency cesarean delivery, and general anesthesia were significant intrapartum risk factors for neonatal encephalopathy (Table 3.2). Such things as general anesthesia and emergency cesarean are not believed to be causative in themselves but by association with the reasons for these interventions. They concluded that 70% of term or near-term neonates with neonatal encephalopathy had only antepartum risk factors with no evidence of adverse intrapartum events, 25% had evidence of

TABLE 3.2 **Risk factors for neonatal encephalopathy**

Preconceptional factors	Antepartum factors	Intrapartum factors	Decreased risk
Increasing maternal age	Maternal thyroid disease	Intrapartum fever	Elective C/S
Unemployed, unskilled worker, or housewife	Severe preeclampsia	Prolonged rupture of membranes	
No private health insurance	Bleeding in pregnancy	Thick meconium	
Family history of seizures	Viral illness during pregnancy	Malpresentation and malposition	
Family history of neurologic disorders	Postdate pregnancy	Intrapartum hypoxia	
Infertility treatment	Growth restriction in the fetus	Acute intrapartum events	
	Placental abnormalities	Forceps delivery or emergency C/S	

C/S, cesarean section.

Indicates risk factors that are significant by multiple logistic regression analysis of term infants with neonatal encephalopathy compared with term infants without neonatal encephalopathy.

Adapted from Manning FA, Bondaji N, Harman CR, et al. Fetal assessment based on fetal biophysical profile scoring. VIII. The incidence of cerebral palsy in tested and untested perinates. *Am J Obstet Gynecol.* 1998;178(4):696-706.

antepartum risk factors and intrapartum hypoxia, and only 4% had only intrapartum hypoxia as a risk factor.[18] A problem with this analysis assumes that if any antepartum risk factor is present, the cause cannot be only intrapartum. For example, if a patient has antepartum preeclampsia and enters labor with normal electronic fetal monitoring (EFM) and subsequently has a prolapsed cord with prolonged deceleration or bradycardia and profound metabolic acidemia at birth, this would not be an isolated intrapartum event. The small contribution of intrapartum asphyxia as a cause of CP probably accounts largely for the fact that intrapartum FHR monitoring has been disappointing as a strategy to prevent CP,[19,20] but the epidemiologic analysis of Badawi probably underestimates the actual intrapartum contribution. A recent population-based study of children with CP in California revealed that about one-third of 7242 children with CP had an adverse intrapartum identifiable event compared to 12.9% in controls without CP.[21] The effect was more pronounced in children born prematurely (36.8%) than children born at term (28.3%). Maternal and neonatal infections were also significantly more common in birth records of children with CP. In a recent study from Japan that looked at CP in the setting of chorioamnionitis, 50% had an obstetric event leading to bradycardia and acute acidemia.[22] While the various estimates of the contribution of acute intrapartum events to the development of CP continue to vary between 5% and 50%, it is clear that adverse intrapartum events are a definite contributor to later CP.

FORMS OF CONGENITAL NEUROLOGIC DAMAGE RELATED TO FETAL HYPOXIA

Cerebral Palsy

CP caused by intrapartum fetal hypoxia will always have evidence of encephalopathy in the neonatal period and will be of the spastic quadriparetic or dyskinetic type. Unilateral brain lesions are not likely to be caused by global hypoxia as is seen in intrapartum asphyxia.[23,24] A large population-based survey placed the incidence of neonatal encephalopathy at 3.8 per 1000 term infants and the incidence of hypoxic-ischemic encephalopathy at 1.9 per 1000 term infants.[25] In the collaborative project, the incidence of neonatal encephalopathy was 5.4 per 1000 births weighing more than 2500 g. CP, defined as "a persistent but not changing disorder of movement and posture, appearing in the early years of life and owing to a nonprogressive disorder of the brain,"[15] will develop in approximately 5 infants per 1000 births, with a prevalence of one to two per 1000 school-age children. As a result, CP affects 350,000 children in the United States today.[14,26,27] Approximately 50% have mild intellectual retardation (IQ <70), and one-fourth are severely affected (IQ <50). One-fourth of children with CP have a seizure disorder.[26] CP is classified according to the distribution of extremities involved (diplegia, paraplegia, tetraplegia, and hemiplegia) and the type of movement disorder. Diplegia, a commonly used term, implies bilateral lower extremity involvement. Motor symptom classification describes the dominant movement disorder and includes spasticity, dyskinesia (athetosis), and ataxia.

Spastic diplegia is the abnormality most commonly associated with prematurity.[28] Infants born prematurely are also more likely to have periventricular white matter damage (periventricular leukomalacia [PVL]) than infants born at or near term. PVL is frequently associated with intraventricular hemorrhage and ventriculomegaly.[29] One study showed that abnormalities of the umbilical cord and frequent moderate variable decelerations seen in premature infants were more common in infants that were shown to have PVL.[30] There is no evidence that intervention for moderate variable decelerations in a premature fetus is indicated in that PVL did not develop in more than one-fourth of premature fetuses that also had frequent moderate variable decelerations.

Mental Retardation

Estimates of severe mental retardation are surprisingly uniform from country to country at about 3.5 per 1000 population.[31] Mild retardation is somewhat more variable, occurring in 23 to 31 per 1000, probably because of testing inaccuracy, predilection for testing, and the effect of environment in this group.[31] Mental retardation is a much less specific result of perinatal asphyxia than is CP. Perinatal causes are estimated to be responsible for approximately 10% of cases of mental retardation[32,33]; chromosome abnormalities and various hereditary disorders, 65%; infection, 5%; prenatal causes such as toxins and maternal disease, 10%; and the rest are unknown.[34] Many studies, including the Collaborative Perinatal Project,[35] have conducted prospective analyses of children determined to be asphyctic at birth, examining several criteria including Apgar score, neonatal apnea, shock, or acidosis. The vast majority (generally >90%) have normal IQs, and the mean IQ is usually only 5 to 10 points below average. Mental retardation without associated CP is not believed to be caused by fetal asphyxia.[36]

Epilepsy

Although the potential for hypoxia to cause seizures in both newborns and adults is acutely clear, there is not a strong relationship between perinatal events and epilepsy. The Collaborative Perinatal Project did not demonstrate an increase in epilepsy in low-birth-weight infants or in depressed infants[37]; however, epilepsy is found more commonly in infants with CP and mental retardation. Epilepsy without CP is not attributable to fetal asphyxia.[36]

Behavioral and Learning Disorders

Because most depressed neonates do not have demonstrable intellectual impairment, many have questioned whether indeed such infants do eventually reach their full intellectual potential. The data suggest the opposite because many children born hypoxic and acidotic, with demonstrated intellectual impairment in infancy and preschool periods, will test in normal ranges later on. Whether this implies dissipation of the effects of hypoxia with catch-up intellectual growth or limitations of testing is open to question. Some of Windle's severely asphyxiated monkeys had structural brain defects despite apparent normal behavior. The subtleties of behavioral difficulties and learning disorders make the problem very difficult to analyze. One study found that hyperactivity and learning disorders correlated weakly and inconsistently with perinatal asphyxia.[38] Thus, current knowledge does not consistently link isolated behavioral or learning disorders to fetal hypoxia.

OTHER FACTORS ASSOCIATED WITH NEONATAL ENCEPHALOPATHY AND CEREBRAL PALSY

Asphyxia is one cause of prenatal and perinatal neurologic damage. Other factors may be causative or contributive, or indeed, as pointed out by Freud,[10] in babies apparently distressed and hypoxic at birth, there may have been precedent damage or anomaly unrelated to hypoxia.

Prematurity

The association of prematurity and perinatal neurologic insults and their sequelae have long been recognized. Shakespeare's King Richard III, then Duke of Gloucester, proclaimed:

> I that am curtailed of this fair proportion, Cheated of feature by this dissembling nature, Deformed, unfinished, sent before my time Into this breathing world, scarce half made up—And that so lamely and unfashionable That dogs bark at me as I halt by them— ....

Little pointed out this passage in presenting his paper and documented a high association between spastic rigidity and prematurity.

Of all perinatal factors that are identifiable as being related to CP, prematurity has the highest correlation.[11] In a recent cohort study, this was reinforced in that prematurity was more predictive of CP than birth asphyxia.[39] Improvements in neonatal care have decreased the incidence of neurologic damage in very low-birth-weight babies, but survival rates have increased so much that the contribution of prematurity to CP rates continues to be significant. In several recent studies, the rates of long-term neurologic disabilities at the earlier gestations from 22 to 26 weeks have not appreciably decreased, but as survival rates have increased, there is likely a greater contribution from periviable births to CP cases.[40]

Prolonged Pregnancy

The risk for neonatal encephalopathy increases progressively after 39 weeks gestational age at birth. One study[18] found that the risk at 40 weeks was increased 1.41 times; at 41 weeks, 3.34 times; and at 42 weeks, 13.2 times. Causally, there were higher rates of perinatal asphyxia in post-term as compared to term infants identified in a cohort study of CP cases. The impact of post-term delivery was less when controlled for small gestational age and maternal age.[41,42]

Fetal Growth Restriction

Fetal growth restriction (FGR), also known as intrauterine fetal growth retardation, may be caused by perinatal infections, teratogens, congenital anomalies, inadequate nutrition, or uteroplacental insufficiency which is associated with birth asphyxia. In a cohort study of 96 full-term growth-restricted infants (excluding anomalies and congenital infections) up to eight years of age, CP occurred in 1% and epilepsy in 6%.[43] However, "minimal cerebral dysfunction (learning difficulties, hyperactivity, and poor coordination) were found in 25%." Of these infants, 30% had speech problems and 40% had poor school performance. In a case-controlled study, FGR was the most significant antepartum risk factor for the development of neonatal encephalopathy with an odds ratio of 4.37 between the third and ninth percentiles and 38.23 for FGR below the third percentile.[44] Because this group of fetuses/newborns is known to have a high incidence of perinatal asphyxia, it is difficult to determine whether a long-term antepartum respiratory and/or nutritional deficiency, intrapartum asphyctic insult, or some combination is responsible for such neurologic damage.

Traumatic Birth

The relatively high incidence of midforceps, high forceps, and breech deliveries in retrospective studies of neurologically damaged babies[14,15] suggests that birth trauma may have played a contributing role. For some mid- and high-forceps, it may also be an association with the indication for the delivery, known as confounding by indication. In breech births, further evidence is provided by the reduced incidence of these problems with elective cesarean delivery.[45] However, even delivered by cesarean delivery, breech neonates have a higher risk of long-term neurodevelopmental disorders, so the long-term outcomes would not all be related to traumatic birth. Because difficult operative vaginal deliveries have decreased over the past three decades, they are probably a less frequent cause of neurologic damage.

Prolonged Labor

Friedman et al,[46-48] in their series of studies concerning the effects of prolonged labor on adverse developmental outcomes, have demonstrated that this also may have contributed to sublethal CNS damage but that this may not be as important as the means of delivery (ie, midforceps). Because Friedman's work was largely done before EFM, it is difficult to know if the association with prolonged labor was because of fetal hypoxia or other causes such as infection. More recently, the association between prolonged labor and neonatal acidemia itself has been questioned with some studies finding no association between the two.[49]

Anesthesia and Analgesia

Drugs and anesthesia may contribute to neurologic damage in one of two ways. Regional analgesia may cause maternal hypotension with resultant fetal hypoxemia from decreased uterine perfusion.[50] Depressants, whether anesthetic agents or narcotics, may cause neonatal apnea. In a setting with the availability of good, appropriate neonatal resuscitation, this should contribute little to hypoxic-ischemic damage.

Genetic Factors

Congenital anomalies are associated with high incidences of CP, mental retardation, epilepsy, and developmental disabilities. Generally, researchers evaluating mental retardation report higher incidences of associated congenital defects than those studying CP. In a series of 1410 autopsies from three hospitals for the mentally retarded, Malamud reports a 61% incidence of anomalies, with Down syndrome the most frequent single cause.[51] Fetuses with a family history of neurologic disease or seizures had a twofold to threefold increase in neonatal encephalopathy[36] and CP.[11] This suggests a relation to genetic or early developmental causes. Some inherited metabolic abnormalities also are causes of neonatal encephalopathy and CP.[52] Recently, with the advent of whole exome and whole genome screening, a variety of genetic causes for CP have been identified. In a recent systematic review, 31% of CP cases had an identified genetic abnormality that may have been related.[53]

Fetal Infections

Congenital infections can be associated with CNS damage with or without microcephaly or hydrocephaly. Rubella, cytomegalovirus, syphilis, and toxoplasmosis (TORCH infections) are among well-known causes. As in anomalies, congenital TORCH infections are more likely to contribute to mental retardation and somatic growth retardation than to CP. They are estimated to account for 10% of mentally retarded children in developed countries.[31] Recently, there was an outbreak of the Zika virus in Brazil and several other countries that led to vertical infections of fetuses with long-term neurodevelopmental injury. Similar to CMV infections, even in those offspring who had normal antenatal ultrasounds, there was evidence for long-term in the setting of intrauterine the Zika virus infection.[54]

The fetal inflammatory response associated with maternal fever during labor, chorioamnionitis, and funisitis has been implicated as a cause of later CP.[55-57] It is believed that inflammatory cytokines can cause cerebral ischemia resulting in damage to the paraventricular area of premature fetal brains.[58-62] These lesions appear as PVL and intraventricular hemorrhage. The relation between chorioamnionitis and CP in term fetuses has been demonstrated.[63,64] Cytokines have also been implicated in term fetuses.[65] As our knowledge of infectious causes of CP increases, it may account for some of the large percentage of CP with unknown causes, and strategies for intervention may become evident.

Coagulation and Autoimmune Disorders

Infants whose blood contains indicators of coagulation or autoimmune disorders have a higher incidence of neonatal encephalopathy, stroke, and, later, CP, especially of the hemiparetic subtype.[63,66,67] One study looking at the placentas of children in whom CP developed showed that thromboses were the most frequent finding.[68] This study also showed that some of these mothers had a history of pregnancy loss and some had histories of autoimmune disorders. Thyroid disorders in mothers are a potent risk factor for neonatal encephalopathy and may be related to autoimmune mechanisms.[69] Neonatal encephalopathy resulting from cerebral infarcts caused by coagulation disorders may closely resemble hypoxic-ischemic encephalopathy. Neonates with encephalopathy should be evaluated for thrombophilias and autoimmune disease.

Toxins

Fetal neurotoxins may be the least understood causative factor in neurologic congenital diseases. Certainly, there are examples of environmental toxins (methyl mercury), drugs (folic acid antagonists such as methotrexate), and food and drink substances (alcohol) that are known to affect fetal neurologic development and cause serious mental retardation and even spasticity. Other environmental toxins may be responsible for a portion of the large group of cases of CP and mental retardation of unknown cause.

Antenatal Factors

The contributing role of antenatal factors is perhaps the most controversial and difficult to analyze of the factors involved in neurologic damage. Antenatal insult probably contributes to FGR, and when one observes the high incidence of antepartum bleeding and toxemia in the histories of children with neurologic damage, the contribution of antepartum damage seems likely. These babies often appear depressed at birth and have intrapartum FHR tracings that indicate fetal hypoxemia, but the damage may have occurred before the onset of labor.

Factors other than intrapartum hypoxia do seem very important in the pathogenesis of congenitally acquired neurologic damage. In assessing what contribution can be made with intrapartum assessment techniques, consideration must be given to such insults that may have occurred before the onset of labor. As described earlier, many cases of CP have no history of neonatal depression or perinatal insults. Furthermore, a large percentage of neonates with encephalopathy and CP have causes other than global hypoxia. Therefore, the abnormally developing child with features consistent with CP should not be assumed to have suffered antenatal or perinatal asphyxia.

OTHER ORGANS AFFECTED BY HYPOXIC-ISCHEMIC DAMAGE

Redistribution of blood flow in response to fetal hypoxia affects non-CNS organs acutely. Neurologic damage is not the only sublethal result of intrauterine fetal hypoxemia. It is well known that the lungs, kidney, and gastrointestinal tract are also sensitive to hypoxic ischemia and that newborn sequelae may result; however, non-neurologic damage usually repairs itself.[70]

Respiratory Distress Syndrome

Respiratory distress syndrome (RDS) is the leading cause of neonatal death and serious morbidity in prematurity. The primary etiologic factor is generally thought to be inadequate pulmonary surfactant. The synthesis of pulmonary lecithin (the major component of surfactant) is significantly diminished by hypoxia and acidosis.[71] Even in infants with mature ratios of lecithin to sphingomyelin, depressed and acidotic babies are more likely to have RDS.[72-74] It has been previously demonstrated that premature newborns, acidotic babies, and those with abnormal heart rate patterns suggesting hypoxia had both higher incidences of and higher mortalities from RDS.[73] Furthermore, in another study ominous FHR patterns were more predictive of RDS than Apgar scores.[74] In a recent study of neonates delivered at term by cesarean, neonatal acidemia was associated with a number of outcomes including RDS.[75]

Renal Damage

The association between hypoxia and renal damage, that is, anuria and renal failure similar to that in the adult, has been known since 1920. Animal data suggest such ischemic damage may be the result of the decreased renal blood flow after blood redistribution with hypoxia.[76,3,77] In a recent study, nearly half of the neonates with hypoxic-ischemic encephalopathy had acute kidney injury.[78] In a long-term follow-up study, the large majority of those with AKI did not have long-term renal dysfunction.[79]

Gastrointestinal Damage

Similarly, when blood flow is redistributed during periods of fetal hypoxia, blood flow to the fetal gastrointestinal tract is particularly diminished. Alward et al[80] have shown that in animal fetuses, asphyxia could lead to decreased blood flow to the gastrointestinal tract, thus resulting in dilation of segments of the large and small bowel and scattered mucosal necrosis. Towbin and Turner,[81] in looking at autopsies with other hypoxic-ischemic damage, found intestinal injuries caused by venous stasis and infarction, with lesions ranging from focal mucosal necrosis to massive gross intestinal infarction. Necrotizing enterocolitis (NEC), seen most frequently in premature infants, may at least in part be the result of such damage. Preliminary data suggest abnormal FHR patterns are often seen in fetuses destined to develop NEC.[82]

EVIDENCE FOR THE ASSOCIATION OF ABNORMAL FETAL HEART RATE PATTERNS WITH INTRAUTERINE HYPOXIA-ISCHEMIA AND METABOLIC ACIDOSIS

Knowing the association between intrauterine fetal hypoxia, ischemia and metabolic acidosis, and other intrapartum events with sublethal neurologic damage, one must demonstrate the relationship of abnormal FHR patterns with hypoxia and metabolic acidosis. If Apgar scores are used to measure neonatal depression, one must show the association of neonatal depression with fetal hypoxia and acidosis. The latter was well demonstrated by Modanlou et al.[83] Biochemical changes, especially pH and base deficit, have a statistically significant correlation with depressed newborns.[84]

Although it is not within the realm of this chapter to discuss the mechanisms responsible for the genesis of FHR patterns, it has been established that many FHR changes are triggered by fetal hypoxemia, which can progress to metabolic acidemia and have been associated with neonatal depression. Barcroft[85] first demonstrated the typical variable-type deceleration caused by umbilical cord occlusion in the fetal goat. Subsequently, Lee and Hon[86] were able to reproduce this in the human fetus. Myers et al[9] were able to reproduce late decelerations in the rhesus monkey by precipitating uterine artery hypotension.

Kubli et al[87] described the relationship of human fetal scalp pH with various FHR patterns and demonstrated that the more severe the pattern, the more likely the fetus is to be acidemic. However, the correlation between pH and severity of FHR pattern abnormality had a large standard deviation. The correlation with fetal base deficit was much tighter. Paul et al[88] further refined this work. They found that, with both acidosis and depressed Apgar scores, the FHR variability associated with late decelerations had a higher correlation than the amplitude of the late decelerations. Many subsequent

TABLE 3.3 Relationship between FHR pattern and 1-minute Apgar score

				Apgar 4-6 (moderate depression)		Apgar 0-3 (marked depression)	
FHR pattern	**Number**	**Percent**	**Mean Apgar**	**Number**	**Percent**	**Number**	**Percent**
Normal	322	45.0	8.2	16	5.0	3	.9
Uncomplicated baseline tachycardia	24	3.4	7.9	1	4.2	1	4.2
Uncomplicated baseline bradycardia	38	5.3	8.1	3	7.9	0	0
Uncomplicated loss of beat-to-beat variation	40	5.6	7.2	7	17.5	2	5.0
Complicated loss of beat-to-beat variation	11	1.5	6.7	2	18.2	2	18.2
Acceleration	52	7.3	8.4	1	1.9	0	0
Early deceleration	122	17.1	8.0	6	4.9	1	.8
Late deceleration	20	2.8	5.4	7	35.0	5	25.0
Variable deceleration with normal baseline	71	9.9	7.7	9	12.7	2	2.8
Variable deceleration with abnormal baseline	14	2.0	5.9	0	0	7	50.0

FHR, fetal heart rate.
From Bisonette JM. Relationship between continuous fetal heart rate patterns and Apgar score in the newborn. *Br J Obstet Gynaecol.* 1975;82(1):24, with permission.

studies have supported the parallel relationship of the abnormal FHR patterns and metabolic acidemia.

Many studies have linked FHR patterns to Apgar scores, showing generally that abnormal tracings are more likely to result in a depressed baby at birth. Because there are really no studies in which fetal monitor patterns are blinded and not acted upon, intervention may have decreased the degree of correlation because, in most patterns, a certain time is necessary from the onset of hypoxemia to the development of metabolic acidemia. Bisonette[89] has produced one of the most detailed retrospective analyses of FHR patterns and Apgar scores (Table 3.3). In a study that attempted to predict Apgar scores from FHR patterns obtained within 30 minutes of delivery without regard to clinical circumstances during labor demonstrated varied success.[90] When a normal baby was predicted, they were nearly always right; when a depressed baby was predicted, they were more often wrong, but when a baby was born depressed, it was nearly always predicted (Fig. 3.1). Clearly, neonates with intrapartum hypoxia sufficient to cause death or damage will always have FHR patterns reflecting the severe hypoxia. Because there are other causes of neonatal depression besides intrapartum hypoxia-asphyxia, one would not expect to find a 100% correlation between a predicted healthy baby and a normal Apgar score.

Normal Apgar Predicted
1 Min – 93% Correct
5 Min – 99% Correct

Low Apgar Predicted
1 Min – 43% Correct
5 Min – 20% Correct

Low Apgar Baby Delivered
1 Min – 54% Predicted
5 Min – 83% Predicted

Figure 3.1. Reliability of prediction of Apgar score from fetal heart rate tracings. (From Schifrin BS, Dame L. Fetal heart rate patterns. Prediction of Apgar score. *JAMA.* 1972;219(10):1322.)

It can be concluded, therefore, that FHR patterns suggesting fetal hypoxia and/or acidosis do correlate with depression at birth. One must be careful to point out that (a) not all abnormal patterns are associated with poor outcomes, (b) the extent to which intervention ameliorates or prevents adverse outcomes is unknown, (c) EFM corresponds best and is most valuable when the pattern is normal, and (d) FHR patterns, by themselves, are not predictive of later neurologic outcome.[91]

CRITERIA NECESSARY TO ASSIGN ACUTE INTRAPARTUM ASPHYXIA AS A CAUSE OF NEONATAL BRAIN DAMAGE

The criteria necessary to assign acute intrapartum hypoxia-asphyxia as a cause for neonatal brain damage have historically been derived from a 1992 American College of Obstetricians and Gynecologists (ACOG) technical bulletin, the Task Force on Cerebral Palsy and Neonatal Asphyxia of the Society of Obstetricians and Gynecologists of Canada, the Perinatal Society of Australia and New Zealand. In 2003, the ACOG and AAP published a revised statement[92] in a publication entitled Neonatal Encephalopathy and Cerebral Palsy: Defining the Pathogenesis and Pathophysiology, also known as the Green Book (as the cover is green). This publication was endorsed by

- The CDC
- The Child Neurology Society
- The March of Dimes
- The NICHD
- The Royal Australian and New Zealand College of Obstetricians and Gynecologists
- The Society of Maternal and Fetal Medicine
- The Society of Obstetricians and Gynecologists of Canada

The criteria published in this monograph were similar to those in the prior references, there were some changes based on the most recent evidence, however, which follow.

CRITERIA TO DEFINE AN ACUTE INTRAPARTUM HYPOXIC EVENT AS SUFFICIENT TO CAUSE CEREBRAL PALSY

Essential Criteria (must meet all four)

1. Evidence of metabolic acidosis in fetal umbilical cord arterial blood obtained at delivery (pH <7 and base deficit >12 mmol per L)
2. Early onset of severe or moderate neonatal encephalopathy in infants born at 34 or more weeks of gestation
3. CP of the spastic quadriplegic or dyskinetic type
4. Exclusion of other identifiable etiologies such as trauma, coagulation disorders, infectious conditions, or genetic disorders

Criteria that Collectively Suggest an Intrapartum Timing (Within Close Proximity to Labor and Delivery, eg, 0-48 hours) but Are Nonspecific to Asphyxial Insults

1. A sentinel (signal) hypoxic event occurring immediately before or during labor
2. A sudden or sustained fetal bradycardia or the absence of FHR variability in the presence of persistent, late, or variable decelerations, usually after a hypoxic sentinel event when the pattern was previously normal
3. Apgar scores of 0 to 3 beyond 5 minutes
4. Onset of multisystem involvement within 72 hours of birth
5. Early imaging study showing evidence of acute nonfocal cerebral abnormality

If the damaging hypoxic insult occurred prior to labor or during labor with full recovery from the hypoxic period, these criteria may not apply. It should also be noted that hypoxia and a fetal inflammatory insult may act synergistically. It is important to understand that these criteria may not all hold depending on the exact clinical situation. For example, there could be a hypoxic, bradycardic event that the fetus recovers from, leading to acute injury, but relatively normal cord gases and Apgar scores. Such a neonate might be readily resuscitated at birth, but develop seizures in the first 24 hours of life and demonstrate the other hallmarks of an acute, hypoxic injury.

THE IMPACT OF INTRAPARTUM ELECTRONIC FETAL MONITORING

Early studies of EFM indicated a correlation between FHR patterns and fetal pH, Apgar scores, and intrapartum death. Since the clinical introduction of intrapartum electronic FHR monitoring in the late 1960s and early 1970s, there have been a large number of both retrospective and prospective nonrandomized studies.[93-105] Initially, the nonrandomized, largely retrospective studies indicated a decrease in fetal and neonatal deaths with electronic intrapartum FHR monitoring compared with intermittent auscultation, as was done in the early 1970s. Some studies showed better outcomes in high-risk EFM fetuses than in low-risk fetuses monitored by intermittent auscultation. At that time, the intrapartum period was regarded as an especially vulnerable time for the fetus, and it was generally believed that most cases of CP were caused by intrapartum asphyxia.

In one of the first randomized prospective trials of intrapartum electronic FHR monitoring,[106] to the surprise of many, when compared to a one-on-one nurse listening every 15 minutes in the first stage of labor and every 5 minutes in the second stage of labor, outcomes including fetal and neonatal death, Apgar scores, and cord pH values were not different, with excellent results in both groups. The incidence of cesarean birth, however, was significantly increased in the EFM group. A follow-up study,[107] using fetal scalp blood pH before operative intervention, revealed that the excess cesarean birth rate decreased. Since then, there have been a number of prospectively randomized trials that have not shown any advantage to intrapartum EFM over intermittent auscultation with a one-on-one nurse listening every 15 minutes in the first stage of labor and every 5 minutes in the second stage of labor.[108-112] One randomized prospective trial,[113] done in Greece, suggested a benefit to intrapartum EFM with no hypoxic perinatal deaths and nine per thousand in the intermittent auscultation group. This was compared to 0.4 per thousand in the combined auscultation groups from the other prospectively randomized trials, suggesting either a different patient population or different auscultation techniques.

When these randomized prospective trials were completed, long-term neurologic outcome was evaluated in some of the study patients. In the Dublin study with excellent follow-up, while there were more neonatal seizures in the auscultation group, the incidence of CP was not different between groups.[114] A randomized prospective trial was then done[115] in preterm fetuses weighing between 700 and 1750 g found no difference in immediate outcome measures was noted. A three-year follow-up study on these infants[116] interestingly found that the EFM group actually had more cases of CP. This could have been owing to the study protocol that required documentation of acidotic fetal scalp pH before intervention in the EFM group, resulting in a longer delay to delivery after recognition of the abnormal pattern than in the auscultation group where no pH documentation was required.

The increased cesarean birth rate seen in some of the randomized trials with EFM without apparent benefit continues to be a concern. Because a high percentage of abnormal FHR strips are not associated with poor outcomes or metabolic acidemia, a technique that will safely reduce the cesarean birth rate among patients with FHR patterns that are concerning would be highly desirable. Fetal scalp blood pH sampling was such a technique, but because of the technical difficulty of this method, it has been largely abandoned in the US fetal pulse oximetry was a promising technique but with a large trial finding no differences in outcomes has been widely abandoned.[117,118] Fetal ST segment analysis is discussed later in this book, and although it appeared to be promising as a secondary technique to aid in the management of questionable FHR patterns, the large NICHD-funded trial demonstrated no benefit.[119] In the INFANT trial, a computer-based FHR interpretation tool found no benefit to short- or long-term neonatal outcomes.[120] One issue was that a significant proportion of providing clinicians disregarded the computer recommendations, so it is unclear whether the tool might work better in an environment with more compliant clinicians.

There have been no trials comparing intrapartum EFM to no monitoring. Another way to look at intrapartum EFM is to point out that it appears to be as good as having a one-on-one nurse listening every 15 minutes in the first stage of labor and every 5 minutes in the second stage of labor. Clearly, most busy labor and delivery units cannot provide that type of coverage for all laboring patients. It is the knowledge gained from EFM that is used to do intermittent auscultation, and, in fact, when auscultation is concerning, electronic monitoring is virtually always used before an intervention decision is made.

Thus, today we are left with a technique that clearly detects fetal hypoxia even in its earliest stages, but it appears to show no better outcome than intermittent auscultation with a one-on-one nurse listening every 15 minutes in the first stage of labor and every 5 minutes in the second stage. This then leaves us with some questions. Could most fetal asphyxia occur before labor, resulting in an abnormal pattern from the time of admission and a good correlation with the outcome but no benefit from the intervention? With sudden onset acute intrapartum hypoxia, perhaps fetal damage or death can occur so rapidly that even rapid intervention is not sufficient. Finally, perhaps neurologically abnormal fetuses are more likely to become hypoxic during labor, resulting in FHR patterns that detect the hypoxia but provide no benefit from intervention. Clearly, however, acute intrapartum asphyxia can result in fetal death or later neurologic damage, and in the fetus with a previously normal FHR pattern, acute damaging hypoxia with acidemia will be detected by FHR change, and the potential for intervention with prevention of death or damage exists.

The Effect of Electronic Fetal Monitoring and Dedicated Auscultation on Intrapartum Fetal Mortality

Although questions remain regarding the relative value of continuous intrapartum EFM versus intermittent auscultation, it is clear that dedicated electronic or auscultatory fetal monitoring during the intrapartum period reduces the intrapartum fetal death rate when compared to no dedicated auscultation during labor. Intrapartum fetal death is a clear endpoint, which, prior to the adoption of intrapartum EFM, occurred at a rate between one and four per 1000 in most obstetric populations. For this reason, a rather large study population would be required to determine the effect of EFM on the intrapartum death rate when compared to intensive auscultation as occurred in the randomized trials. However, it is clear that since the adoption of EFM and more intensive auscultation for routine fetal evaluation in labor, intrapartum fetal deaths are now relatively rare events. The first clinical studies were retrospective and noncontrolled. These studies included over 135,000 patients, and approximately one-third of these patients were electronically monitored.[95-105] The intrapartum death rate in these studies was 1.76 per 1000 in patients monitored during labor with auscultation and .54 per 1000 in patients monitored with EFM (P <.001). The intrapartum fetal death ratio calculates to 3.26:1 for auscultated versus electronically monitored patients (Table 3.4). These data were restricted to infants who weighed over 1500 g at birth and who were corrected for congenital anomalies. These studies can certainly be criticized on several bases, including different time frames in the EFM versus the auscultated groups and no consistent protocols for the use of auscultation. In most of these studies, the electronically monitored patients were at higher risk than the auscultated patients, and despite this, the intrapartum stillbirth rate was lower in the high-risk group that was electronically monitored. A recent ACOG practice bulletin no. 106 published in 2009[121] indicated that although there is no definitive evidence that EFM reduces perinatal mortality or CP, it is still recommended for all high-risk patients.

In 2010, the ACOG issued another practice bulletin no. 116[122] on the management of intrapartum FHR tracings, which is referred to in later chapters. This publication

TABLE 3.4 Intrapartum fetal death and EFM: nonrandomized trials

Primary author	Year	No EFM	IFD	EFM	IFD	Ratio
Chan et al[95]	1973	5427	17	1162	2	
Kelly and Kulkarni[96]	1973	17,000	15	150	0	
Tutera and Newman[97]	1975	6179	37	608	1	
Edington et al[98]	1975	991	4	1024	0	
Koh et al[99]	1975	1161	4	1080	5	
Shenker et al[100]	1975	11,599	14	1950	1	
Lee and Baggish[101]	1976	4323	15	3529	1	
Paul et al[102]	1977	36,724	34	13,344	6	
Amato[103]	1977	2981	12	4226	1	
Johnstone et al[104]	1978	9099	13	7313	3	
Hamilton et al[105]	1978	4353	11	4399	1	
Total		99,842	176	38,785	21	
Rate		1.76/1000		.54/1000		3.26 (P<.001)
Critical no. of subjects for P<.05 = 18,046						

EFM, electronic fetal monitoring; IFD, intrapartum fetal death.
From Antenatal Diagnosis. Report of a consensus development conference. NIH Publication no. 79-1973, Bethesda, MD, April 1979.

TABLE 3.5 Intrapartum fetal deaths: randomized prospective studies[a]

	Intermittent auscultation		Continuous EFM	
Study author	**Cases**	**Deaths**	**Cases**	**Deaths**
Haverkamp et al[106]	241	0	242	0
Haverkamp et al[107]	232	0	453	0
Renou et al[108]	175	1	175	0
Kelso et al[109]	251	0	252	0
Wood et al[110]	432	0	445	0
McDonald et al[111]	4999	2	4987	3
Totals	6155	3	6554	3

EFM, electronic fetal monitoring.
[a]Does not include the study by Leveno et al,[112] which used selective EFM in the control group and Vintzileos et al,[113] where the hypoxic death rate in the auscultated group was an outlier.

outlines one recommended approach to management based on the three-tiered categorization of FHR tracings delineated in the 2008 NICHD statement.[123]

Eight published randomized controlled trials have compared EFM to auscultation in both high- and low-risk patients and with one exception have shown no difference in intrapartum fetal death.[106-113] In one study,[113] there was a difference favoring electronically monitored patients and the high hypoxic mortality rate in the auscultated group that may not apply as discussed previously. It is significant that in most of the trials, both groups in each randomized controlled trial had a dedicated one-on-one nurse assigned to the patient, and the auscultated groups were followed much more frequently than was commonly practiced in hospitals. This is substantiated by the low combined intrapartum fetal death rate in the auscultated groups: 1.05 per 1000. If the studies without one-to-one nursing are excluded, the intrapartum fetal death rate drops to 0.4 per 1000 (Table 3.5). Furthermore, in these studies, abnormal auscultative heart rates were often backed up by electronic FHR monitoring. It is thus evident that either EFM or dedicated auscultation will reduce the intrapartum fetal death rate compared to less stringent monitoring.

What Are the Risks of Electronic Fetal Monitoring?

There has been much written about the risk of invasive EFM with a fetal scalp electrode (FSE) and infection of the fetus and/or mother. Fetal infections have consisted almost exclusively of small scalp infections characterized by erythema and induration requiring no more than local medication and are reported in from 0.3% to 4.5%[124-129] of internally monitored labors. Despite this, there is a theoretical risk of vertical transmission of HIV, so FSE is generally advised against in such patients.[130]

Maternal infection in patients with internal EFM via FSE during labor has been said to be increased in several studies,[106,125-127] whereas other studies have indicated no increased risk of maternal infection.[95,108] When one examines the reports, it becomes obvious that infection is most pronounced if the patient is monitored and then delivered by cesarean, as opposed to the patient who is monitored and then delivered vaginally. Scrutiny will reveal that the patient with long labor, many vaginal examinations, prolonged ruptured membranes, and obstructed labor requiring cesarean section is also the most likely patient to be internally monitored for a prolonged time. This association is probably responsible for the presumed cause-effect relationship between EFM and infection following cesarean section, but it is unlikely that the monitoring itself is responsible for the infections. Gibbs et al[128] looked at all associated factors with postcesarean infection and, using multivariate analysis, found that internal monitoring had little or no effect on infection. In medical-legal cases, poor-quality external fetal monitoring can be a deviation from the standard of care that results in plaintiff decisions. The reluctance to use a FSE and/or intrauterine pressure monitoring device can contribute to this problem.

Effect of Electronic Fetal Monitoring on the Cesarean Section Rate

Perhaps the most discussed risk of EFM is the increase in the cesarean rate that some have attributed to EFM (Table 3.6). Determining the exact contribution, if any, that EFM makes to the overall cesarean section rate is complicated by the fact that many other practices, such as routine cesarean section for breech presentations and abandoning midforceps, have changed during the same period that EFM has been on the increase. However, five of the seven randomized controlled trials have shown an increase in the cesarean section rate in the EFM group.

Clearly, there are patients who are allowed to labor because of the fetal monitor, whereas before EFM, they would not have even been given a trial of labor. In our practice, this has been best demonstrated in diabetics, patients with clinical abruptions, elderly gravidas, and certain patients with previous intrapartum fetal death where the monitoring reassures both the patient and the physician.

An early study examined the impact of EFM on the cesarean section rate in California during 1977.[131] They surveyed 324,085 births and determined that about half the patients in California had electronically monitored labors. They determined the expected perinatal mortality rates for each hospital based on the risk of the population served. They then determined those medical care factors that favorably or unfavorably affected those mortality rates. The most significant factors that favorably affected perinatal mortality were a high cesarean rate and a high incidence of fetal monitoring. Other factors favorable to an improved perinatal outcome included a neonatal intensive care unit in the hospital, delivery by a trained obstetrician, a perinatal morbidity committee in the hospital, and the occurrence of the birth in a nonprofit community hospital with a teaching program. The data, which included a large number of deliveries over a one-year period from all types of hospitals, suggest that the overall impact of high technology with its probably higher rate of intervention would seem to be justified on the basis of improved perinatal mortality. However, since 1977, the cesarean section rate has more than doubled, and it has increased by 50% since 1996. It is hard to say this rise has been associated with additional benefit.[132]

TABLE 3.6 Impact of EFM on cesarean section rates: randomized prospective studies[a]

Study author	C-sections (%) Intermittent auscultation	Continuous EFM
Haverkamp et al[106]	7	17
Haverkamp et al[107]	6	11
Renou et al[108]	14	22
Kelso et al[109]	4	10
Wood et al[110]	2.1	4
McDonald et al[111]	2.2	2.4

C-sections, cesarean sections; EFM, electronic fetal monitoring.
[a]Does not include study by Leveno et al,[112] which used selective EFM in the control group.

THE IMPACT OF ANTEPARTUM FETAL HEART RATE MONITORING

There have been several randomized prospective trials comparing primary antepartum fetal surveillance using the nonstress test to no nonstress test surveillance, which have shown no benefit to this form of testing alone.[133-136] None of these trials involved long-term follow-up. There is only one prospective randomized trial of antepartum surveillance that showed benefit. This study was of fetal movement counting that showed a decrease in antepartum fetal deaths in patients instructed in fetal movement counting compared with patients with no fetal movement counting instructions.[137] A 1983 study[138] demonstrated that when a nonreactive positive spontaneous contraction stress was found, there was a 28% perinatal mortality rate, and 27% of surviving infants were found to have a neurologic handicap. Manning looked retrospectively at patients studied with biophysical profile surveillance and found fewer cases of CP when these cases were compared with patients not monitored with biophysical profiles (1.33 vs 4.74 per 1000).[139,140] Dayal, Manning et al[141] reported that among 86,955 patients studied with the biophysical profile fetal-maternal hemorrhage was the most common cause of a false-negative test. In August of 2007, the NICHD convened a workshop titled Antenatal Testing: A Reevaluation.[142] A summary based on this workshop was published in Seminars in Perinatology in 2008, which pointed out the possible benefits and the problems with antenatal testing. The conclusion was that further research was indicated regarding

- The epidemiology of antepartum stillbirth and neurologic injury
- Normal fetal physiology and fetal responses to intrauterine insults
- The technology and utility of existing and emerging fetal assessment methods
- Maternal and fetal indications for antenatal testing
- Cost and benefits of antenatal testing

Certainly, the potential for benefit of antepartum surveillance would seem high because a majority of stillbirths occur before labor, and even those fetuses with intrapartum hypoxia, more often than not, have evidence of antepartum risk factors. However, because of the high incidence of normal outcomes in patients with abnormal antepartum testing, the predictive value of antepartum testing remains poor.

SUMMARY

Intrapartum fetal hypoxemia that progresses to metabolic acidemia is a clear although infrequent cause of fetal mortality and morbidity that may lead to long-term neurologic damage. Electronic fetal monitoring and dedicated intrapartum auscultation decrease the intrapartum fetal death rate when compared to practices before the introduction of either technique. Most cases of neonatal encephalopathy and CP are attributed to causes other than intrapartum hypoxia alone. Electronic FHR monitoring appears to be associated with an increased cesarean section rate in some settings. Our current understanding of fetal monitoring patterns shows substantial agreement with respect to patterns consistent with normal fetal oxygenation and with respect to patterns consistent with ongoing fetal hypoxia and acidosis. There is, however, much disagreement with respect to patterns in between.[143-145]

REFERENCES

1. Yudkin PL, Johnson A, Clover LM, Murphy KW. Clustering of perinatal markers of birth asphyxia and outcome at age five years. *Br J Obstet Gynecol.* 1994;101(9):774-781.
2. Behrman RE, Lees MH, Petersen EN, De Lannoy CW, Seeds AE. Distribution of circulation in the normal and asphyxiated fetal primate. *Am J Obstet Gynecol.* 1970;108(6):956-969.
3. Cohn EH, Sacks EJ, Heymann MA, Rudolph AM. Cardiovascular responses to hypoxemia and acidemia in fetal lambs. *Am J Obstet Gynecol.* 1974;120(6):817-824.
4. Peeters LL, Sheldon RE, Jones MD, Makowski EL, Meschia G. Blood flow to organs as a function of arterial oxygen content. *Am J Obstet Gynecol.* 1979;135(5):637-644.
5. Little WJ. On the influence of abnormal parturition, difficult labours, premature birth and asphyxia neonatorum, on the mental and physical condition of the child, especially in relation to deformities. *Trans Obstet Soc London.* 1862;3:293.
6. Windle WF, Becker RF. Asphyxia neonatorum: an experimental study in the guinea pig. *Am J Obstet Gynecol.* 1943;45(2):183-200.
7. Windle WF. Neuropathology of certain forms of mental retardation. *Science.* 1963;140(3572):1186-1189.
8. Myers RE. Two patterns of perinatal brain damage and their conditions of occurrence. *Am J Obstet Gynecol.* 1972;112(2):246-276.
9. Myers RE, Mueller-Huebach E, Adamsons K. Predictability of the state of fetal oxygenation from a quantitative analysis of the components of late decelerations. *Am J Obstet Gynecol.* 1973;115(8):1083-1094.
10. Freud S. *Die Infantile Cerebrallahmung.* A. Hoelder; 1897.
11. Nelson KB, Ellenberg JH. Antecedents of cerebral palsy: multivariate analysis of risk. *N Engl J Med.* 1986;315(2):81-86.
12. Torfs CP, van den Berg BJ, Oechsli FW, Cummins S. Prenatal and perinatal factors in the etiology of cerebral palsy. *J Pediatr.* 1990;116(4):615-619.
13. Lilienfeld AM, Pasamanick B. The association of maternal and fetal factors with the development of cerebral palsy and epilepsy. *Am J Obstet Gynecol.* 1955;70(1):93-101.
14. Eastman NJ, DeLeon M. The etiology of cerebral palsy. *Am J Obstet Gynecol.* 1955;69(5):950-961.
15. Eastman NJ, Kohl SG, Maisel JE, Kavaler F. The obstetrical background of 753 cases of cerebral palsy. *Obstet Gynecol Surv.* 1962;17:459-500.
16. Steer CW, Bonney W. Obstetric factors in cerebral palsy. *Am J Obstet Gynecol.* 1962;83:526-531.
17. Quilligan EJ, Paul RH. Fetal monitoring: is it worth it? *Obstet Gynecol.* 1975;45(1):96-100.
18. Badawi N, Kurinczuk JJ, Keogh JM, et al. Intrapartum risk factors for newborn encephalopathy: the Western Australia case control study. *BMJ.* 1998;317(7172):1554-1558.
19. Paneth N. Birth and the origins of cerebral palsy [Editorial]. *N Engl J Med.* 1986;315(2):124-126.
20. Freeman RK. Intrapartum fetal monitoring—a disappointing story. *N Engl J Med.* 1990;322(9):624-626.
21. Gilbert WM, Jacoby BN, Xing G, Danielsen B, Smith LH. Adverse obstetrics events are associated with significant risk of cerebral palsy. *Am J Obstet Gynecol.* 2010;203(4):328-331.
22. Yamaguchi-Goto T, Ohashi M, Kodama Y, Sameshima H. Fetal heart rate patterns complicated by chorioamnionitis and subsequent cerebral palsy in Japan. *J Obstet Gynaecol Res.* 2023;49(2):625-634. doi: 10.1111/jog.15508.
23. Michelis R, Rooschuz B, Dopfer R. Prenatal origin of spastic hemiparesis. *Early Hum Dev.* 1980;4(3):243-255.
24. Nelson KB, Grether JK. Potentially asphyxiating conditions and spastic cerebral palsy in infants of normal birth weight. *Am J Obstet Gynecol.* 1998;179(2):507-513.

25. Badawi N, Kurinczuk JJ, Hall D, Field D, Pemberton PJ, Stanley FJ. Newborn encephalopathy in term infants: three approaches to population based investigation. *Semin Neonatol.* 1997;2(3):181-188.
26. Nelson KB, Ellenberg JH. Epidemiology of cerebral palsy. In: Schoenberg BS, ed. *Advances in Neurology*, vol. 19. Raven Press; 1979.
27. Alberman E. Main causes of major mental handicap: prevalence and epidemiology. In: *CIBA Foundation Symposium 59: Major Mental Handicap: Methods and Costs of Prevention.* Elsevier-Excerpta Medica; 1978.
28. Hagberg G, Hagberg B, Olow I. The changing panorama of cerebral palsy in Sweden, 1954-1970. I. Analysis of the general changes. *Acta Paediatr Scand.* 1975;64(2):187-192.
29. Kunban C, Sanocka U, Leviton A, et al. White matter disorders of prematurity: association with intraventricular hemorrhage and ventriculomegaly. *J Pediatr.* 1999;134(5):539-546.
30. Ito T, Kadowaki K, Takahashi H, Nagata N, Makio A, Terakawa N. Clinical features and cardiotocographic findings for premature infants with antenatal periventricular leukomalacia. *Early Hum Dev.* 1997;47(2):195-201.
31. Stein Z, Susser M. Mental retardation. In: Last JM, ed. *Public Health and Preventive Medicine.* Appleton-Century-Crofts; 1980.
32. McDonald AD. Severely retarded children in Quebec: prevalence, causes and care. *Am J Ment Defic.* 1973;78(2):205-215.
33. Drillien CM. Studies in mental handicap. II. Some obstetric factors of possible aetiological significance. *Arch Dis Child.* 1968;43(229):283-294.
34. Warkany J. Mental retardation. In: *Congenital Malformations.* Year Book Medical Publishers, Inc.; 1971:262-267.
35. Drage JS, Kennedy S, Berendes H, Schwarz BK, Weiss W. The Apgar score as an index of infant morbidity: a report from the collaborative study of cerebral palsy. *Dev Med Child Neurol.* 1966;8(2):141-148.
36. American College of Obstetricians and Gynecologists. Fetal and neonatal neurologic injury. ACOG Technical Bulletin 163. Washington, DC: ACOG; 1992.
37. Ellenberg J, Nelson K. Birth weight and gestational age in children with cerebral palsy or seizure disorders. *Am J Dis Child.* 1979;133(10):1044-1048.
38. Nichols PL, Chen TC. *Minimal Brain Dysfunction: A Prospective Study.* Erlbaum Associates; 1981.
39. Sukhov A, Wu Y, Xing G, Smith LH, Gilbert WM. Risk factors associated with cerebral palsy in preterm infants. *J Matern Fetal Neonatal Med.* 2012;25(1):53-57. doi: 10.3109/14767058.2011.564689.
40. Younge N, Goldstein RF, Bann CM, et al. Survival and neurodevelopmental outcomes among periviable infants. *N Engl J Med.* 2017;376(7):617-628.
41. Campbell MK, Truls-Ostbye MD, Lorentz M. Post-term birth: risk factors and outcomes in a 10 year cohort of Norwegian births. *Obstet Gynecol.* 1997;89(4):543-548.
42. Frank R, Garfinkle J, Oskoui M, Shevell MI. Clinical profile of children with cerebral palsy born term compared with late- and post-term: a retrospective cohort study. *BJOG.* 2017;124(11):1738-1745.
43. Fitzhardinge PM, Steven EM. The small for date infant. II. Neurological and intellectual sequelae. *Pediatrics.* 1972;50(1):50-57.
44. Badawi N, Kurinczuk JJ, Keogh JM, et al. Antepartum risk factors for neonatal encephalopathy: the Western Australia case-control study. *BMJ.* 1998;317(7172):1549-1553.
45. Hannah ME, Hannah WJ, Hewson SA, Hodnett ED, Saigal S, Willan AR. Planned cesarean section versus planned vaginal birth for breech presentation at term: a randomized multicentre trial. Term breech trial collaborative group. *Lancet.* 2000;356(9239):1375-1383.
46. Friedman EA, Niswander KR, Sachtleben MR, Naftaly N. Dysfunctional labor. X. Immediate results to infant. *Obstet Gynecol.* 1969;33(6):776-784.
47. Friedman EA, Niswander KR, Sachtleben MR. Dysfunctional labor. XI. Neurologic and developmental effects on surviving infants. *Obstet Gynecol.* 1969;33(6):785-791.
48. Friedman EA, Sachtleben MR, Bresky PA. Dysfunctional labor. XII. Long term effects on infant. *Am J Obstet Gynecol.* 1977;127(7):779-783.
49. Cheng YW, Hopkins LM, Caughey AB. How long is too long: does a prolonged second stage of labor in nulliparous women affect maternal and neonatal outcomes? *Am J Obstet Gynecol.* 2004;191(3):933-938.
50. Rimsza RR, Perez WM, Babbar S, O'Brien M, Vricella LK. Time from neuraxial anesthesia placement to delivery is inversely proportional to umbilical arterial cord pH at scheduled cesarean delivery. *Am J Obstet Gynecol.* 2019;220(4):389.e1-389.e9.
51. Malamud N. Neuropathology. In: Stevens HA, Heber R, eds. *Mental Retardation.* The University of Chicago Press; 1964.
52. Leviton A, Nelson KB. Problems with definitions and classifications of newborn encephalopathy. *Pediatr Neurol.* 1992;8(2):85-90.
53. Gonzalez-Mantilla PJ, Hu Y, Myers SM, et al. Diagnostic yield of exome sequencing in cerebral palsy and implications for genetic testing guidelines: a systematic review and meta-analysis. *JAMA Pediatr.* 2023;177(5):472-478.
54. Pool KL, Adachi K, Karnezis S, et al. Association between neonatal neuroimaging and clinical outcomes in Zika-exposed infants from Rio de Janeiro, Brazil. *JAMA Netw Open.* 2019;2(7):e198124.
55. Dammann O, Leviton A. Role of the fetus in perinatal infection and neonatal brain damage. *Curr Opin Pediatr.* 2000;12(2):99-104.
56. Lieberman E, Richardson DK, Lang J, Frigoletto FD, Heffner LJ, Cohen A. Intrapartum maternal fever and neonatal outcome. *Pediatrics.* 2000;105(1 Pt 1):8-13.
57. Impey L, Greenwood C, MacQuillan K, Reynolds M, Sheil O. Fever in labour and neonatal encephalopathy: a prospective cohort study. *Br J Obstet Gynecol.* 2001;108(6):594-597.
58. Yoon BH, Jun JK, Romero R, et al. Amniotic fluid inflammatory cytokines (interleukin 6, interleukin 1B, and tumor necrosis factor α), neonatal white matter lesions, and cerebral palsy. *Am J Obstet Gynecol.* 1997;177(1):19-26.

59. Yoon BH, Romero R, Park JS, et al. Fetal exposure to an intraamniotic inflammation and the development of cerebral palsy at the age of three years. *Am J Obstet Gynecol.* 2000;182(3):675-681.
60. Naccasha N, Hinson R, Montag A, Ismail M, Bentz L, Mittendorf R. Association between funisitis and elevated interleukin-6 in cord blood. *Obstet Gynecol.* 2001;97(2):220-224.
61. Dammann O, Leviton A. Maternal intrauterine infection, cytokines, and brain damage in the preterm newborn. *Pediatr Res.* 1997;42(1):1-8.
62. Steinborn A, Niederhut A, Solbach C, Hildenbrand R, Sohn C, Kaufmann M. Cytokine release from placental endothelial cells, a process associated with preterm labour in the absence of intrauterine infection. *Cytokine.* 1999;11(1):66-73.
63. Grether JK, Nelson LB. Maternal infection and cerebral palsy in infants of normal birth weight. *JAMA.* 1997;278(3):207-211.
64. Eschenbach DA. Amniotic fluid infection and cerebral palsy (Editorial). *JAMA.* 1997;278(3):247-248.
65. Nelson KB, Dambrosia JM, Grether JK, Phillips TM. Neonatal cytokines and coagulation factors in children with cerebral palsy. *Ann Neurol.* 1998;44(4):666-675.
66. Kraus FT, Acheen VI. Fetal thrombotic vasculopathy in the placenta: cerebral thrombi and infarcts, coagulopathies and cerebral palsy. *Hum Pathol.* 1999;30(7):759-769.
67. Redline RW, Wilson-Castillo D, Borawski E, Fanaroff AA, Hack M. Placental lesions associated with neurologic impairment and cerebral palsy in very low birth weight infants. *Arch Pathol Lab Med.* 1998;122(12):1091-1099.
68. Kraus FT. Cerebral palsy and thrombi in placental vessels of the fetus. *Hum Pathol.* 1997;28(2):246-248.
69. Badawi N, Kurinczuk JJ, Mackenzie CL, et al. Maternal thyroid disease: a risk factor for newborn encephalopathy in term infants. *Br J Obstet Gynecol.* 2000;107(6):798-801.
70. Perlman JM, Tack EC. Renal injury in the asphyxiated newborn infant: relationship to neurological outcome. *J Pediatr.* 1998;113(5): 875-879.
71. Merritt TA, Farrell PM. Diminished pulmonary lecithin synthesis in acidosis: experimental findings as related to the respiratory distress syndrome. *Pediatrics.* 1976;57(1):32-40.
72. Cruz AC, Bohi WC, Birk SA, Spellacy WN. Respiratory distress syndrome with mature lecithin/sphingomyelin ratios: diabetes mellitus and low Apgar scores. *Am J Obstet Gynecol.* 1976;126(1):78-82.
73. Hobel CJ, Hyvarinen M, Oh W. Abnormal fetal heart rate patterns and fetal acid-base balance in low birth weight infants in relation to respiratory distress syndrome. *Obstet Gynecol.* 1972;39(1):83-88.
74. Martin CB, Siassi B, Hon EH. Fetal heart rate patterns and neonatal death in low birthweight infants. *Obstet Gynecol.* 1974;44(4):503-510.
75. Bligard KH, Cameo T, McCallum KN, et al. The association of fetal acidemia with adverse neonatal outcomes at time of scheduled cesarean delivery. *Am J Obstet Gynecol.* 2022;227(2):265.e1-265.e8.
76. Ikeda T, Murata Y, Quilligan E, Parer JT, Murayama T, Koono M. Histologic and biochemical study of the brain, heart, kidney and liver in asphyxia caused by occlusion of the umbilical cord in near term fetal lambs. *Am J Obstet Gynecol.* 2000; 182(2):449-457.
77. Perlman JM, Tack EK. Renal injury in the asphyxiated newborn infant: relationship to neurological outcome. *J Pediatr.* 1988;113(5):875-879.
78. Modisett AK, Patel RM, Jernigan SM, Figueroa J, Sewell EK, Hamrick SEG. Patterns of acute kidney and hepatic injury and association with adverse outcomes in infants undergoing therapeutic hypothermia for hypoxic ischemic encephalopathy. *J Perinatol.* 2022;42(10):1361-1367.
79. Robertsson GK, Vishnevskaya L, Diaz RS, et al. Kidney outcomes in early adolescence following perinatal asphyxia and hypothermia-treated hypoxic-ischaemic encephalopathy. *Pediatr Nephrol.* 2023;38(4):1205-1214.
80. Alward CT, Hook JB, Helmrath TA, Mattson JC, Bailie MD. Effects of asphyxia on cardiac output and organ blood flow in the newborn piglet. *Pediatr Res.* 1978;12(8):824-827.
81. Towbin A, Turner GL. Obstetric factors in fetal-neonatal visceral injury. *Obstet Gynecol.* 1978;52(1):113-124.
82. Braly P, German J, Garite T. Fetal heart rate patterns in infants who develop necrotizing enterocolitis. *Arch Surg.* 1980;115(9): 1050-1053.
83. Modanlou H, Yeh SY, Hon EH, Forsythe A. Fetal and neonatal biochemistry and Apgar scores. *Am J Obstet Gynecol.* 1973;117(7):942-951.
84. Low JA, Victory R, Derrick EJ. Predictive value of electronic monitoring for intrapartum fetal asphyxia with metabolic acidosis. *Obstet Gynecol.* 1999;93(2):285-291.
85. Barcroft J. *Researches on Perinatal Life.* Blackwell Scientific Publications Ltd.; 1946:124.
86. Lee ST, Hon EH. Fetal hemodynamic response to umbilical cord compression. *Obstet Gynecol.* 1963;22:533-562.
87. Kubli FH, Hon EH, Khazin AF, Takemura H. Observations on fetal heart rate and pH in the human fetus during labor. *Am J Obstet Gynecol.* 1969;104(8):1190-1206.
88. Paul RH, Suidan AK, Yeh SY, Schifrin BS, Hon EH. Clinical fetal monitoring. VII. The evaluation and significance of intrapartum FHR variability. *Am J Obstet Gynecol.* 1975;123(2):206-210.
89. Bissonnette JM. Relationship between continuous fetal heart rate patterns and Apgar score in the newborn. *Br J Obstet Gynaecol.* 1975;82(1):24.
90. Schifrin BS, Dame L. Fetal heart rate patterns: prediction of Apgar score. *JAMA.* 1972;219(10):1322-1325.
91. Nelson KB, Dambrosia JM, Ting TY, Grether JK. Uncertain value of electronic fetal monitoring in predicting cerebral palsy. *N Engl J Med.* 1996;334(10):613-618.
92. American College of Obstetricians and Gynecologists and American Academy of Pediatricians. Neonatal encephalopathy and cerebral palsy. Washington, DC: Author, 2003.
93. Tejani N, Mann L, Bhakthavathsalan A, Weiss RR. Correlation of fetal heart rate-uterine contraction patterns with fetal scalp blood pH. *Obstet Gynecol.* 1975;46(4):392-396.
94. Banta HD, Thacker SB. Costs and benefits of electronic fetal monitoring: a review of the literature. Department of HEW Publication no. (PHS) 79-3245, Washington, DC.

95. Chan WH, Paul RH, Toews J. Intrapartum fetal monitoring maternal and fetal morbidity and perinatal mortality. *Obstet Gynecol.* 1973;41(1):7-13.
96. Kelly VC, Kulkarni D. Experiences with fetal monitoring in a community hospital. *Obstet Gynecol.* 1973;41(6):818-824.
97. Tutera G, Newman RL. Fetal monitoring: its effect on the perinatal mortality and caesarean section rates and its complications. *Am J Obstet Gynecol.* 1975;122(6):750-754.
98. Edington PT, Sibanda J, Beard RW. Influence on clinical practice of routine intrapartum fetal monitoring. *BMJ.* 1975;3(5979):341-343.
99. Koh KS, Greves D, Yung S, Peddle LJ. Experience with fetal monitoring in a university teaching hospital. *Can Med Assoc J.* 1975;112(4):455-456.
100. Shenker L, Post RC, Seiler JS. Routine electronic monitoring of fetal heart rate and uterine activity during labor. *Obstet Gynecol.* 1975;46(2):185-189.
101. Lee WK, Baggish MS. The effect of unselected intrapartum fetal monitoring. *Obstet Gynecol.* 1976;47(5):516-520.
102. Paul RH, Huey JR, Yaeger CF. Clinical fetal monitoring—its effect on cesarean section rate and perinatal mortality: five-year trends. *Postgrad Med.* 1977;61(4):160-166.
103. Amato JC. Fetal monitoring in a community hospital: a statistical analysis. *Obstet Gynecol.* 1977;50(3):269-274.
104. Johnstone FD, Campbell DM, Hughes GJ. Antenatal care: has continuous intrapartum monitoring made any impact on fetal outcome? *Lancet.* 1978;311(8077):1298-1300.
105. Hamilton LA, Gottschalk W, Vidyasagar D, Horn C, Wynn RM. Effects of monitoring high-risk pregnancies and intrapartum FHR monitoring on perinates. *Int J Gynecol Obstet.* 1978;15(6):483-490.
106. Haverkamp AD, Thompson HE, McFee JG, Cetrulo C. The evaluation of continuous fetal heart rate monitoring in high risk pregnancy. *Am J Obstet Gynecol.* 1976;125(3):310-320.
107. Haverkamp AD, Orleans M, Langendoerfer S, McFee J, Murphy J, Thompson HE. A controlled trial of the differential effects of intrapartum fetal monitoring. *Am J Obstet Gynecol.* 1979;134(4):399-412.
108. Renou P, Chang A, Anderson I, Wood C. Controlled trial of fetal intensive care. *Am J Obstet Gynecol.* 1976;126(4):470-476.
109. Kelso IM, Parsons RJ, Lawrence GE, Arora SS, Edmonds DK, Cooke ID. An assessment of continuous fetal heart rate monitoring in labor: a randomized trial. *Am J Obstet Gynecol.* 1978;131(5):526-532.
110. Wood C, Renou P, Oates J, Farrell E, Beischer N, Anderson I. A controlled trial of fetal heart rate monitoring in a low-risk population. *Am J Obstet Gynecol.* 1981;141(5):527-534.
111. MacDonald D, Grant A, Sheridan-Pereira M, Boylan P, Chalmers I. The Dublin randomized control trial of intrapartum fetal heart rate monitoring. *Am J Obstet Gynecol.* 1985;152(5):524-539.
112. Leveno KJ, Cunningham FG, Nelson S, et al. A prospective comparison of selective and universal electronic fetal monitoring in 34,995 pregnancies. *N Engl J Med.* 1986;315(10):615-619.
113. Vintzileos AM, Antsaklis A, Varvarigos O, Papas C, Sofatzis I, Montgomery JT. A randomized trial of electronic fetal heart rate monitoring versus intermittent auscultation. *Obstet Gynecol.* 1993;81(6):899-907.
114. Grant A, O'Brien N, Joy MT, Hennessy E, MacDonald D. Cerebral palsy among children born during the Dublin randomized trial of intrapartum monitoring. *Lancet.* 1989;2(8674):1233-1236.
115. Luthy DA, Shy KK, van Belle G, et al. A randomized trial of electronic fetal monitoring in pre-term labor. *Obstet Gynecol.* 1987;69(5):687-695.
116. Shy KK, Luthy DA, Bennett FC, et al. Effects of electronic fetal heart rate monitoring a compared with periodic auscultation on the neurologic development of premature infants. *N Engl J Med.* 1990;322(9):588-593.
117. Garite TJ, Dildy GA, McNamara H, et al. A multicenter controlled trial of fetal pulse oximetry in the intrapartum management of nonreassuring fetal heart rate patterns. *Am J Obstet Gynecol.* 2000;183(5):1049-1058.
118. Bloom SL, Spong CY, Thom E, et al. Fetal pulse oximetry and cesarean delivery. *N Engl J Med.* 2006;355(21):2195-2202.
119. Belfort MA, Saade GR, Thom E, et al. A randomized trial of intrapartum fetal ECG ST-segment analysis. *N Engl J Med.* 2015;373(7):632-641.
120. INFANT Collaborative Group. Computerised interpretation of fetal heart rate during labour (INFANT): a randomised controlled trial. *Lancet.* 2017;389(10080):1719-1729.
121. Intrapartum fetal heart rate monitoring: nomenclature, interpretation, and general management principles. American College of Obstetricians and Gynecologists 2009: practice bulletin no. 106.
122. Management of intrapartum fetal heart tracings. American College of Obstetricians and Gynecologists 2009: practice bulletin no. 116 Nov. 2010.
123. Macones GA, Hankins GD, Spong D, Hauth J, Moore T. The 2008 NICHD workshop report on electronic fetal monitoring: update on definitions, interpretation, and research guidelines. *Obstet Gynecol.* 2008;112(3):661-666.
124. Cordero L, Hon EH. Scalp abscess: a rare complication of fetal monitoring. *J Pediatr.* 1971;78(3):533-537.
125. Gassner CB, Ledger WJ. The relationship of hospital-acquired maternal infection to invasive intrapartum monitoring techniques. *Am J Obstet Gynecol.* 1976;126(1):33-37.
126. Hagen D. Maternal febrile morbidity associated with fetal monitoring and cesarean section. *Obstet Gynecol.* 1975;46(3):260-262.
127. Wiechetek WJ, Horiguchi T, Dillon TF. Puerperal morbidity and internal fetal monitoring. *Am J Obstet Gynecol.* 1974;119(2):230-233.
128. Gibbs RS, Jones PM, Wilder CJY. Internal fetal monitoring and maternal infection following cesarean section: a prospective study. *Obstet Gynecol.* 1978;52(2):193-197.
129. Paul RH. Clinical fetal monitoring: experience on a large clinical service. *Am J Obstet Gynecol.* 1972;113(5):573-577.
130. Maiques V, García-Tejedor A, Perales A, Navarro C. Intrapartum fetal invasive procedures and perinatal transmission of HIV. *Eur J Obstet Gynecol Reprod Biol.* 1999;87(1):63-67.
131. Williams RL, Hawes W. Cesarean section, fetal monitoring and perinatal mortality in California. *Am J Public Health.* 1979;69(9):864-870.

132. Kuehn BN. Study probes increase in Cesarean Section rate. *JAMA.* 2010;304(15):1658.
133. Kidd LC, Patel N, Smith R. Non-stress antenatal cardiotocography: a prospective randomized clinical trial. *Br J Obstet Gynecol.* 1985;92(11):1156-1159.
134. Flynn A, Kelly J, Mansfield H, Needham P, O'Conor M, Viegas O. A randomized controlled trial of antepartum non-stress cardiotocography. *Br J Obstet Gynecol.* 1982;89(6):427-433.
135. Brown V, Sawyers S, Parsons R, Duncan SL, Cooke ID. The value of antenatal cardiotocography in the management of high risk pregnancy: a randomized controlled trial. *Br J Obstet Gynecol.* 1982;89(9):716-722.
136. Lumley J, Lester A, Anderson I, Renou P, Wood C. A randomized trial of weekly cardiotocography in high-risk obstetrical patients. *Br J Obstet Gynecol.* 1983;90(11):1018-1026.
137. Neldam S. Fetal movements as an indicator of fetal well-being. *Lancet.* 1980;1(8180):1222-1224.
138. Beischer NA, Drew JH, Ashton PW, et al. Quality of survival of infants with critical reserve detected by cardiotocography. *Am J Obstet Gynecol.* 1983;146(6):662-670.
139. Manning FA, Bondagji N, Harman CR, Casiro O, Menticoglou S, Morrison I. Fetal assessment based on the fetal biophysical profile score: relationship of last BPS result to subsequent cerebral palsy. *J Gynecol Obstet Biol Reprod (Paris).* 1997;26(7):720-729.
140. Manning FA, Bondaji N, Harman CR, et al. Fetal assessment based on fetal biophysical profile scoring. VIII. The incidence of cerebral palsy in tested and untested perinates. *Am J Obstet Gynecol.* 1998;178(4):696-706.
141. Dayal AK, Manning FA, Bereck DJ, et al. Fetal death after normal biophysical profile score: an eighteen year experience. *Am J Obstet Gynecol.* 1999;181(5 Pt 1):1231-1236.
142. Signore C, Spong CY. Antenatal testing: a re-evaluation. *Semin Perinatol.* 2008;32(4):231-321.
143. Policy Statement—Task Force on Cerebral Palsy and neonatal asphyxia (part I). SOGC 1267-1279, 1996.
144. MacLennan A, for the International Cerebral Palsy Task Force. A template for defining a causal relationship between acute intrapartum events and cerebral palsy—an international consensus statement. *BMJ.* 1999;319(7216):1054-1059.
145. National Institute of Child Health and Human Development Research Planning Workshop. Electronic fetal heart rate monitoring: research guidelines for interpretation. *Am J Obstet Gynecol.* 1997;177(6):1385-1390.

CHAPTER 4

Instrumentation and Artifact Detection Including Fetal Arrhythmias

Lauren Theilen

INSTRUMENTATION AND ARTIFACT DETECTION

Instrumentation

For the obstetrician or obstetric nurse to interpret fetal monitor tracings correctly, it is necessary to have some understanding of the processes involved in the acquisition and processing of data relating to fetal heart rate (FHR) and uterine activity. Electronic fetal monitors are designed to interpret accurately in most situations, but there are times when their output can be misleading unless the instruments' limitations are understood. Most errors we see in FHR interpretation are related to the quality of the data acquisition and presentation, and, for this reason, an understanding of this chapter is critical for the clinician using electronic fetal monitoring in the treatment of obstetric patients.

Fetal Heart Rate Derived by Direct (Internal) Fetal Electrocardiography

The FHR monitor acquires, processes, and displays an electronic signal. To understand the significance of the FHR display, it is important to understand what the monitor can and cannot count. FHR tracings from a fetal scalp electrode (FSE) are obtained by measuring the interval between consecutive fetal R waves. Therefore, the fetal electrocardiogram (ECG) signal provides the clinician with a measure of the electrical activity of the fetal heart. It does not necessarily represent mechanical activity. The fetal ECG signal is acquired through a bipolar electrode that penetrates the skin of the fetal scalp (first pole) and that has a second conductor residing in the secretions of the maternal vagina (second pole). It is believed that the circuit is completed through the fetal umbilical cord, placenta, and maternal circulation and that the potential difference (voltage) being measured is between the two poles. The original electrode was a modified skin clip, but now a spiral electrode is used.

The raw fetal ECG signal is amplified and fed into a beat-to-beat cardiotachometer (Fig. 4.1). The amplifier uses an automatic gain control circuit to boost the fetal ECG signal to a predetermined voltage before electronic counting. All electronic signals are equally strengthened noise as well as fetal ECG. Once the fetal ECG signal has been amplified, it is filtered, and the interval between R-wave peaks is measured. The interval between R waves is processed to a rate in beats per minute (bpm) by computing the reciprocal of the interval. With internal FHR monitors, a new rate is set each time an R wave is detected; as each new wave arrives, the rate is recalculated from the reciprocal of the previous R-R interval. The result of this rate calculation is the plotting of a series of square waves (Fig. 4.2). The minute rate differences between beats are referred to as beat-to-beat or short-term variability and can only be appreciated when the FHR is computed instantaneously by means of a beat-to-beat cardiotachometer. FHR changes with a cyclicity of 3 to 5 per minute are referred to as long-term variability, and those occurring in response to uterine contractions (UCs) or fetal movement are referred to as periodic changes. Long-term variability and periodic changes can be detected with Doppler systems, but true short-term variability can be measured only with direct or abdominal fetal ECG systems. The newer fetal monitors have advanced technology, utilizing autocorrelation techniques, allowing for Doppler-derived signal data of significantly improved quality such that, although not exact, the FHR recording

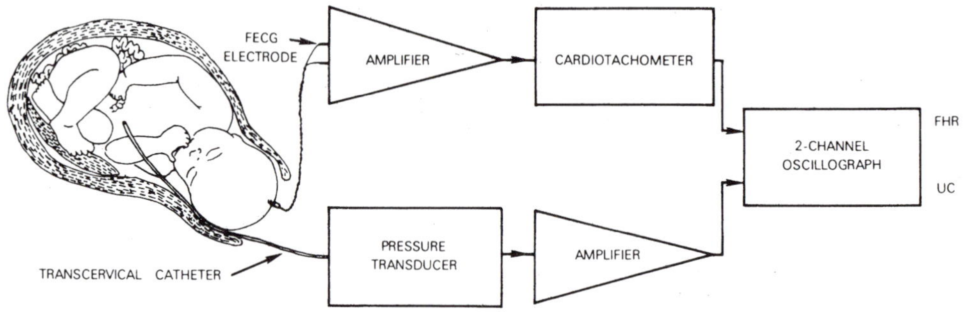

Figure 4.1. Schematic diagram of a direct fetal monitoring system. The fetal heart rate is obtained from a fetal scalp electrode and counted in a cardiotachometer. The actual uterine pressure is recorded directly from a transcervical intrauterine catheter. FHR, fetal heart rate; UC, uterine contraction.

is very close to that obtained from direct fetal ECG and visually approximates true short-term variability in many patients.

Most fetal ECG systems will not record R-R intervals less than 250 milliseconds, which corresponds to a rate of 240 bpm. If the FHR exceeds 240 bpm, not even a direct fetal ECG system will count every beat and may halve or not print such rates. This occurs only with fetal supraventricular tachyarrhythmias (paroxysmal atrial tachycardia, atrial fibrillation, or atrial flutter), intermittent premature atrial contractions (PACs), or premature ventricular contractions (PVCs) (Fig. 4.3).

An additional instance that may cause confusion is in the patient with a cardiac pacemaker. If the transmitted maternal pacemaker pulse is at a higher voltage than the fetal R wave, the scalp electrode may record the pacemaker signal.[1,2]

In the absence of the fetal ECG signal, such as with a dead fetus, there will usually be no tracing. However, depending on the monitor and the existing maternal R wave, amplification of the incoming signal may continue until, on occasion, counting of the maternal heart rate (MHR) from the scalp of the dead fetus results (Fig. 4.4).[3,4] This can obviously lead to confusion. When there is any doubt, fetal demise should be confirmed with real-time ultrasound or comparison to maternal ECG or pulse oximeter signal. In all instances of monitoring, there needs to be documentation of maternal pulse rate as different from the FHR.

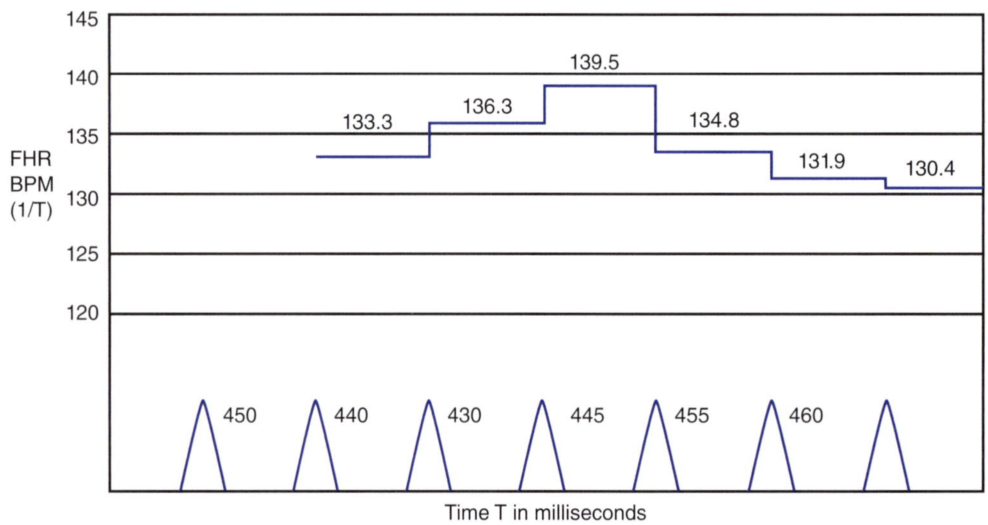

Figure 4.2. This schematic represents an enlarged segment of the fetal heart rate tracing. A new rate is set with the arrival of each R wave in the fetal electrocardiogram. This generates a series of square waves that indicate beat-to-beat changes.

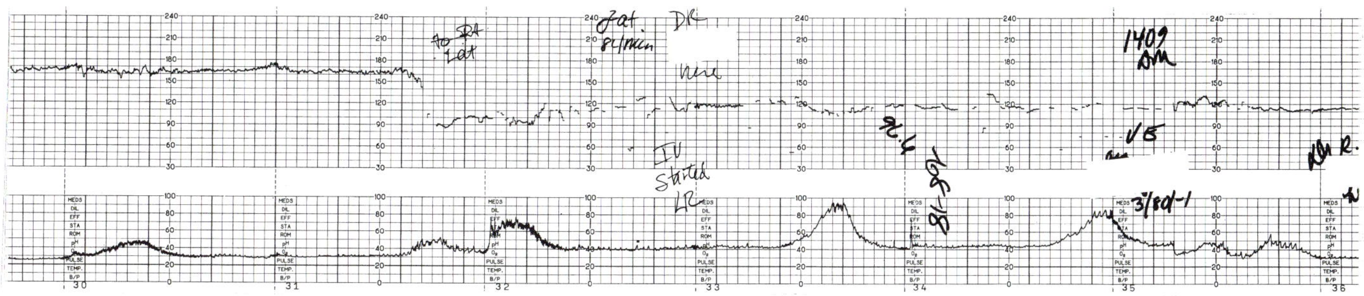

Figure 4.3. This is an example of a change in the atrial pacemaker. The fetus is known to have multiple cardiac abnormalities and presented in supraventricular tachycardia with nonimmune hydrops. Cardioversion was achieved successfully with digoxin and quinidine. This tracing is from early labor.

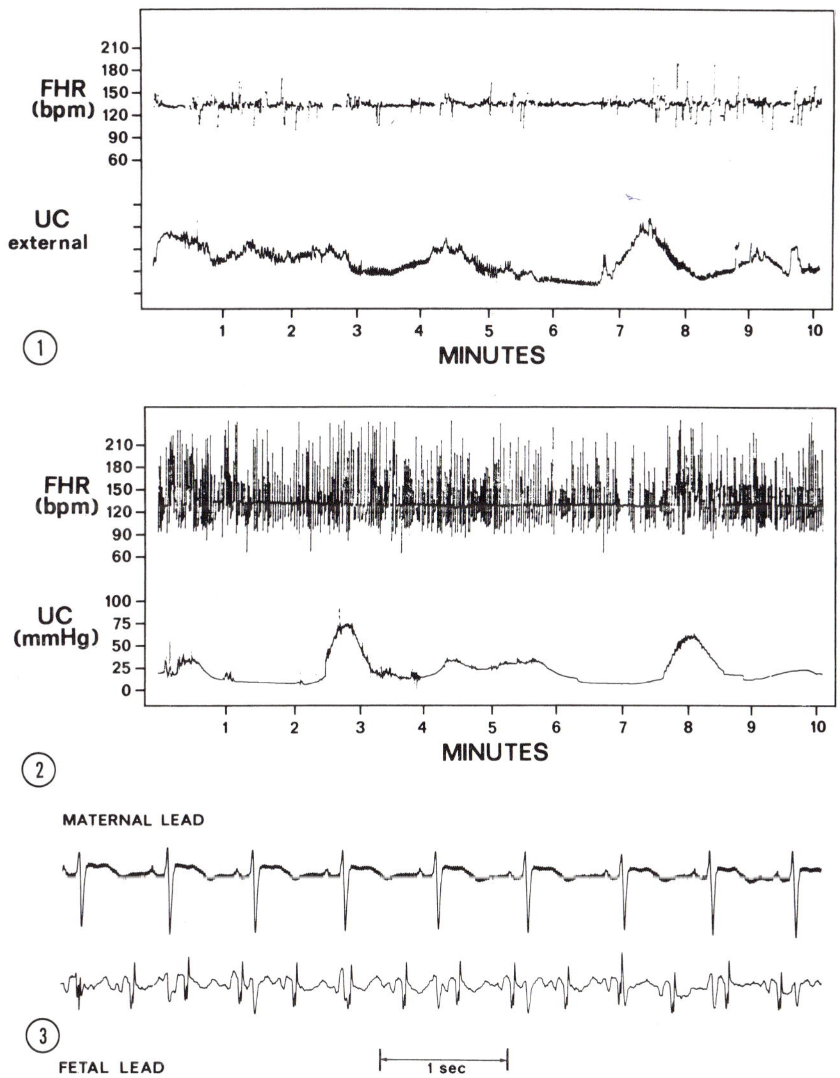

Figure 4.4. The **upper panel** shows the heart rate from a fetal scalp electrode (FHR) and maternal leads (MHR) with a dead fetus. Note the two rates are identical in detail. The **lower panel** shows the fetal scalp lead and the maternal lead electrocardiogram (ECG) tracing indicating that the dead fetus is transmitting the maternal ECG to the fetal lead. UC, uterine contraction. (From Klapholz H, Schifrin BS, Myrick R. Role of maternal artifact in fetal heart rate pattern interpretation. *Obstet Gynecol.* 1974;44(3):373-378, with permission.)

Fetal Heart Rate Derived by Indirect (External) Doppler Ultrasound

In the antepartum period, and often during the intrapartum period, it is neither feasible nor always necessary to use the direct fetal ECG signal to record the FHR. External monitoring using various biophysical modalities has evolved to a point where it currently represents the most frequent form of FHR monitoring. Doppler ultrasound is the method most commonly used to indirectly record FHR (Fig. 4.5).

The principles underlying the use of Doppler FHR monitoring are described.

Ultrasonic signals can penetrate human tissue. When the transmitted ultrasonic beam encounters an interface of increased density, a portion of the signal is reflected. The angle of reflection varies according to the angle of incidence of the beam. A portion of the signal will be transmitted to the next interface. If the interface is moving, the reflected signal undergoes a frequency change (Doppler shift). The frequency increases if the reflecting interface is moving toward the signal source and decreases if the reflecting interface is moving away from the signal source. An example commonly used to describe the Doppler shift is the audible change in pitch (frequency) noticed by a stationary observer of the whistle from a rapidly moving train. As the train approaches, the whistle gets both louder and higher in frequency. As the train passes and moves away, both loudness and pitch rapidly decline.

The fetal monitor Doppler transducer contains a transmitter, or signal source, and receiver. With all of the first-generation fetal monitors and many second-generation monitors, the signal is transmitted and the reflected signals are received continuously by multiple crystals contained in the transducer. A transducer innovation employed by second-generation monitors is pulsed Doppler. The pulsed Doppler transducer alternates the emission of ultrasound waves with the reception of the reflected waves, resulting in a decrease in both the amount and time of exposure of the fetus to ultrasound energy. Ultrasound waves of sufficient intensity will generate heat. Intensities of less than 100 mW/cm^2, regardless of the length of exposure, generate no heat. The amount of energy generated by fetal monitors is only a small fraction of this, with the continuous ultrasound transducers generating intensities of 5 to 12 mW/cm^2 and pulsed ultrasound transducers generating 1.5 to 5 mW/cm^2. Thus, neither first- nor second-generation FHR monitor Doppler transducers generate heat even during prolonged continuous use.

As long as the reflecting interfaces are not in motion, the reflected signal has the same frequency as the transmitted signal. However, if the reflecting interface is the surface of a moving organ such as the fetal heart, there will be a frequency change (Doppler shift) in the reflected signal. The electronic circuitry of the fetal monitor senses this frequency change and converts it to an electronic signal. This signal can then be used as a marker of the fetal heartbeat as well as for the creation of fetal heart sounds produced by the monitor. This is the sound that is heard using a Doppler device. A similar shift is created if the Doppler signal is being reflected by any movement such as fetal blood, maternal vessels, or fetal movement. It is important to understand that with Doppler technology, it is not the actual fetal heart being heard but rather a sound that is created by the device in response to frequency changes generated by a moving interface.

This biphasic signal is immersed in the noise created by fetal movements, arterial blood flow, maternal movements, and random muscle contractions. The signal actually received is a composite consisting of bursts with various amplitudes and frequencies. In addition, the actual signal created by the fetal cardiac motion is

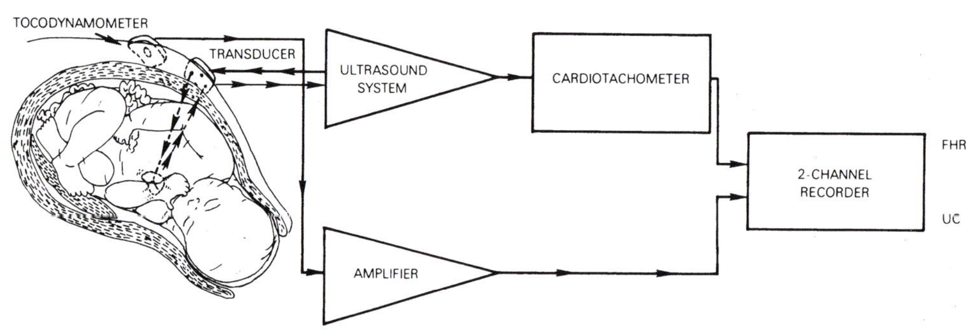

Figure 4.5. Schematic diagram of an indirect fetal monitoring system. The fetal ultrasonogram is obtained from an abdominal wall transducer, conditioned, and then counted by a cardiotachometer. The semiquantitative uterine activity is measured by an external tocodynamometer. FHR, fetal heart rate; UC, uterine contraction.

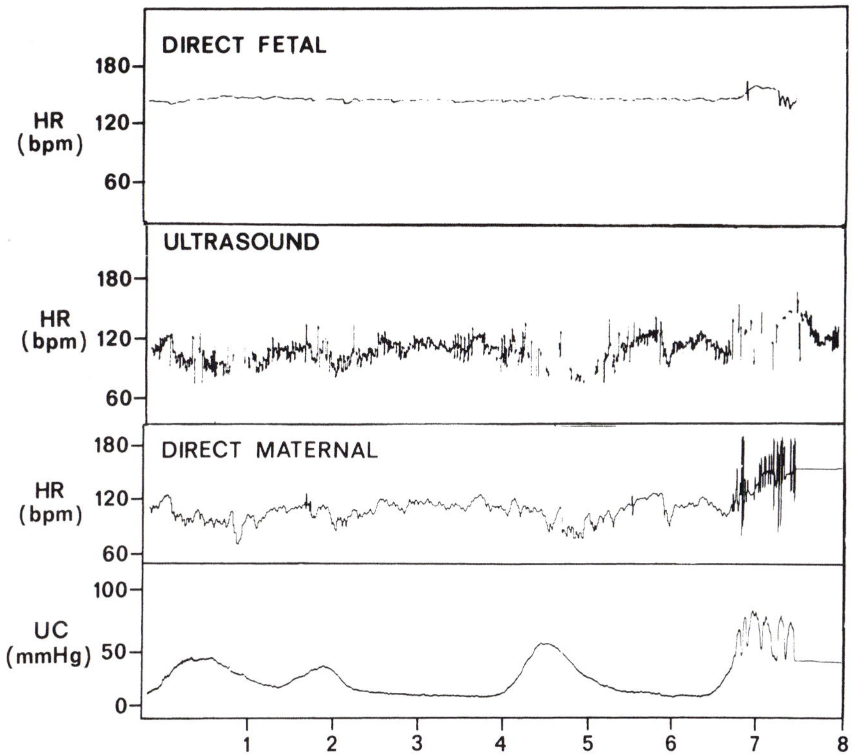

Figure 4.6. Simultaneous recording of heart rate (HR) from the direct fetal scalp electrode **(upper tracing)**, abdominal Doppler **(middle tracing)**, and direct maternal **(lower tracing)**. Note that the abdominal Doppler signal is recording the maternal heart rate from a maternal vessel in the abdomen. UC, uterine contraction. (From Klapholz H, Schifrin BS, Myrick R. Role of maternal artifact in fetal heart rate pattern interpretation. *Obstet Gynecol.* 1974;44(3):373-378, with permission.)

greatly affected by the position and movement of the transducer with respect to the fetus. With older monitors, the quality of the Doppler-created FHR tracing is directly related to the orientation of the signal to the fetal heart, the amount of fetal movement, and the degree of constant attention by nursing personnel to maintaining an adequate signal while caring for the patient. One potential source of error occurs when the Doppler signal is actually maternal and not fetal (Fig. 4.6). The maternal pulse should be checked to confirm the correct recording of FHR at the initiation of fetal monitoring, with any switching of FHR modes or any abrupt decrease in FHR, especially in a setting of noncontinuous tracings. Newer monitors sometimes do not produce noncontinuous tracings when the signal switches from fetal to maternal, making the transition more difficult to identify (see the section on signal ambiguity).

With the evolution of autocorrelation in many of the newer monitors, great advances have been made in both signal quality and continuity. Although new wide-beam ultrasound transducers decrease signal loss because of fetal movement, they increase the chance of recording MHR (see the section on signal ambiguity).

First-Generation Signal Processing

Fetal monitors obtain the FHR indirectly by use of Doppler ultrasound. To produce an FHR tracing, several modulations of the reflected signal need to be used. As previously discussed, amplification and filtering of the incoming signal within certain frequencies extracts FHR signals from those produced by other moving structures. The filtered signal is converted to an electrical waveform by the transducer, and it is this waveform that is used to generate and display the FHR. Detection of fetal motion with a Doppler signal is the same with both the older and newer monitors. It is the process of signal conversion to FHR that differs.

First-generation monitors calculate heart rate by electronic integration and peak detection of the returning Doppler signal. The highest point of the waveform is detected and recorded as a heartbeat, even though it may not appear at the same time in each waveform. Despite various electronic logic and filtering processes, this often results in an apparent increase in short-term variability caused by a false reproduction of the actual interval from one heartbeat or R wave (contraction) to the next (Figs. 4.7–4.9). With signal fading, inconsistent

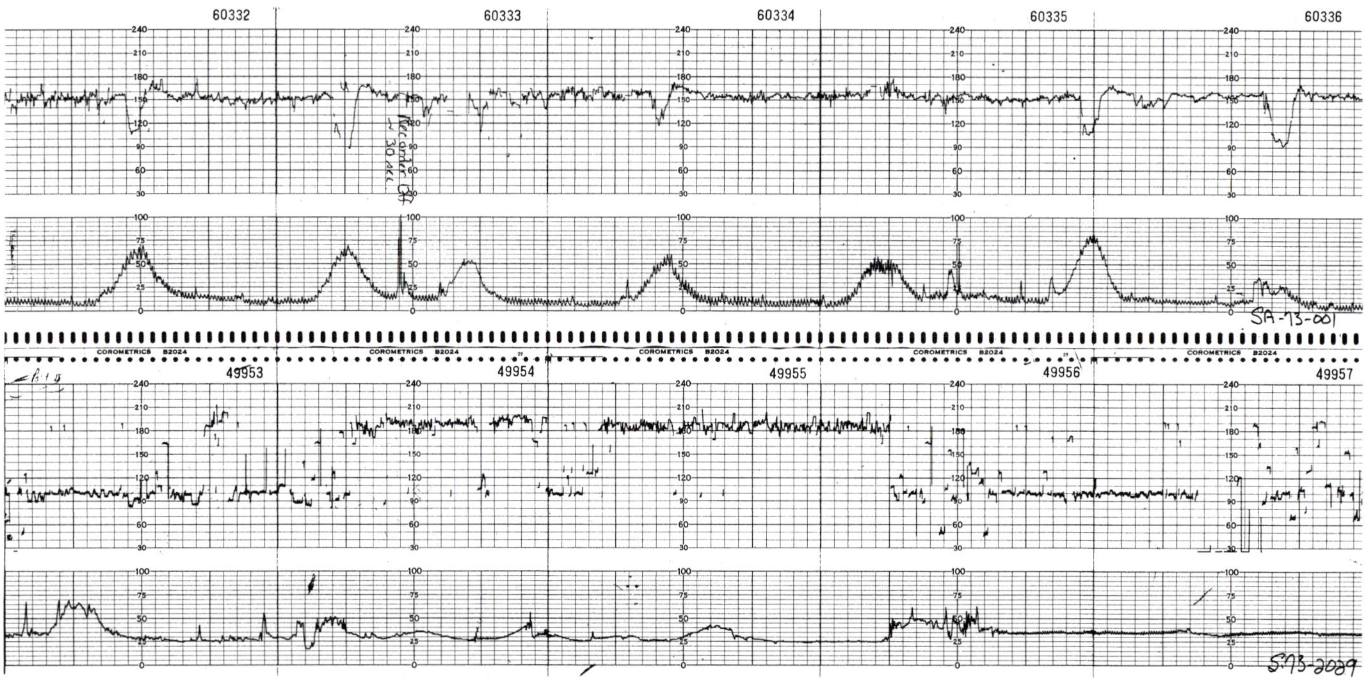

Figure 4.7. Tracing from a Doppler system showing the halving of the fetal heart rate at rates over 180 bpm.

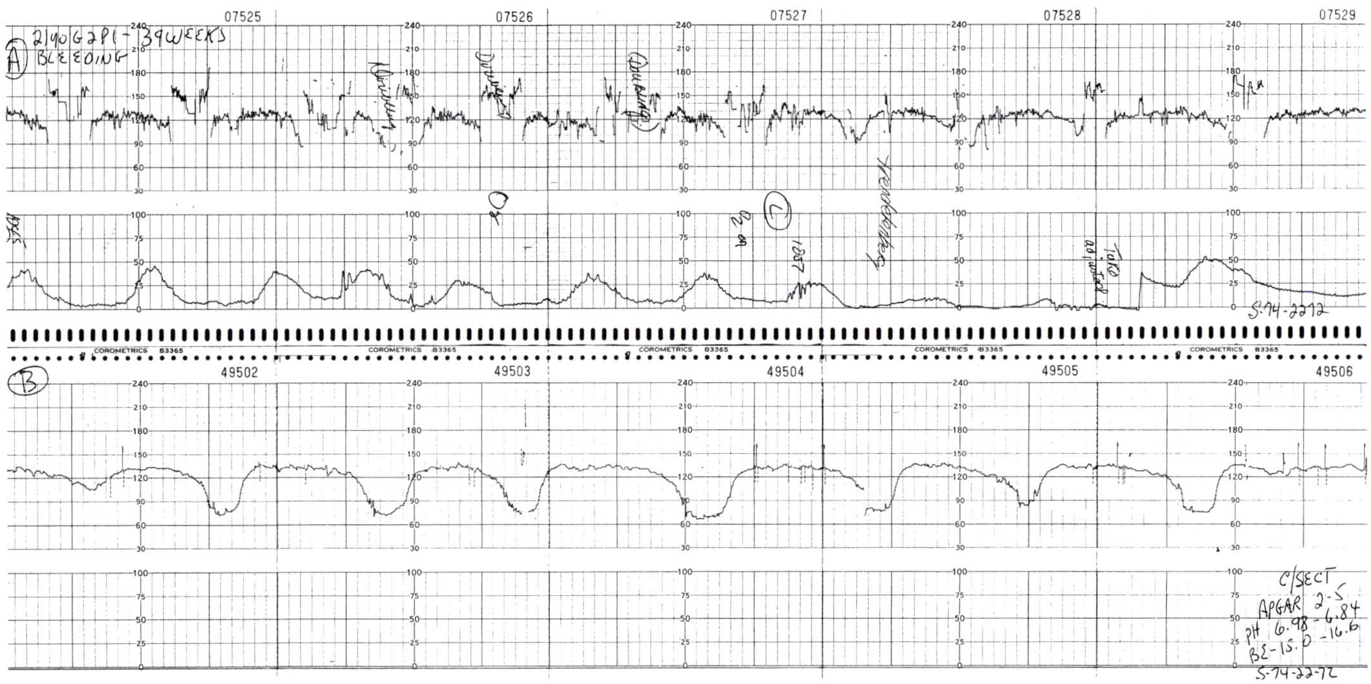

Figure 4.8. The **upper tracing** is taken from a Doppler signal source. At first glance, it appears to be a poor-quality erratic tracing, but upon closer examination, the late decelerations can be seen. The fetal heart rate (FHR) doubles whenever it goes below 90 beats per minute, putting the trough of the late decelerations above the baseline. The **lower tracing**, a continuation of the **upper tracing** after the fetal scalp electrode signal source was begun, shows the deep decelerations that were previously unrecognized because of the artifactual doubling of the FHR by the Doppler logic system.

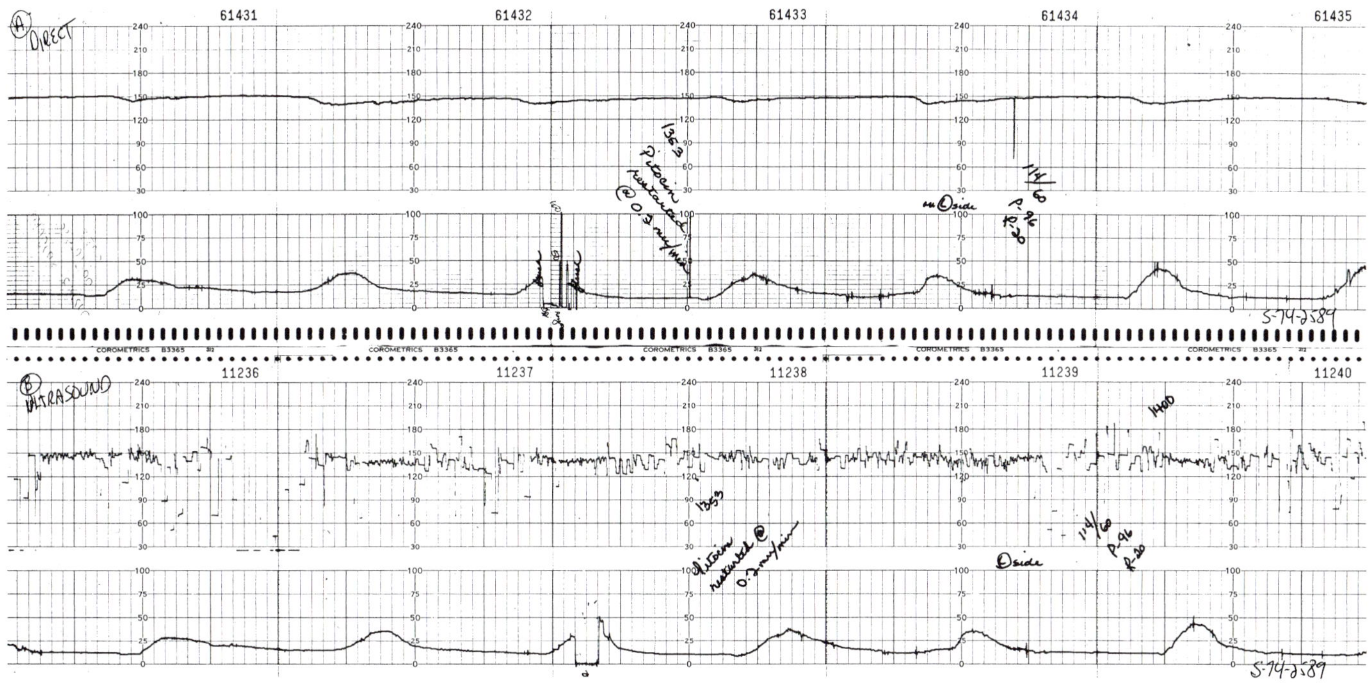

Figure 4.9. Simultaneous recordings with Doppler **(lower tracing)** and direct fetal electrocardiogram **(upper tracing)** signal sources. Note the apparent increased variability and obscuring of periodic changes on the Doppler tracing.

signal shape, and changing signal peaks, the resultant FHR may be, at best, a poor reflection of the true variability of consecutive R-wave intervals. The beat-to-beat variability of the FHR calculated from the fetal ECG usually averages 1 bpm or less,[5,6] but the Doppler signal using the first-generation monitor technology often displays a variability much greater than that and can be very misleading.

Autocorrelation

Although not new in concept, the application of autocorrelation to FHR technology has been made possible by the introduction of high-speed microprocessor, integrated circuitry. The received pattern is broken into very short second envelopes of time made up of 200 to 300 digitalized points (Fig. 4.10). With each

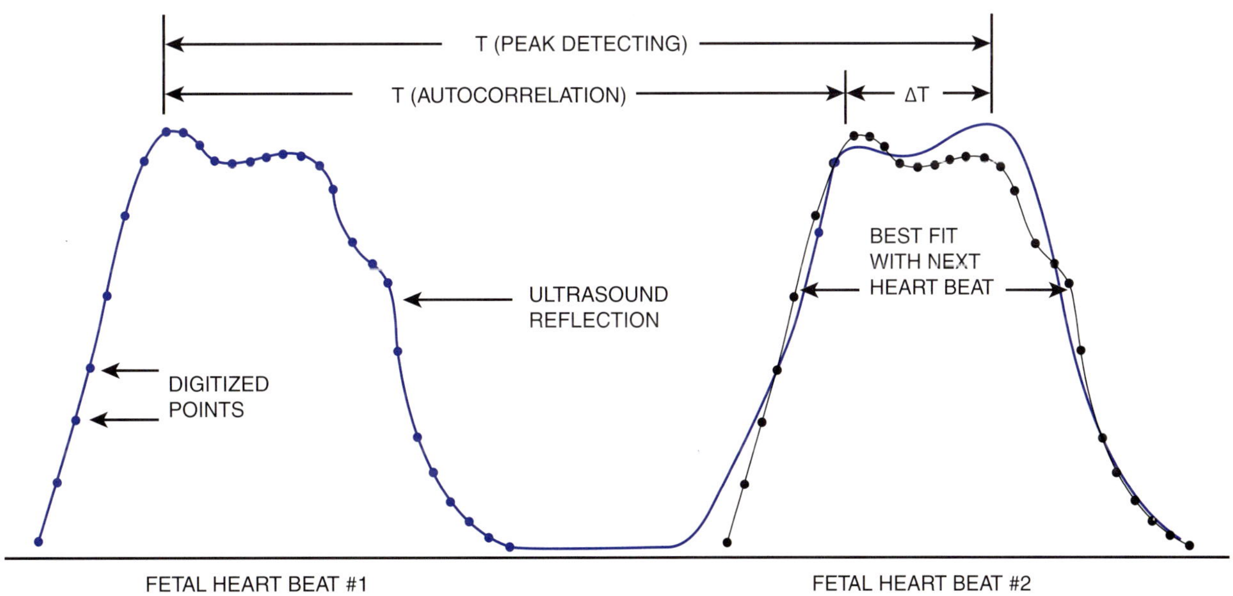

Figure 4.10. Schematic representation of consecutive fetal heartbeat waveforms demonstrating autocorrelation versus peak detection. (Reproduced with permission of Hewlett Packard Corporation, Boeblingen, Germany.)

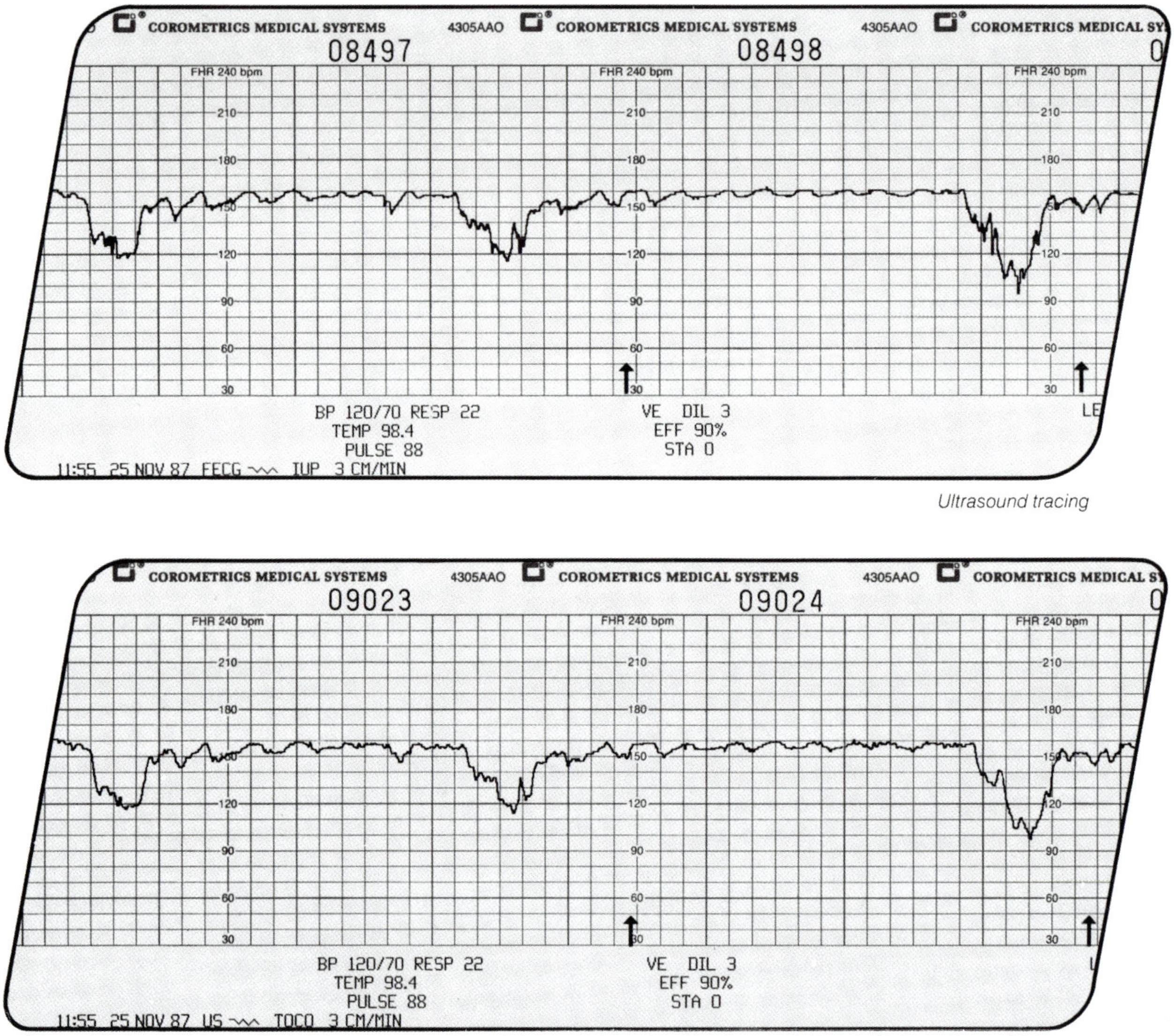

Figure 4.11. Example of simultaneous intrapartum fetal heart rate tracings comparing the external monitor with the direct fetal electrocardiogram internal monitor. Autocorrelation has improved the quality of the tracing and eliminated much of the signal loss or error present with many older monitors. (Courtesy of Corometrics Medical Systems, Wallingford, CT.)

consecutive new heartbeat waveform, the microprocessor compares the digitalized points to the equivalent points in the preceding envelope. Essentially, autocorrelation is a signal-processing scheme that compares the incoming signal with a time-delayed version of previous signals. Important information has a regular form repeated over time, whereas random noise has no such regularity. Artifactual waveforms and older points are discarded. The resultant tracing represents a point in each cardiac cycle more accurately than can be done with first-generation monitors. Varying waveform amplitude problems are, therefore, minimized, and markedly less false variability is produced (Fig. 4.11).

As with first-generation monitors, interpretation of the FHR from newer monitors using autocorrelation must be done cautiously. Despite apparent improvement in signal interpretation, autocorrelation is still not a true measure of short-term variability. The possibility for signal loss, doubling, halving, or recording of MHR or other movements must be kept in mind when reading changes in FHR monitor strips.[6,7] Because autocorrelation enhances signal-to-noise levels and periodic phenomena, in the absence of fetal cardiac motion, it may produce a false signal and resultant "heart rate" (Fig. 4.12). When doubt is present, confirmation with auscultation, visualization of fetal heart motion via ultrasound, or direct FSE must be done.

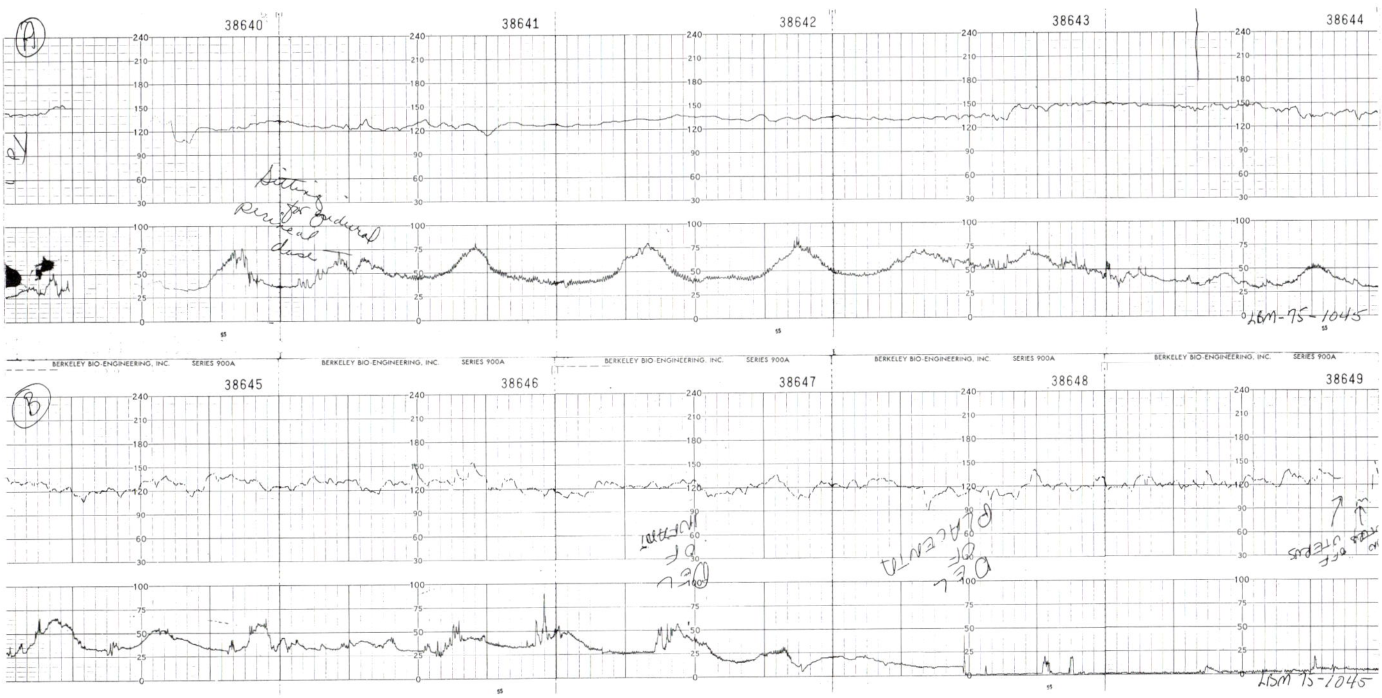

Figure 4.12. This tracing shows a Doppler record from a monitor with an excessive amount of electronic logic. Note in the **lower panel** that, even after the delivery of the baby and placenta, an apparent fetal heart rate can still be seen on the tracing.

Abdominal Fetal Electrocardiographic-Derived Fetal Heart Rate Tracings

Abdominal fetal ECG signals were first recorded by Cremer in 1906.[8] The original application of this method was to diagnose fetal life. Later, Larks and Dasgupta[9] and Hon and Hess[10] showed that the presentation of the fetus could be predicted by the polarity of the fetal QRS complex in relation to the maternal abdomen. With a breech presentation, the fetal ECG complex would be similar in polarity to that of the mother; with a cephalic presentation, the R wave would be opposite that of the maternal polarity. In addition, abdominal fetal ECG tracings could be used to diagnose twins by comparing the fetal complexes and determining two separate rate patterns among the fetal complexes. From the maternal abdomen, the fetal ECG complex is much smaller than the maternal ECG (Fig. 4.13). Often, if the electrical noise level is high, one may not be able to see a fetal ECG signal.

Because of the weakness of the fetal ECG signal before 30 weeks gestation, the interference created by the electromyographic muscle noise of the maternal abdominal wall, and the frequency of coincidence of maternal and fetal ECG signals, abdominal ECG plays little role in modern FHR monitoring other than in arrhythmia detection. However, before the introduction of autocorrelation and improved Doppler

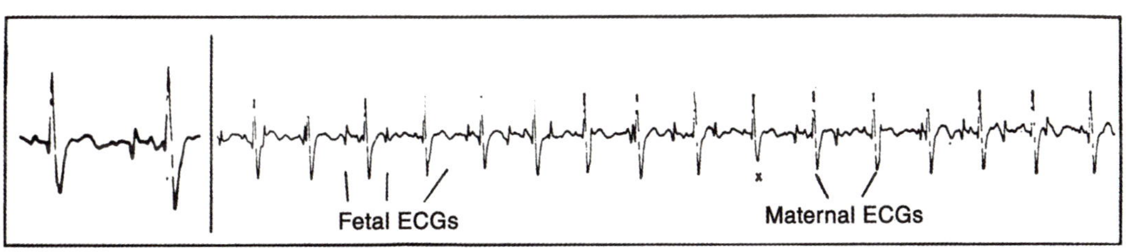

Figure 4.13. An abdominal tracing showing the large maternal electrocardiogram complexes and the clear but much smaller fetal complexes. (From Hon EH, Lee ST. The fetal electrocardiogram. I. The electrocardiogram of the dying fetus. *Am J Obstet Gynecol.* 1963;87:804-813, with permission.)

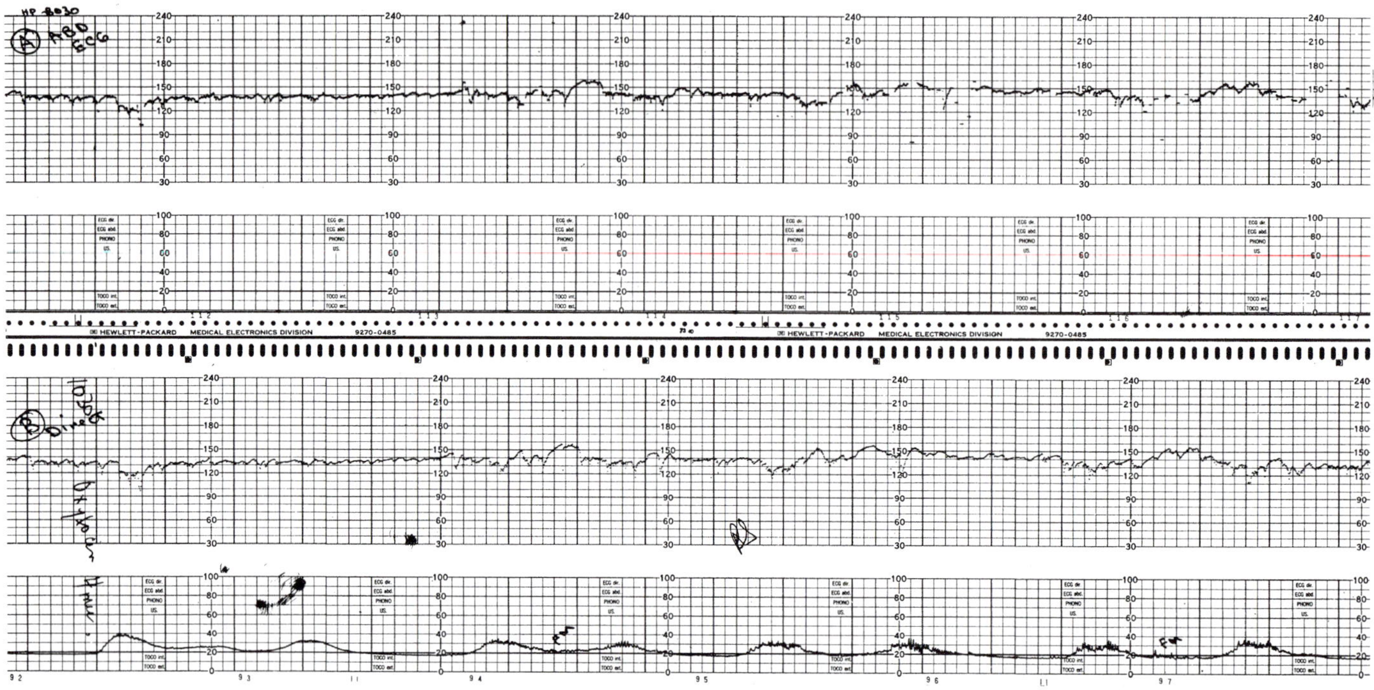

Figure 4.14. Simultaneous fetal heart rate tracings derived from abdominal electrocardiogram (ECG) **(upper panel)** and scalp ECG **(lower panel)**.

technology with the newer monitors, abdominal fetal ECG-derived tracings were the most accurate recordings of FHR signals in many patients (Fig. 4.14). Several attempts have been made, with varying degrees of success, to reliably obtain FHR variability indirectly using the abdominal fetal ECG modality.[5,11] There has been some renewed interest in fetal ECG as the incidence and degree of maternal abdominal obesity increases because the pads on the maternal abdomen are expected to require less frequent adjustment compared to standard external Doppler FHR monitoring. The Novii® Wireless Patch System (GE Healthcare, Chicago, United States) uses fetal ECG, maternal ECG, and uterine electromyogram signals with suggested benefits including reliable tracings on individuals with abdominal obesity.[12] One randomized trial found that fetal ECG via the Novii® system performed similarly to standard external Doppler monitoring in obese women in terms of the percentage of intrapartum FHR tracing that was interpretable.[13] Still, the abdominal FECG signal source for FHR tracings is not widely used in the United States.

Phonocardiographically Derived Fetal Heart Rate

Phonocardiography was the first method used to record FHR electronically. As the fetal heart beats, the closure of the valves may be detected by listening with a suitable stethoscope through the mother's abdominal wall. With ventricular systole, the closure of the atrioventricular (AV) valves produces the first heart sound. This mechanical energy may be sensed by a microphone and amplified, producing an electrical signal that may then be reconverted to sound or used to produce a phonocardiogram, an oscillographic tracing of the heart sounds. The amplified electrical signal can also be used as a counting source for an FHR monitor. The phonocardiographic signal is clearer than the Doppler signal, resulting in less artifactual "jitter." For this reason, phonocardiography historically was widely used for antepartum FHR monitoring.

The main drawback to phonocardiographically derived FHR systems is that they are extremely sensitive to ambient noise such as maternal bowel sounds, voices in the room, certain air-conditioning systems, and, especially, the noise produced by any motion of the microphone or of the bed clothing against the microphone. In addition, any fetal kicking or motion produces a very loud noise that will saturate the automatic gain system on the monitor's amplifier, resulting in a complete loss of recording for several seconds while waiting for the amplifier to reopen. For this reason, manual gain control offers a great advantage when using abdominal fetal phonocardiography for recording heart rate. Also, because of the high sensitivity to

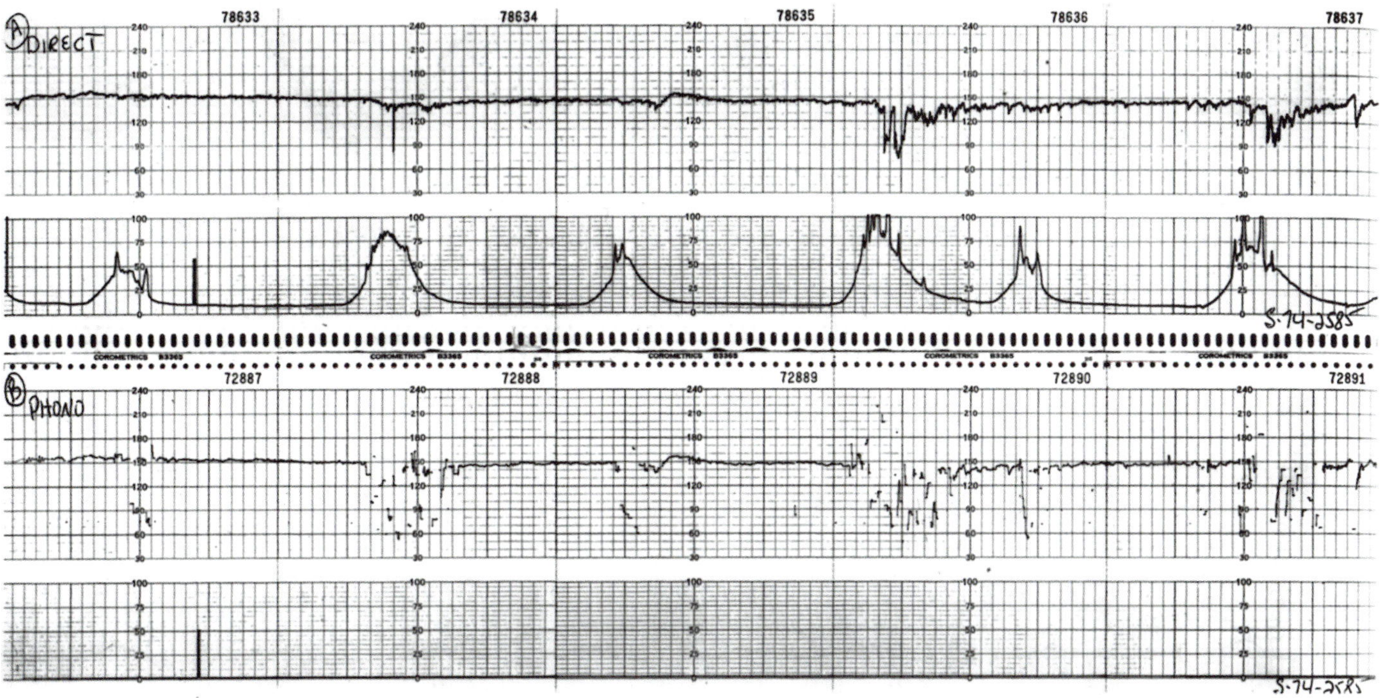

Figure 4.15. Simultaneous fetal heart rate tracings derived from phonocardiographic **(lower panel)** and scalp electrocardiogram **(upper tracing)**. Note the signal loss during contractions with the phono recording.

ambient noise, the technique is unsatisfactory for monitoring during the active phase of labor (Fig. 4.15). The current role of phonocardiographic FHR recording is quite limited but should be considered if abdominal fetal ECG and Doppler do not produce satisfactory recordings. Today, it would have to be considered below Doppler in a ranking of preferred methods of antepartum FHR recording. Both abdominal fetal ECG and phonocardiographic FHR are rarely employed means of fetal monitoring, but they are of historic significance.

Scaling Factors

The choice of vertical and horizontal scaling directly affects the appearance of the FHR and UC tracings. In the United States, the standard factors are 30 bpm/cm on the vertical scale and 3 cm/minute on the horizontal scale. In Europe, standard factors are 20 bpm/cm (vertical) and 1 or 2 cm/minute (horizontal). The European scaling factors accentuate apparent FHR variability and tend to make periodic changes appear more abrupt than American scaling factors. Although US clinicians find 1 cm/minute tracings are harder to read than the same tracings at 3 cm/minute, the slower rate of tracing is commonly used in Europe, South America, and certain centers in this country. Figure 4.16 shows how paper speed can significantly alter the appearance of a tracing.

Application of Monitoring Devices

Uterine Contraction Monitors

Clinically, UCs can be monitored by two techniques: external tocodynamometry or intrauterine pressure measurement. Both methods have advantages and disadvantages. This section will deal with the methodology involved in the clinical application of these techniques.

Intrauterine Pressure Monitoring

The pregnant uterus is a closed, fluid-filled space. The hydrostatic pressure within the uterus should be equal at all points. Intrauterine pressure has historically been determined with the use of an open-ended, fluid-filled catheter placed through the cervix and externally attached to a strain gauge transducer. Pascal's law dictates that assuming such a monitoring system is a closed system, the baseline tone as well as the intrauterine pressure during a contraction will be transmitted directly to the external strain gauge pressure transducer. With such a system, both technical and logistic problems exist,

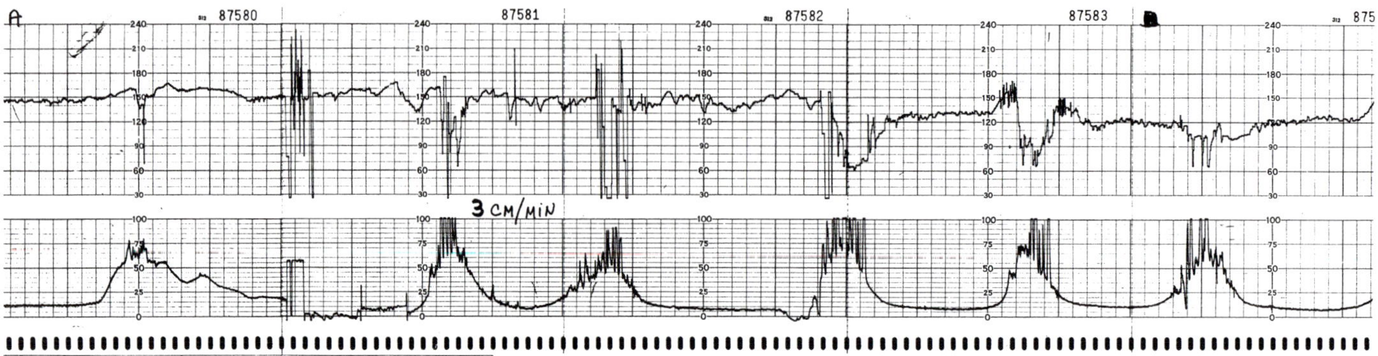

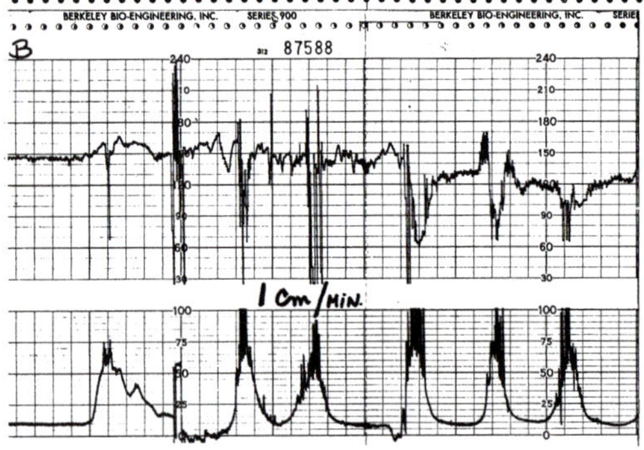

Figure 4.16. Tape-recorded fetal heart rate and uterine contraction patterns were played back simultaneously to monitors running at 3 cm/minute **(upper tracing)** and 1 cm/minute **(lower tracing)**.

such as catheter occlusion by solid matter, kinking or entrapment of catheter between the uterus and the fetus, as well as the introduction of artifact secondary to maternal movement and catheter manipulation.[14] An alternative type of intrauterine pressure device was introduced in 1987. This device has a micropressure transducer located at the tip of the catheter, which is inserted through the cervix into the uterine cavity. Such a device eliminates most of the problems associated with the fluid-filled devices used for uterine pressure monitoring. Most devices currently employed to monitor intrauterine pressure come from one of the manufacturers of these transducer-tipped catheters (see Figs. 5.3 and 5.4).

The pressure within the uterine cavity is directly proportional to the uterine wall tension and inversely proportional to the diameter of the uterus. Thus, the larger the uterus, the lower the intrauterine pressure for a given uterine wall tension. Clinical support of this concept is reflected by the fact that pressure in the nonpregnant uterus may exceed 200 mm Hg during menstrual contractions, whereas intrauterine pressure with twins may never exceed 35 or 40 mm Hg, even in active labor. The usual pressures observed in the pregnant uterus during active labor at term are in the range of 50 to 100 mm Hg at the peak of contractions, with a baseline tone of 5 to 12 mm Hg.

Insertion of the uterine pressure catheter is accomplished by introducing it, while within the sterile introducer tube, just inside the uterine cervix and next to the presenting part (Fig. 4.17). The flexible intrauterine catheter is usually advanced into the uterus quite easily, but on occasion, resistance will be met. In this situation, one should move the introducer 90 degrees in its orientation to the cervix and try again. Usually, one

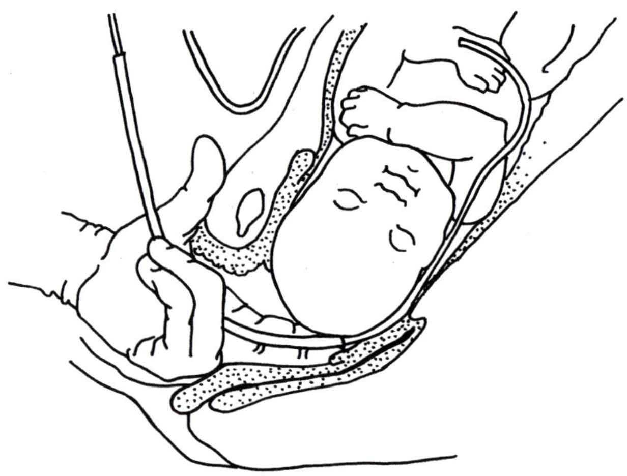

Figure 4.17. The technique of transcervical insertion of the uterine catheter. Note that the introducer is only inserted about 1 cm inside the cervix.

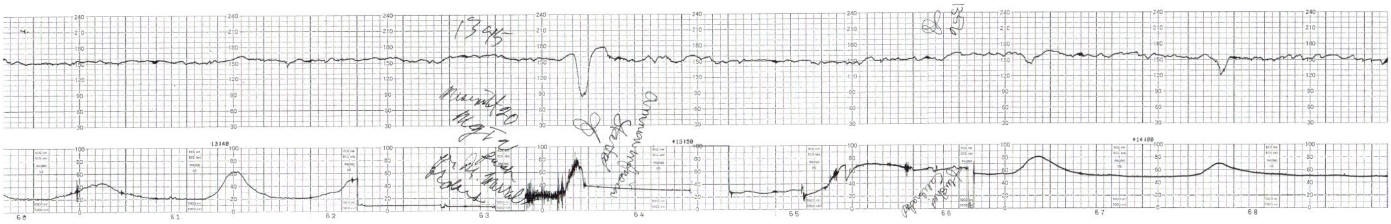

Figure 4.18. Amnioinfusion effect on uterine tone. Note the significant change in the baseline uterine tone associated with the initiation of amnioinfusion. This results from the hydrostatic pressure of the infusate and must be considered in assessing the actual intrauterine pressure.

begins posterior to the presenting part, but the catheter can be inserted anywhere in the 360-degree circumference of the cervix. When the catheter advances easily, it should be inserted to the mark on the catheter that should be just visible at the introitus. All systems for measuring intrauterine pressure must be zeroed, which is the referencing of the pressure to 0 mm Hg while the system is open to air. Any reconnection of the patient to the monitor requires re-zeroing. It is expected that there will be a baseline uterine tone, so if the monitor is registering zero or a negative number, the calibration is incorrect. Replacement of the catheter is necessary if a good recording does not result from simple manipulation.

Another modification of the intrauterine pressure catheter allows for amnioinfusion while simultaneously recording contraction strength. The accuracy of pressure monitoring is not lessened with this catheter and allows for continuous amnioinfusion without artifactual elevation of baseline uterine pressure or a need for the placement of a second catheter for infusion. If one is using a single-lumen catheter for pressure readings and simultaneous amnioinfusion, there is an elevation of the apparent baseline uterine tone (Fig. 4.18). However, this is actually the result of the hydrostatic pressure from the infusion and is readily confirmed by interrupting the infusion and confirming true baseline and peak contraction strength.

The Spiral Fetal Scalp Electrode

The most commonly used fetal electrode consists of a spiral or corkscrew-shaped device placed inside two concentric tubes, with the wires trailing through the center tube. After clearly identifying the presenting part, the whole assembly is inserted through the vagina and cervix against the fetus. The inner tube is then rotated clockwise one full turn so that the electrode tip penetrates the fetal presenting part (Fig. 4.19). The wires are then attached to the leg plate, which is usually placed on the mother's thigh. The leg plate is then attached to the fetal monitor.

If the signal is not adequate, efforts should be made to be certain that the electrode is attached to the fetal presenting part and that the leg plate is appropriately adherent.

Precautions that should be taken when inserting an internal electrode include the following:

1. Use sterile technique.
2. Do not attempt placement if unsure of the exact site of placement.
3. Do not place over facial structures.
4. Avoid the genitalia in a breech position.
5. Never try to reinsert an electrode by twisting manually. Sometimes the spiral is stretched out, and the depth of insertion may exceed the safe depth set on unstretched electrodes.
6. Do not rotate the spiral more than 360 degrees, as tissue injury may result.
7. Do not use in a patient who has active herpes, hepatitis, or human immunodeficiency virus infection.

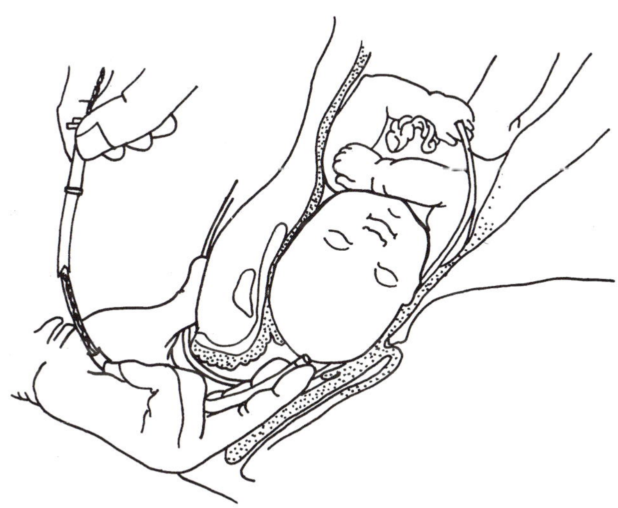

Figure 4.19. Technique for application of the spiral electrode.

When removing the electrode, twist the wires counterclockwise simultaneously. This can be done just before or after delivery of the neonate. At cesarean, the electrode should be removed through the vagina before delivery, if possible, to avoid pulling the contaminated intravaginal portion of the device through the hysterotomy and into the surgical field.

Following delivery, the area of electrode placement in the baby's scalp should be cleaned in the nursery.

The External Tocodynamometer

If the membranes are not yet ruptured, the external tocodynamometer allows the patient's uterine activity to be monitored in a nonquantitative way. This is quite satisfactory for patients who are progressing well. Occasionally, FHR decelerations may be observed in a patient when contractions are not recorded with an external tocotransducer. Intrauterine pressure monitoring may clarify the timing of the decelerations with respect to uterine activity.

External tocotransducers come in many different sizes and shapes and are attached by means of an elastic belt around the patient's abdomen. When the uterus contracts, the change in shape and rigidity slightly depresses a plunger, causing a change in the voltage of a small electrical current. These voltage changes are proportional to the uterine activity and are represented qualitatively by the fetal monitor as contractions. Because this method does not reflect the true intrauterine pressure, avoid detecting only the peaks by adjusting the pen position to set the uterine activity channel at about 25 relative units between contractions. Positioning of the external tocotransducer is important because if not placed over the proper part of the abdomen, uterine activity may not be detected at all. Palpate to find where contractions are the most easily felt abdominally and place the transducer with careful attention to adjustment of the elastic belt to an appropriate tension (Fig. 4.20).

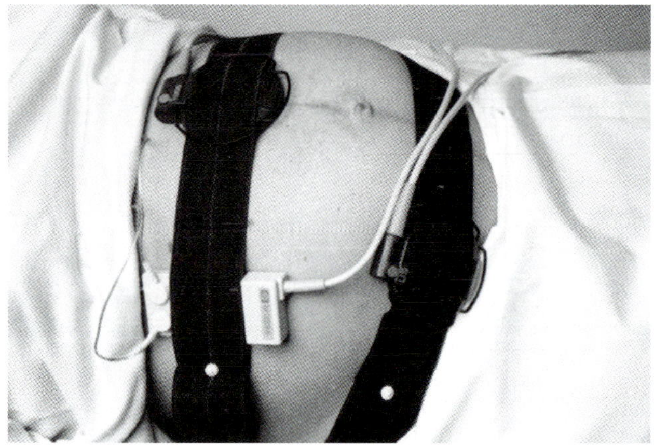

Figure 4.20. Maternal electrocardiogram, external tocodynamometer, and ultrasound fetal heart rate transducer on the patient.

In the presence of maternal obesity or a small uterus, the external tocotransducer may poorly detect uterine activity (Fig. 4.21). Palpate and pay attention to both the patient's complaints of contractions and any evidence of FHR decelerations suggestive of undetected uterine activity. Although the external tocotransducer estimates the frequency and duration of contractions fairly well, the baseline tone and actual contraction amplitude cannot be measured with the external tocotransducer. Monitoring with a tocotransducer provides real-time pressure measurements of uterine activity compared to a baseline. Newer monitors have simplified the technology of establishing a baseline, and this can be accomplished either manually or automatically. One should follow the specific instructions with the type of monitor used in order to obtain as accurate information as possible with external tocotransducers.

The Doppler Transducer

The Doppler transducer is usually secured to the patient with an adjustable elastic strap that encircles the maternal

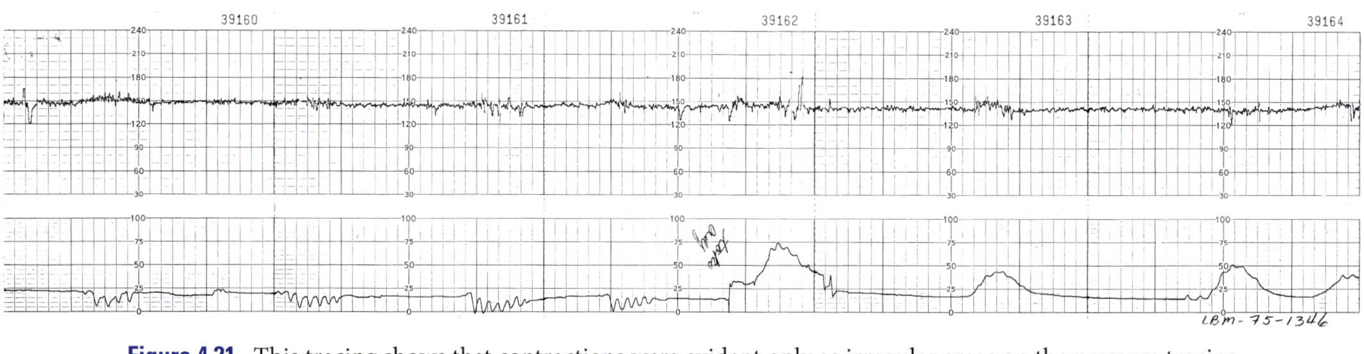

Figure 4.21. This tracing shows that contractions were evident only as irregular areas on the pressure tracing until the tocodynamometer was adjusted and repositioned. Subsequent contraction recording is satisfactory.

abdomen. Selection of the optimum location for the transducer should proceed in the following manner:

1. Place the retaining strap under the patient in the supine position.
2. Place an adequate amount of ultrasonic coupling gel over the transducer face and apply it to the maternal abdomen.
3. Begin searching for the strongest signal by listening with the monitor audio turned on. In cephalic presentation, this is usually found to be below the umbilicus; with a breech, it may be higher on the maternal abdomen. It is often best to locate the fetal back with Leopold's maneuvers and place the transducer over this area. The use of real-time ultrasound can also assist in confirming fetal position and heart location.
4. When the optimal area is located, secure the transducer to the retaining strap and adjust for final placement at the location where the signal is clearest and the monitor is able to record well.

Because the Doppler transducer both transmits ultrasonic beams and receives the reflected signals, the angle of the transducer is important. By the laws of physics, the beam is reflected from a moving interface with the angle of incidence equaling the angle of reflection. Therefore, the beam will only return to the transducer when it is arranged perpendicular to the moving interface. Because of this, the transducer should be tilted (Fig. 4.22) to get the optimal signal, then moved to a point where the tangential placement allows reception of the reflected beam without transducer tilt. Once the transducer placement is optimal, it is necessary to constantly recheck the signal. If the fetus moves or the mother changes position, the signal may be lost and the transducer may have to be repositioned. With newer monitors using wide-beam ultrasound and autocorrelation, obtaining a continuous, reliable fetal cardiac tracing is less problematic, but the possibility of recording MHR is increased.

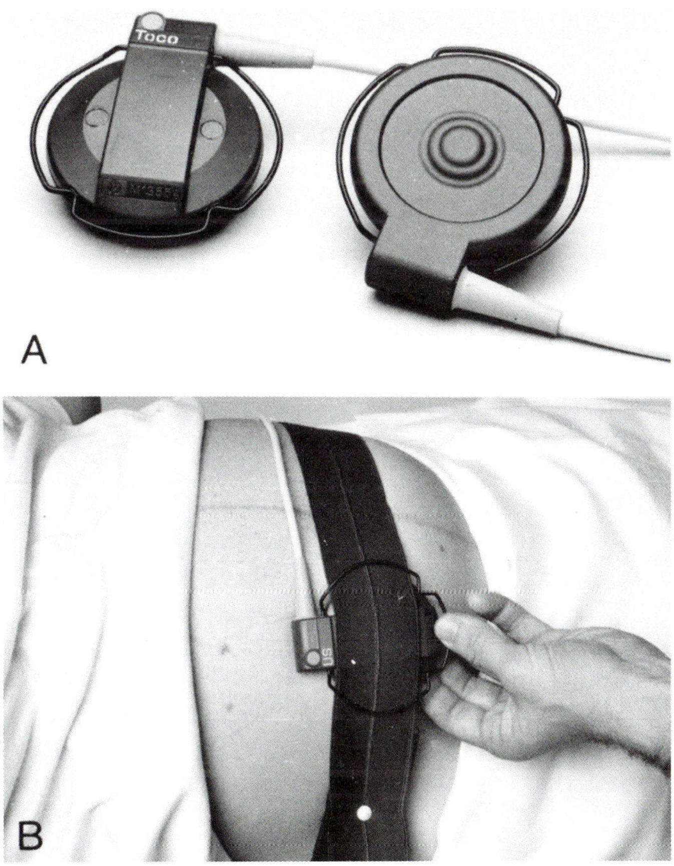

Figure 4.22. Newer monitors have dramatically improved the quality of the external mode. **A.** Both sides of the external tocodynamometer transducer. **B.** Demonstration of the placement of the ultrasound fetal heart rate (FHR) transducer over the area of the maternal abdomen that gives the best FHR signal.

Central Monitoring (Fig. 4.23)

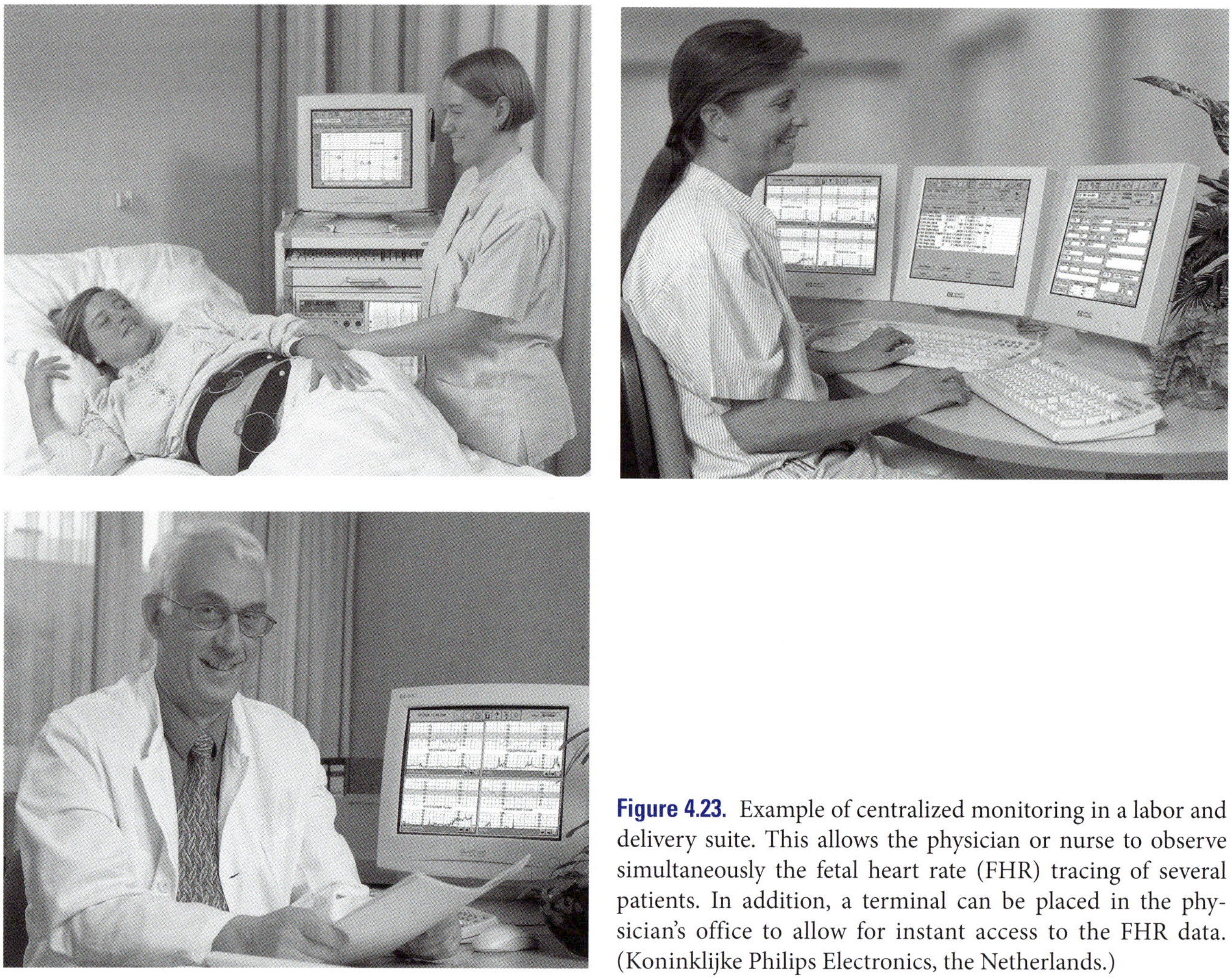

Figure 4.23. Example of centralized monitoring in a labor and delivery suite. This allows the physician or nurse to observe simultaneously the fetal heart rate (FHR) tracing of several patients. In addition, a terminal can be placed in the physician's office to allow for instant access to the FHR data. (Koninklijke Philips Electronics, the Netherlands.)

Twin Monitoring Monitoring twins has always presented a challenge. On fetal monitors with twin monitoring capability, one twin's heart rate is recorded in bold dark style and the other is recorded in thinner light style (Fig. 4.24). The physician/nurse who is monitoring the patient should assign the dark tracing to one twin and the light tracing to the other. Too often, this is not noted in the record, and later on, it is not possible to determine which tracing goes with which twin. When monitoring both twins with Doppler transducers, it is possible to be monitoring the same twin on each transducer. This is referred to as signal coincidence. The easiest way to monitor twins is to have a fetal electrode on the presenting twin and use a Doppler transducer on Twin B.

Because of the difficulty in determining whether there is a signal coincidence (having one twin on both transducers), it is necessary to detect this potentially problematic situation. Newer monitors with twin monitoring capability have built-in logic to detect signal coincidence. Logic in the monitor will compare the two recordings from the two Doppler transducers and, if they are the same, will alarm indicating signal coincidence that indicates the same twin recording on both transducers. On the GE monitor, overlapping hearts above the FHR tracing indicate coincidence. When the coincidence is resolved, the overlapping hearts become side-by-side hearts (Fig. 4.25). On the Philips monitors, question marks above the tracing indicate the same twin on both transducers (Fig. 4.26).

Another problem with twin monitoring occurs when the two twin baseline heart rates are nearly identical. A method that is now available allows the two tracings to be separated by 20 bpm making tracing interpretation less problematic (Fig. 4.27). This can also be done with triplets (Fig. 4.28).

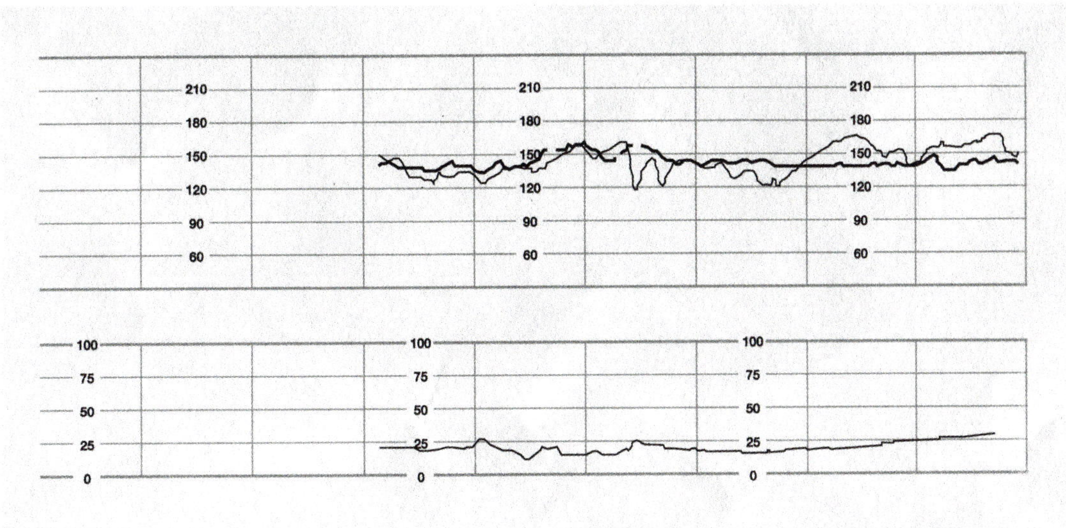

Figure 4.24. Example of twin monitor strip. Note the dark and the light tracing representing the twins. One should note Twins A and B as assigned to dark and light tracing, respectively.

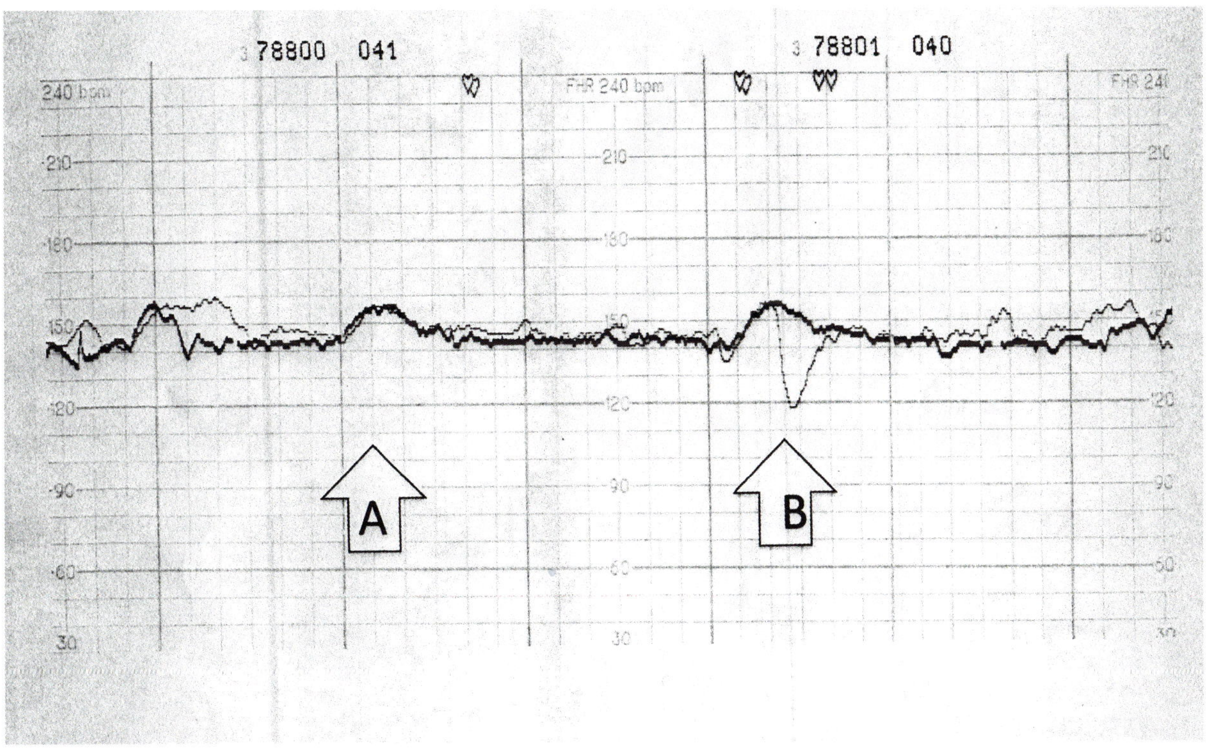

Figure 4.25. With the GE Corometrics monitor, when only one twin is being traced on both transducers, there are overlapping hearts displayed above the tracing (**A**). When the Doppler transducers are each recording different twins, the hearts are separated (**B**).

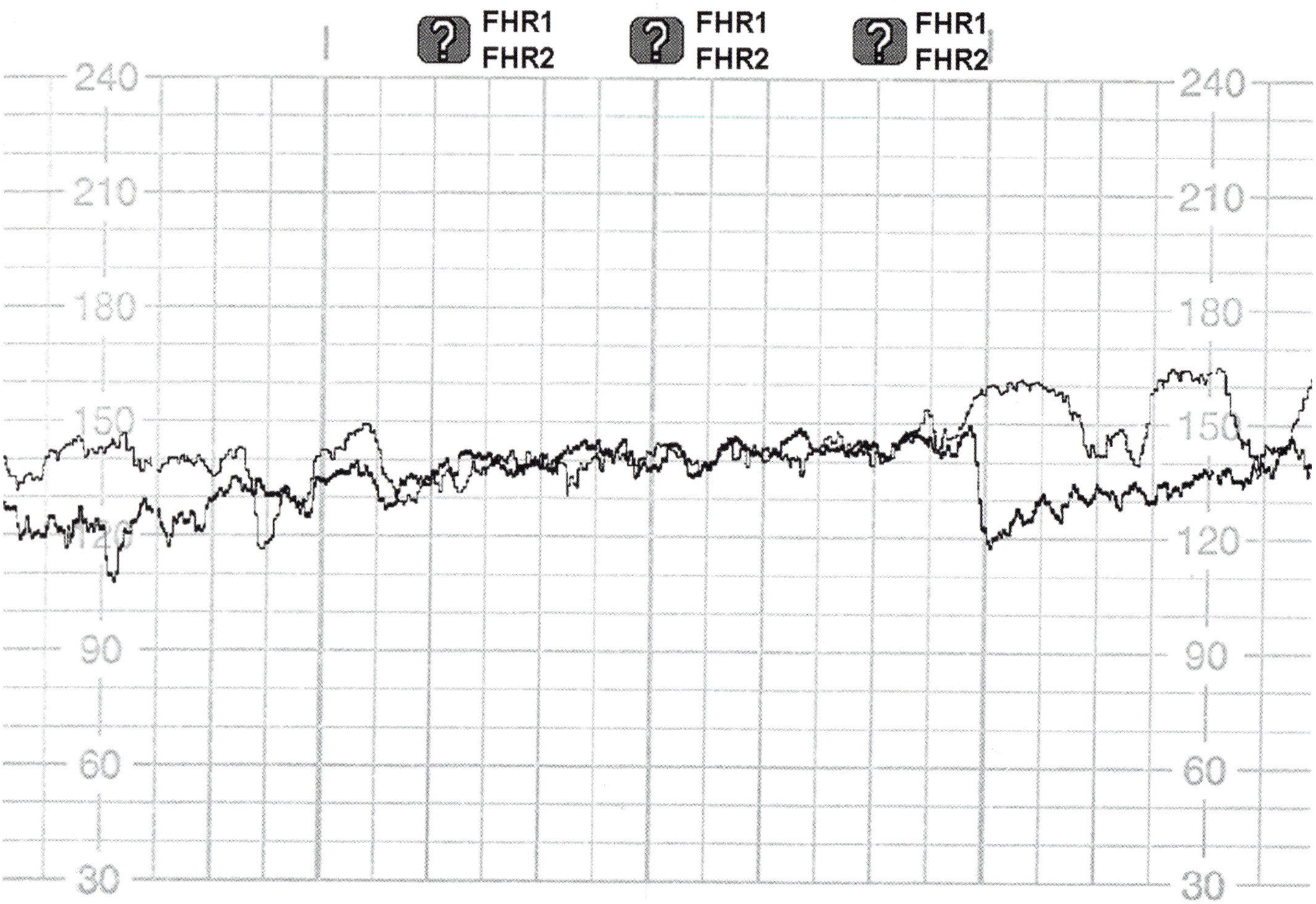

Figure 4.26. On the Philips monitor, when the same twin is being recorded on both transducers, a question mark is printed above the tracing, and when the twins are again separated, the question marks go away.

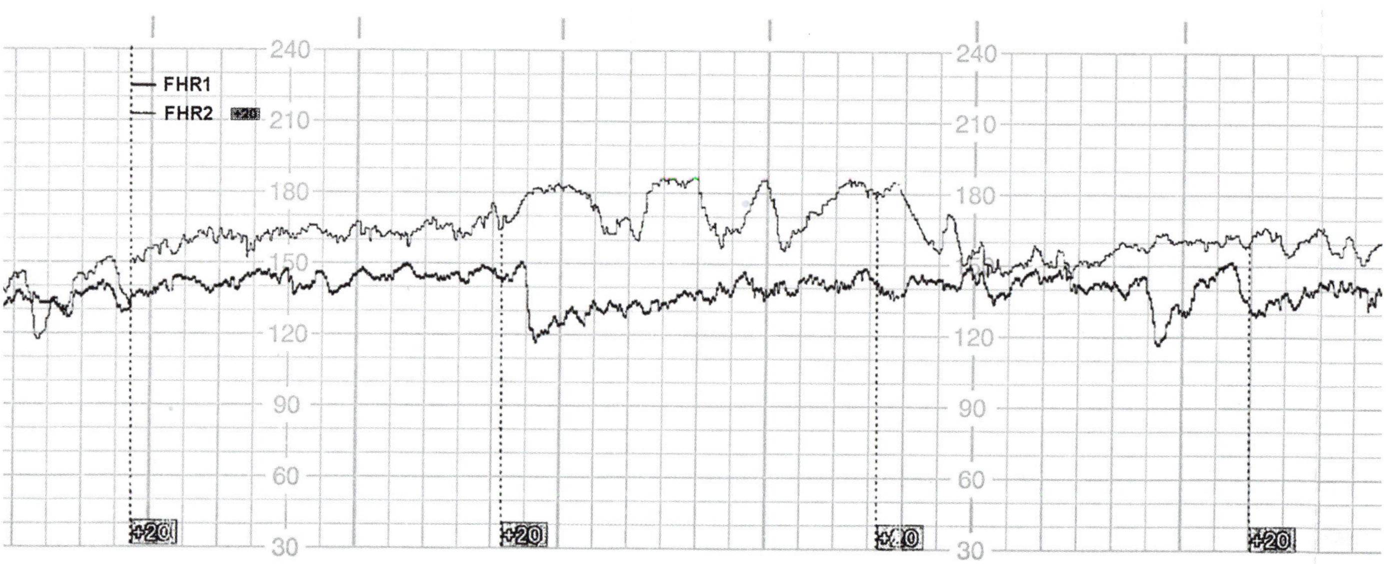

Figure 4.27. There is an option to separate the twins by 20 bpm in order to get a better look at each tracing. On the Philips monitor, a +20 is printed when the separation begins and goes away when the separation is terminated.

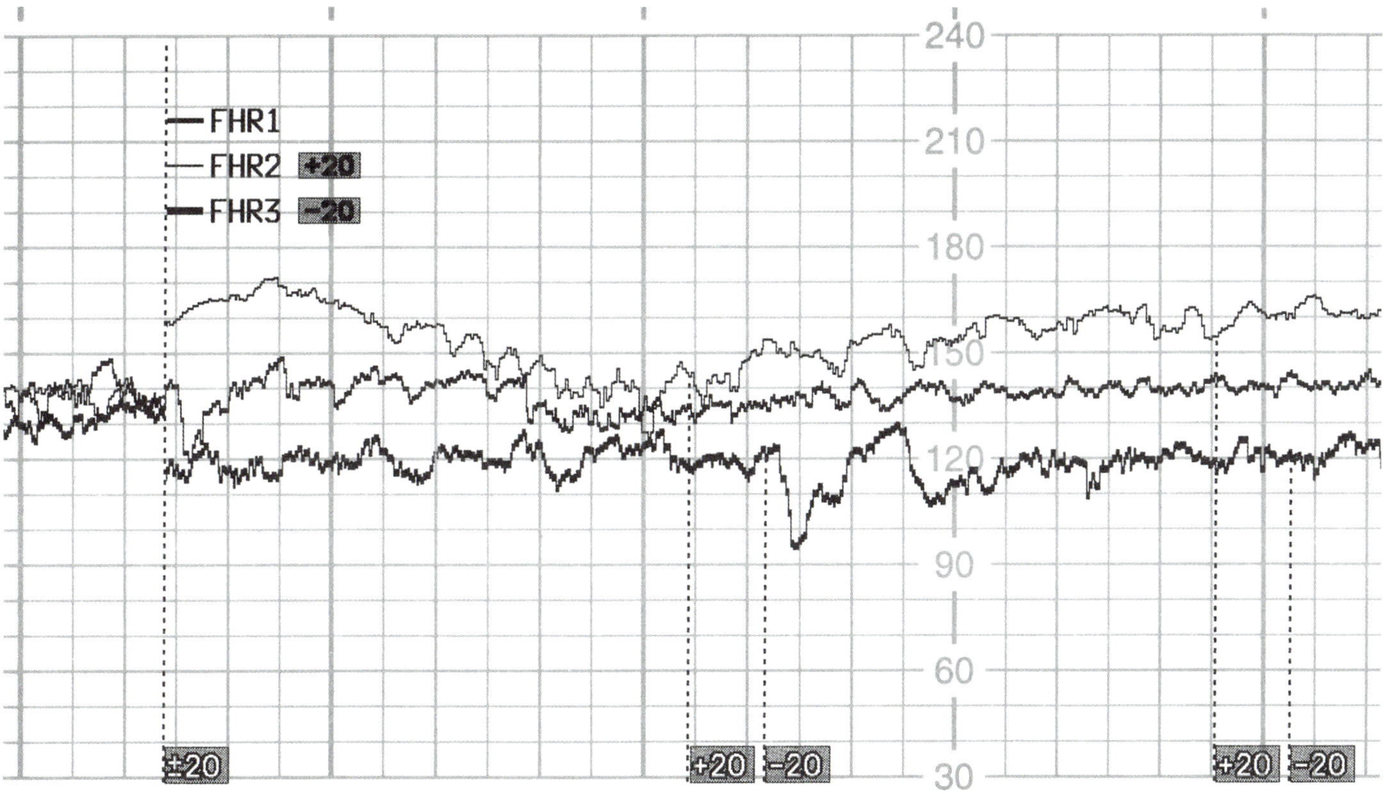

Figure 4.28. With triplets, one fetus may have a 20-bpm increase and another may have a 20-bpm decrease in order to separate the three tracings of the triplets.

Signal Ambiguity from MHR

Figure 4.29 is an example of the transition from fetal to MHR recording while positioning a patient for an epidural with Doppler FHR recording. With newer FHR monitors, the transition from fetal to maternal signal is not always marked by discontinuity of the recording (signal loss) (Fig. 4.30). It is well known that during the second stage of labor, with maternal pushing efforts, the mother becomes tachycardic and accelerates her heart rate with contractions.[15] Erroneous interpretation of this MHR tracing as FHR with accelerations can preclude timely detection of fetal compromise.[16]

The newer monitors have electronic logic that was originally used when monitoring twins (see twin monitoring) to alert if the two Doppler transducers were monitoring the same twin or if there was one twin and the mother's heart rate is recorded. This alerting system compares electronic signals from the two transducers and alerts if they are both recording the same twin or, in the case of MHR recording, comparing the Doppler transducer recording with an MHR source from either a maternal ECG or from maternal pulse oximeter recording. If an MHR source (ECG or pulse oximeter) is fed into the monitor, it will alert, indicating signal coincidence the same as with twins when signal coincidence occurs (Fig. 4.31).

The Philips company developed a solution that involves an optical reflection sensor being placed on the tocotransducer so that there is always an MHR source and presumably such coincidence will always be detected (Fig. 4.32). This Philips system called Smart Pulse was approved by the FDA in August 2011.

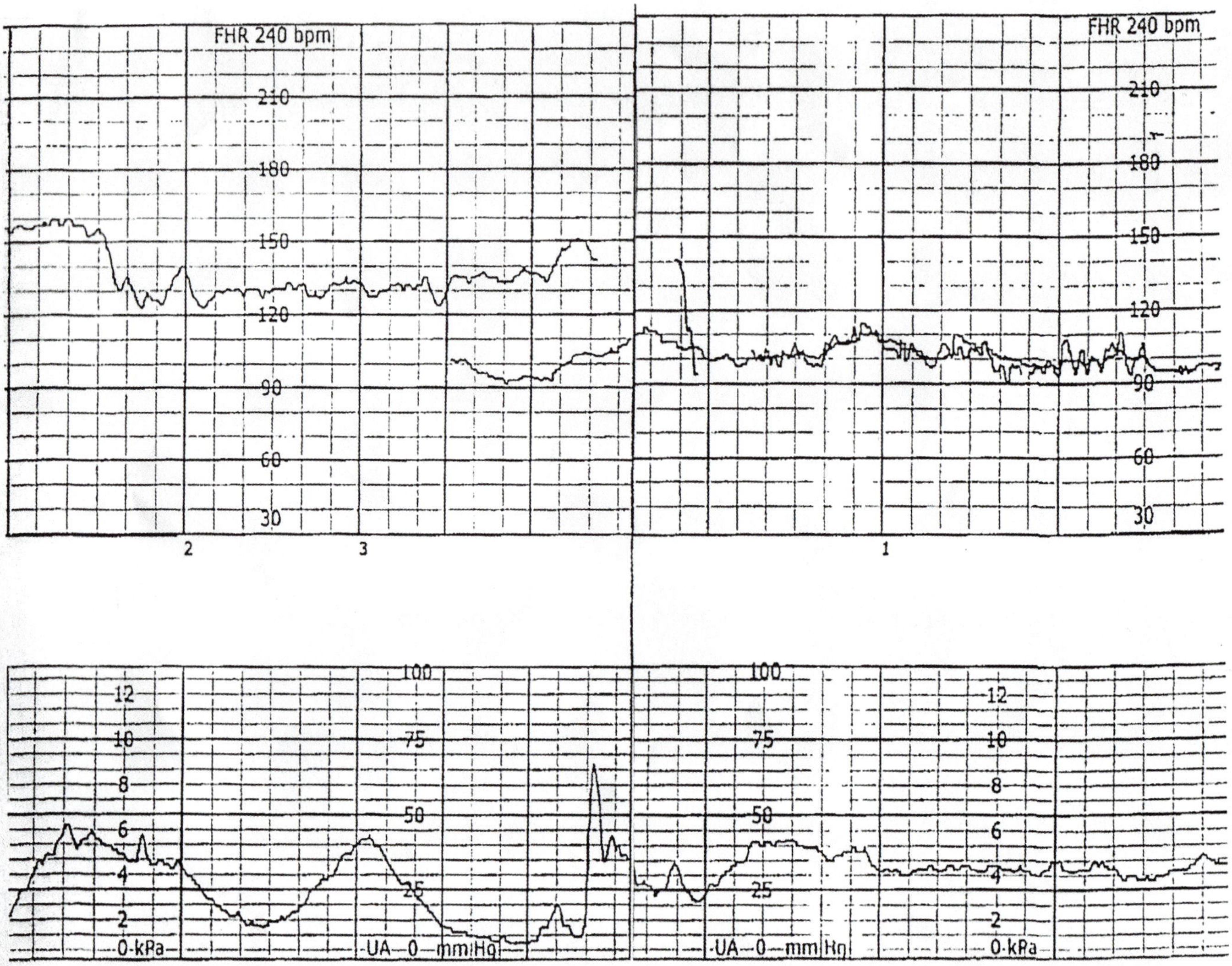

Figure 4.29. When this patient, who was being monitored with a Doppler external transducer, was moved to administer an epidural, the fetal signal was lost and the monitor began recording the maternal heart rate (MHR). The MHR was being recorded from a pulse oximeter just prior to the switch showing that the new heart rate was indeed maternal and not a fetal deceleration. This monitor did not have a signal coincidence warning system in place.

Networking of Fetal Heart Rate Monitoring

Over the years, there have been many advances in our ability to record, store, and transmit fetal monitoring data electronically. Battery-powered devices with Bluetooth capability allow for increased mobility during labor for patients undergoing continuous intrapartum FHR. Technological advances have also allowed for increased mobility for obstetric providers who can now access FHR tracings far from the bedside. Any practitioner who has access to a computer or "smart phone" can observe fetal monitoring data from remote locations, with the appropriate software.

In summary, FHR monitoring instrumentation continues to evolve, and yet the problem of signal ambiguity resulting in MHR recording leading to poor fetal outcomes has not been eliminated. Twin monitoring, even with signal coincidence detection capability, similarly can result in MHR recording from one transducer, thus obscuring one twin's FHR recording.

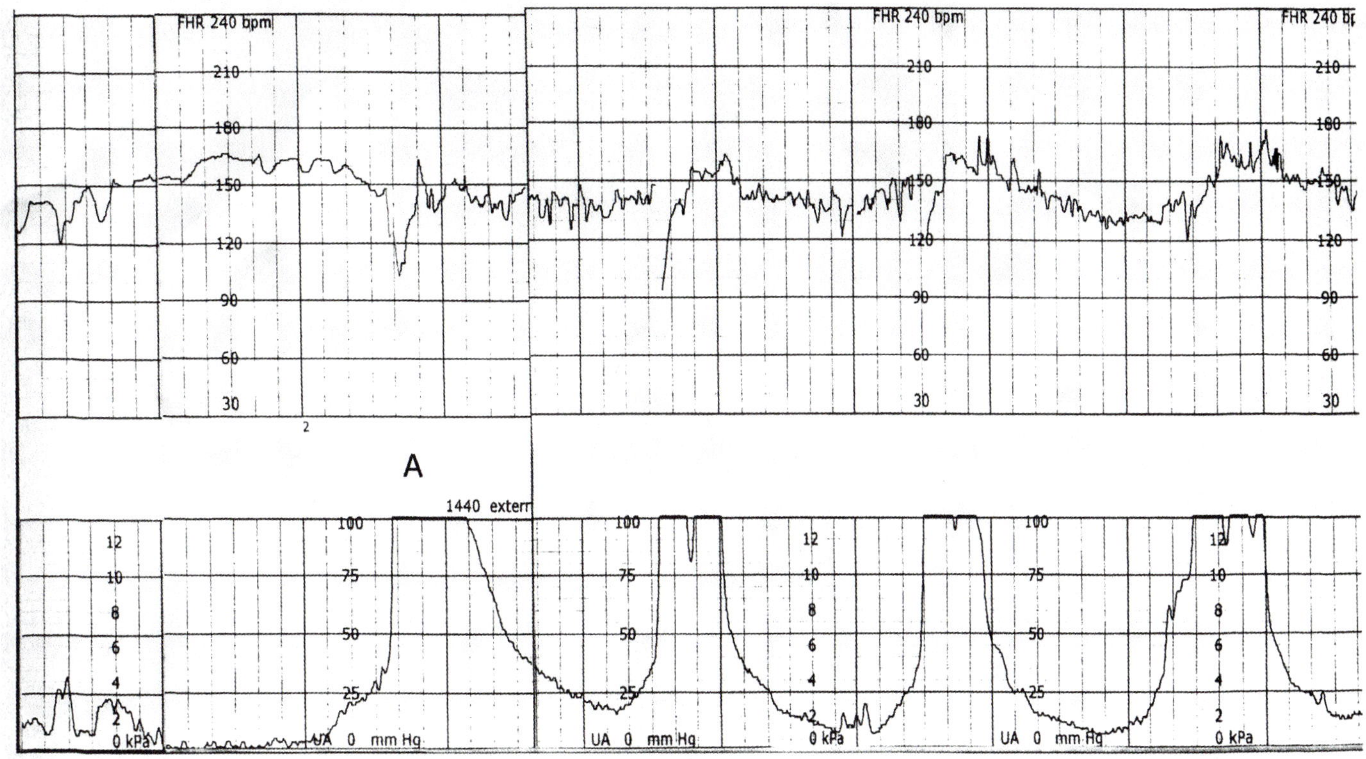

Figure 4.30. This fetus was being monitored with a Doppler external transducer, and at point A, it switched to begin monitoring the maternal heart rate. The switch occurred during a continuous tracing without signal loss as was usually seen on older monitors.

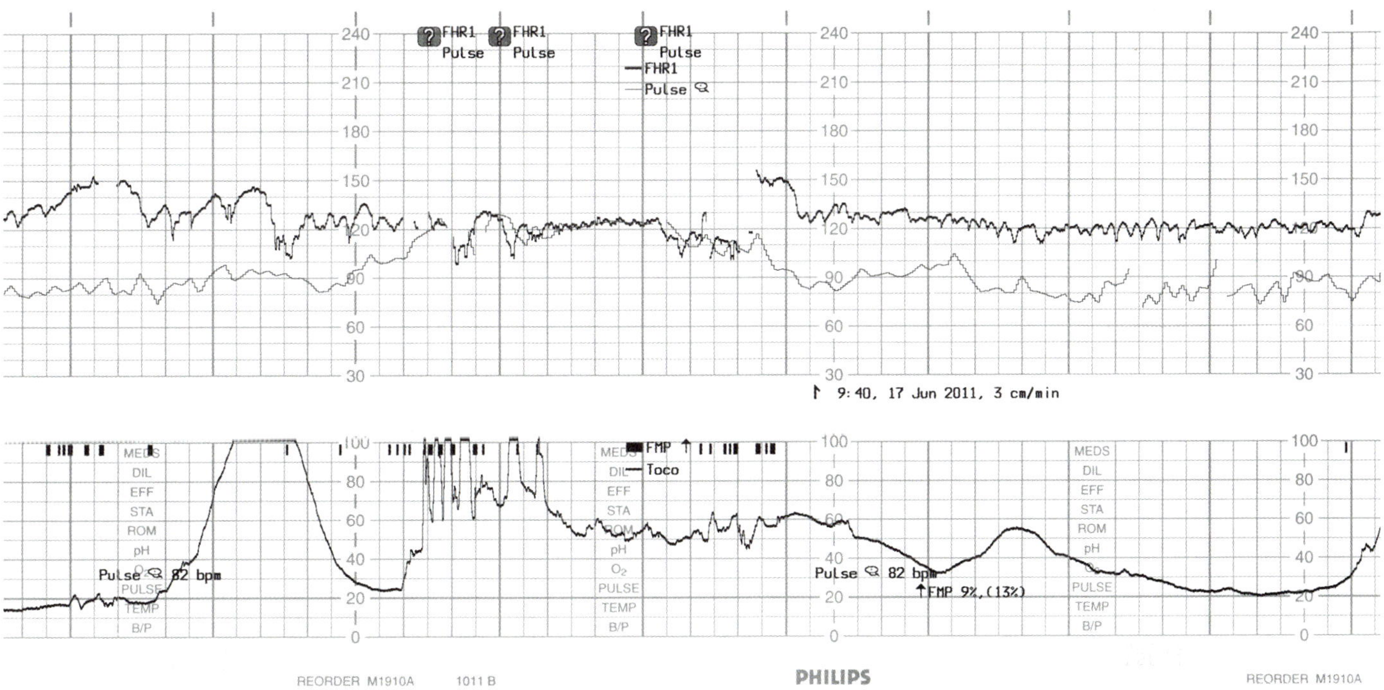

Figure 4.31. This recording begins with the fetal heart rate baseline at about 120 bpm and maternal pulse rate from an optical sensor integrated into the Toco transducer with a baseline of about 80 bpm. When the ultrasound Doppler transducer from the maternal abdomen began to pick up the maternal pulse, the characteristic question marks appear at the upper part of the tracing, indicating coincidence on a Philips monitor.

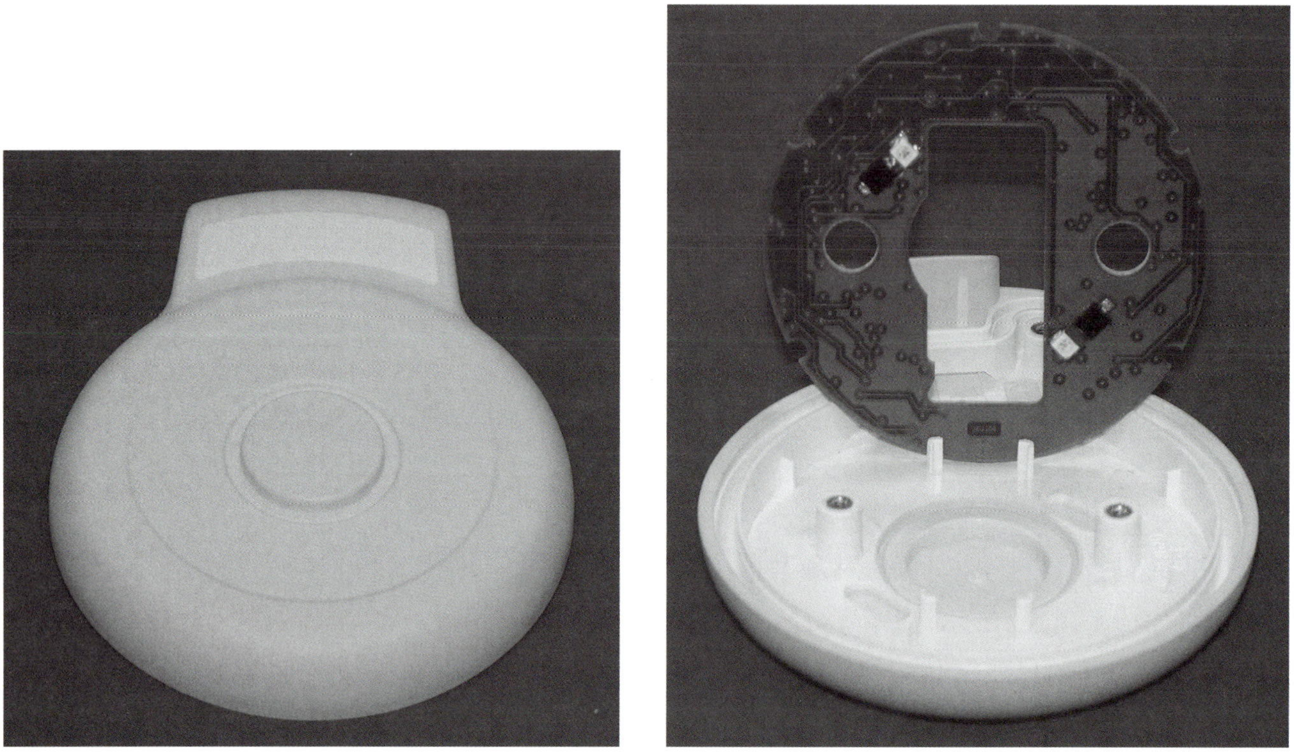

Figure 4.32. This figure shows the new Toco transducer developed by Philips: It has an integrated maternal optical reflection sensor system giving a continuous maternal pulse rate signal that is automatically used to detect fetal/maternal signal coincidence.

FETAL CARDIAC ARRHYTHMIAS

Fetal cardiac arrhythmias occur in one form or another in a significant number of pregnancies. The documentation of various fetal arrhythmias has increased subsequent to the more extensive application of antepartum and intrapartum electronic FHR monitoring. The importance of recognition of an abnormal cardiac rhythm, correct diagnosis of arrhythmia type, associated incidence of underlying heart disease, and the need for appropriate medical intervention depends on the specific type of arrhythmia present. Diagnosis can be established through M-mode and real-time ultrasound.[17,18] In the absence of signs of heart failure (ie, cardiac enlargement or hydrops) or evidence of FHR abnormalities suggestive of hypoxia, most fetal cardiac arrhythmias are benign, do not require immediate delivery, and are not associated with structural fetal cardiac abnormalities. Many arrhythmias, particularly those diagnosed during the intrapartum period, such as PACs and PVCs, do not persist in the neonatal period and rarely require medical therapy. Rarely, PACs and PVCs can be so frequent that they preclude reliable FHR monitoring and interpretation intrapartum, in which case a cesarean may be recommended (similar to a complete heart block below). For the most part, though, PACs and PVCs are benign and do not require any special attention. However, certain types of arrhythmias are of clinical significance for both mother and fetus. Supraventricular tachycardias (SVTs) and fetal heart block may be associated with previously undiagnosed fetal compromise, maternal disease, or both and frequently require active management.

Fetal Tachycardia

The three general types of fetal tachycardia are sinus tachycardia, atrial flutter/fibrillation, and SVT.

Sinus Tachycardia

Sinus tachycardia is defined as FHR above 160 bpm and is usually secondary to maternal fever, drugs (ie, atropine, b-sympathomimetics), amnionitis, congenital infection, or hyperthyroidism (Fig. 4.33). Although usually benign, on occasion, sinus tachycardia accompanied by late or severe variable

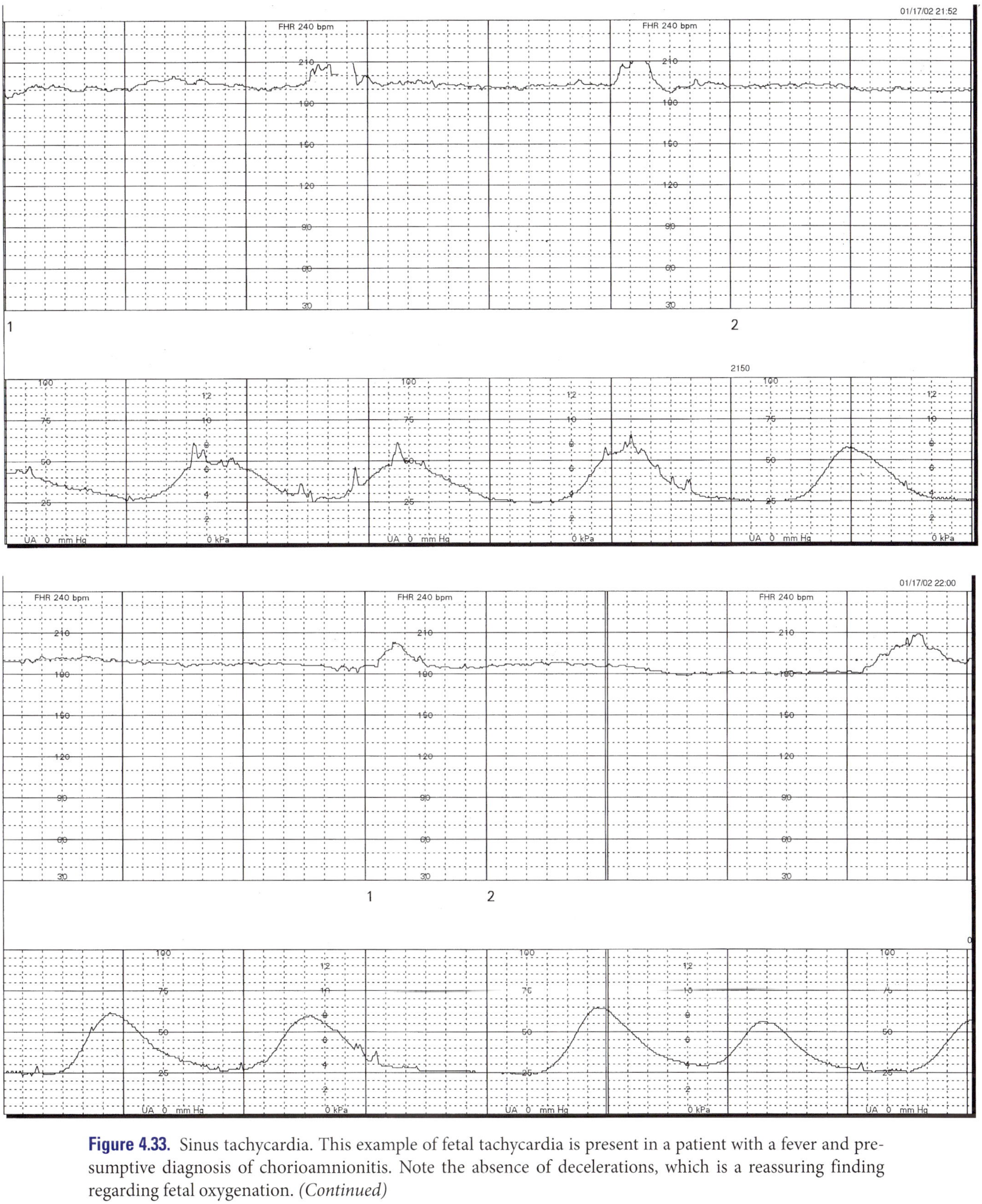

Figure 4.33. Sinus tachycardia. This example of fetal tachycardia is present in a patient with a fever and presumptive diagnosis of chorioamnionitis. Note the absence of decelerations, which is a reassuring finding regarding fetal oxygenation. *(Continued)*

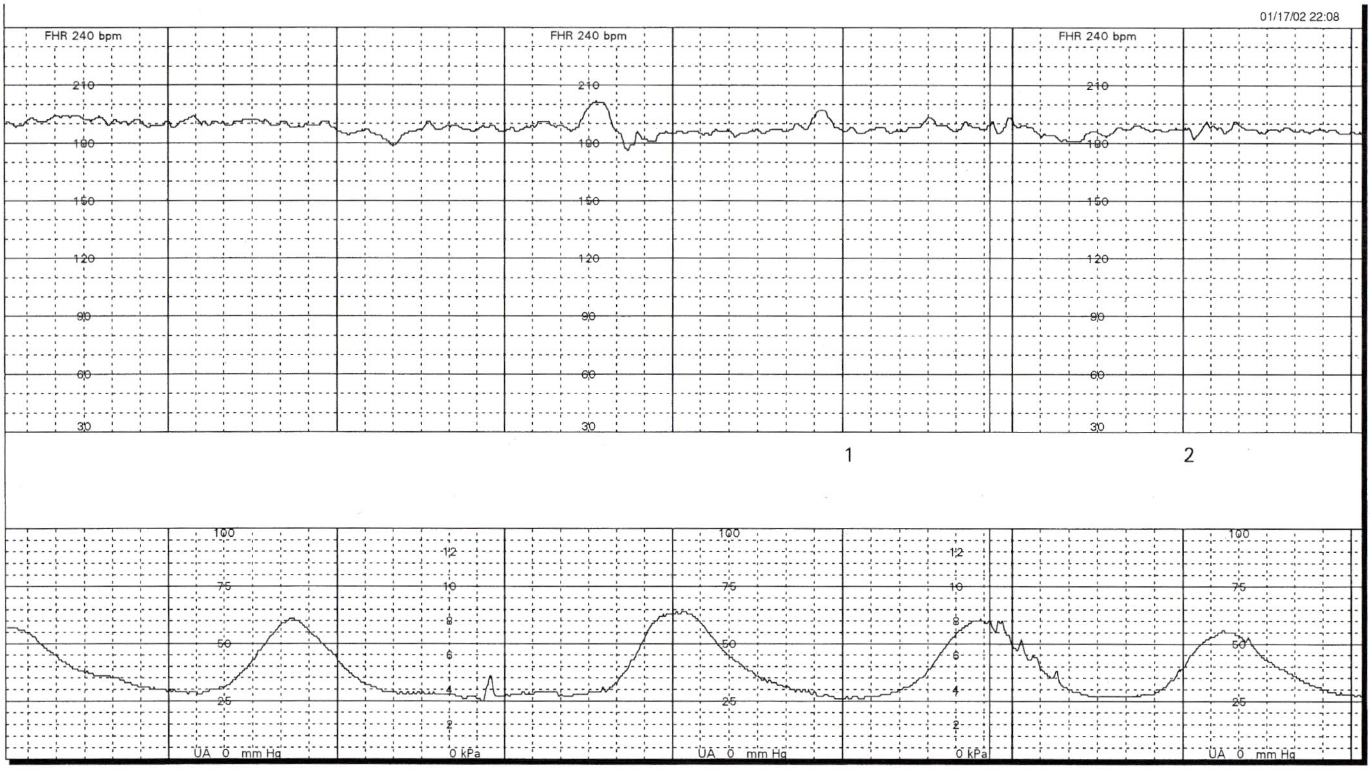

Figure 4.33. *(Continued)*

decelerations may be a sign of early fetal hypoxia.[19] Recognition of the cause of tachycardia and differentiation from SVT are of obvious importance. Tachycardia alone is not a sign of fetal hypoxia unless it is associated with an ominous pattern of decelerations.

Atrial Flutter/Fibrillation

The antepartum diagnosis of atrial flutter or fibrillation is rare. A monotonous atrial rate that varies between 400 and 500 bpm is seen with this form of supraventricular tachyarrhythmia in the fetus. The ventricular rate is much lower because of an accompanying AV block. If the AV block is fixed, a regular ventricular rate of 60 to 200 bpm is seen. If the block is intermittent, the ventricular rate will vary widely. Atrial flutter and fibrillation are serious arrhythmias; nonimmune hydrops can occur, and a concomitant severe congenital heart defect is found in as many as 20% of cases.[20] These arrhythmias are most resistant to in-utero therapy and are associated with a very high fetal and neonatal mortality rate. Atrial fibrillation is rarer in the fetus than atrial flutter. Treatment with digoxin and/or verapamil may increase the degree of AV block but rarely corrects the atrial arrhythmia. However, control of ventricular rate does not necessarily improve fetal hydrops. This may require the restoration of a 1:1 AV conduction. The use of type I antiarrhythmic agents (eg, flecainide, quinidine, and procainamide) should be considered as well in such patients.

Supraventricular Tachycardia

Thought to be the most frequent form of fetal tachyarrhythmia, SVT can occur for short periods and be of no clinical significance, or it can persist for long periods and lead to high output failure, nonimmune hydrops fetalis, and fetal death.[21,22] Defined as an FHR greater than 220 bpm with no variability or conduction abnormality, SVT can be suspected on cardiac auscultation and confirmed with M-mode echocardiography and pulsed-Doppler flow-velocity waveforms.[23] Real-time ultrasound often will demonstrate varying degrees of cardiac failure. Although there may be no evidence of effusions or hydropic changes coexistent with SVT, rapid progression can be seen in as little as 36 hours of continued tachyarrhythmia. More commonly, this is not a continuous but rather an intermittent arrhythmia for which the term paroxysmal atrial tachycardia was used in the past.

SVT may be a manifestation of atrial flutter or fibrillation and, in theory, results from one of two mechanisms. The first is increased automaticity of an ectopic pacemaker (other than the normal sinus nodal pacemaker) above the bundle of His. The second, and more likely, mechanism in fetal and childhood SVT is reentrant tachycardia resulting from a circular "circus movement" of electrical activity, most commonly within the AV node. Less commonly but seen in the Wolff-Parkinson-White (WPW) syndrome, this movement is caused by an accessory conduction pathway (bundle of Kent). Both types of reentrant tachycardia are thought to result from an atrial premature contraction being conducted through or around the AV node down a repolarized but relatively slow pathway. The fast pathway is thought to be in a refractory period following the previously normally timed atrial depolarization. If sufficiently slow conduction occurs, allowing recovery of the fast pathway, ventriculoatrial conduction up the fast pathway results in a sudden re-entrant tachycardia. The initiation and maintenance of this tachycardia depend on the refractory periods and conduction velocities within the slow and fast conduction pathways in the AV node. The timing of the arrival of the premature contraction is the critical factor in the initiation of the arrhythmia.

Treatment of Fetal Tachycardia

Sinus tachycardia is often encountered in the intrapartum period and usually reflects a drug effect, sympathetic fetal response to maternal infection, occult amnionitis, or, rarely, fetal hypoxia. The importance of identifying sinus tachycardia is not to institute a specific therapy but to determine its cause and separate it from SVT (Fig. 4.33). Ventricular tachycardia (VT), as defined by three or more consecutive premature ventricular systoles, is extremely rare in the fetus, and its significance remains unknown. Ventricular fibrillation in the fetus has not been reported.

Treatment of fetal SVT has been extensively reported. In utero pharmacologic therapy utilizing single drugs or various combinations of digoxin, calcium-channel blockers, β-blockers, procainamide, and quinidine have all been reported with varying degrees of success.[24] Once the diagnosis of SVT is made, with or without the associated signs of fetal cardiac failure, delivery of the mature fetus or in utero therapy of the immature fetus must be initiated. Fetal SVT requires urgent management at any gestational age. Digoxin has been the most commonly used drug for the initial treatment, and the combination of rapid digitalization and maintenance of the maternal digoxin level in the middle-to-upper therapeutic range with the addition of a calcium-channel blocker, such as verapamil, or beta-blocker, such as propranolol or atenolol, has been our most successful approach (Figs. 4.34 and 4.35). Quinidine is an alternative drug that, following adequate digitalization, can be of value in controlling fetal SVT. Unfortunately, 30% of patients cannot tolerate this drug because of severe nausea and vomiting. Digoxin should be initiated as a single agent with an intravenous loading dose of 1.0 mg (0.5 mg followed by 0.25 mg at 6-hour intervals) while the patient is hospitalized and on continuous cardiac monitoring. The goal is to achieve a maternal blood level at the upper end of the therapeutic range. If there is no improvement in fetal rhythm after two days with a high therapeutic blood level of digoxin in the mother, a second or even third agent may be required. It is very important to consider that many of these additional antiarrhythmic agents increase both the serum level and bioavailability of digoxin. Consequently, the maternal digoxin dose should be reduced by at least 50% when using such agents as quinidine, verapamil, or amiodarone. When M-mode echocardiography reveals atrial flutter or fibrillation, one of the drugs of choice to control the associated rapid ventricular response caused by AV node bypass is procainamide, following the administration of digoxin, verapamil, or propranolol. The different types of fetal SVT can be controlled most frequently with digoxin and either verapamil or propranolol. When a combination of agents is indicated, the best choice is to combine the use of an agent that affects the fast pathway with one that affects the slow pathway (Tables 4.1 and 4.2). With the exception of digoxin, cardiac antiarrhythmic drugs used to treat reentrant SVT also decrease automaticity with consequent lowering of the incidence of premature beats.

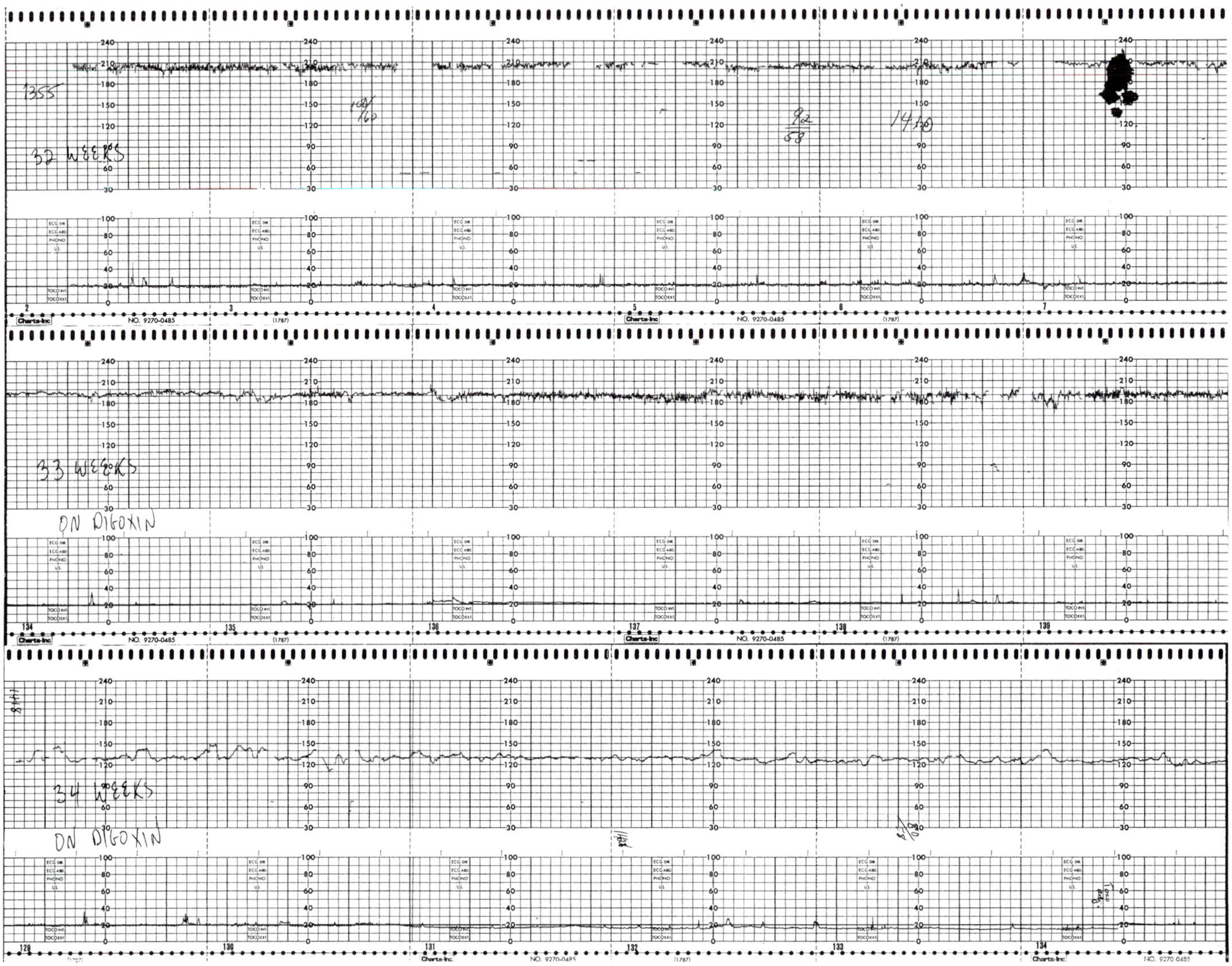

Figure 4.34. Sequential examples of fetal supraventricular tachycardia cardioverted in utero with digoxin treatment of the mother. The fetus was not hydropic during treatment.

Congenital Heart Block

Although most fetal arrhythmias are either extrasystoles or tachyarrhythmias, bradyarrhythmias caused by complete heart block comprise approximately 10% of cases.[25] The forms of heart block are first, second, and third degree (complete). Prolongation of the interval between the P and R waves (first-degree AV block), usually secondary to impaired conduction in the AV junction proximal to the bundle of His, generally requires no treatment. Second-degree or partial AV block, in which some but not all atrial impulses are conducted to the ventricles, is present in most fetuses with SVT. Second-degree AV block presents in two forms, Mobitz types I and II. In Mobitz type I block, the P-R interval increases progressively until complete blockage of an atrial impulse results in a dropped

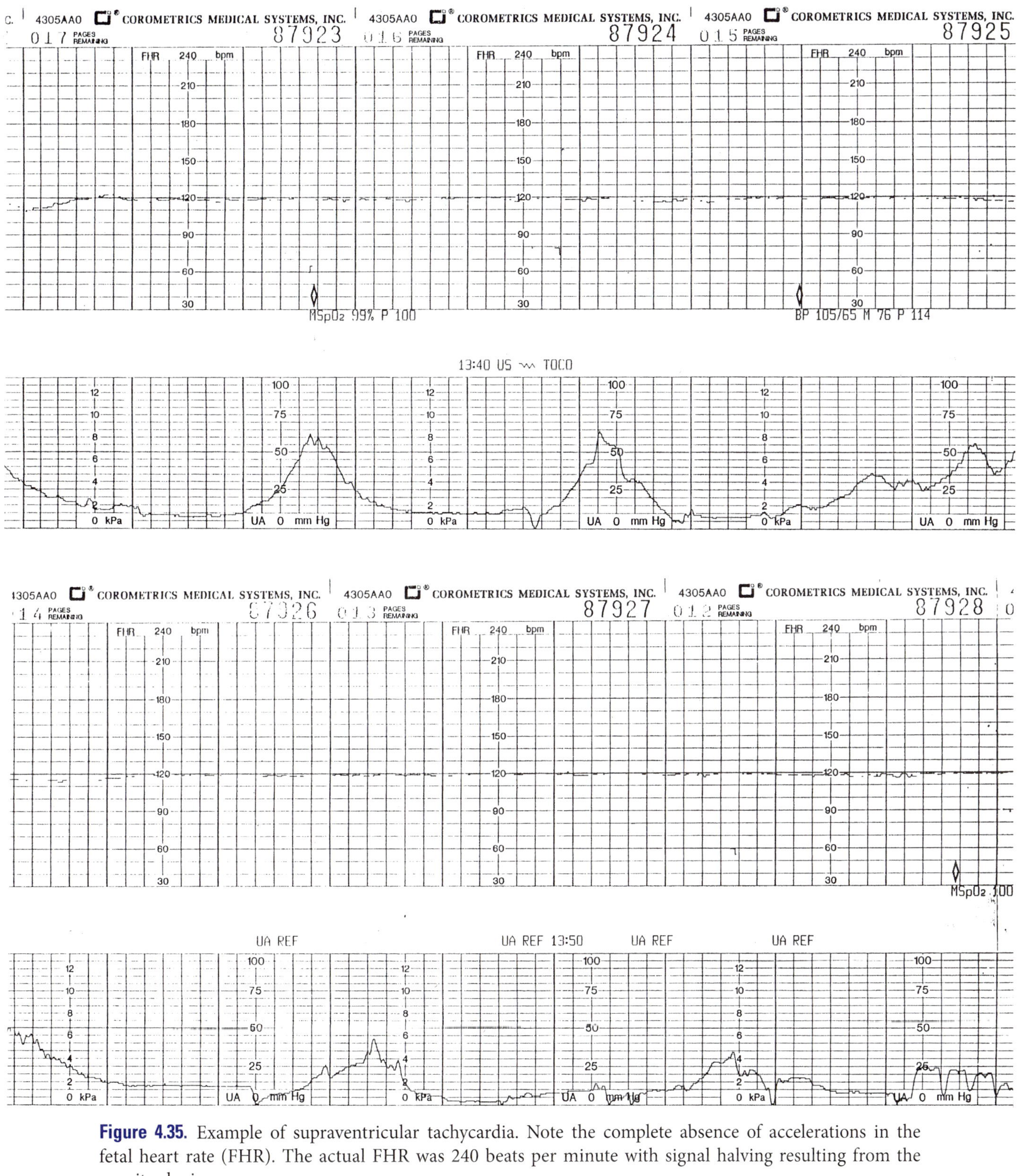

Figure 4.35. Example of supraventricular tachycardia. Note the complete absence of accelerations in the fetal heart rate (FHR). The actual FHR was 240 beats per minute with signal halving resulting from the monitor logic.

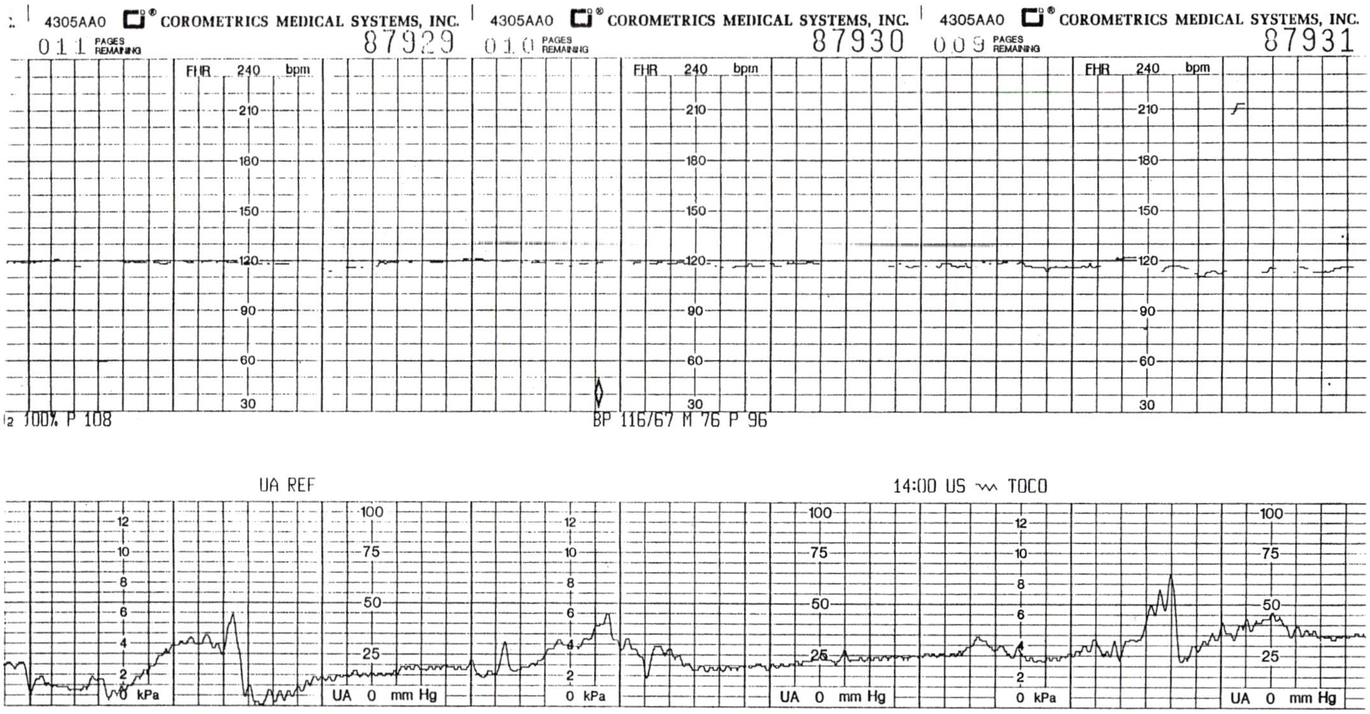

Figure 4.35. *(Continued)*

ventricular beat (Wenckebach type). This cycle is repeated, following anywhere from two to eight consecutive impulses with progressive lengthening of the P-R interval. In the fetus, Mobitz type I second-degree block is rarely either persistent or of any significance.[26] Mobitz type II block occurs infrequently and is more serious. The delay is at a level below the AV junction, and the P-R interval is normal or increased but fixed. This arrhythmia has dropped beats in a regular or irregular frequency and usually results from blockage in the bundle of His or trifascicular block. Mobitz type II second-degree block has been well described in the fetus.[27] This form may precede the development of complete heart block.

Complete, or third-degree, AV block has been the focus of most reports of fetal or neonatal heart block. Thought to be caused by a failure of union of the AV

TABLE 4.1 Antiarrhythmic drug classes

Class	Repolarization	Indications	Drug
IA	Prolongs	Atrial flutter Atrial fibrillation SVT VT	Quinidine Procainamide Disopyramide
IB	Shortens	VT	Lidocaine Mexiletine
IC	Unchanged	VT SVT	Flecainide Encainide
II	Unchanged	Atrial tachycardia VT	β-Blockers
III	Markedly prolongs	VT Atrial flutter Atrial fibrillation SVT	Amiodarone Sotalol
IV	Unchanged	Reciprocating SVT	Verapamil Diltiazem Adenosine

SVT, supraventricular tachycardia; VT, ventricular tachycardia.
From Kleinman CS, Copel JA. Electrophysiological principles and fetal antiarrhythmic therapy. *Ultrasound Obstet Gynecol.* 1991;1(4):286–297, with permission.

TABLE 4.2 Depression of AV nodal conduction—fast and slow pathways

Antegrade (slow) limb	Retrograde (fast) limb
Digitalis	Class IA—quinidine, procainamide
β-Blockers	Class IC—flecainide
Calcium-channel blockers	

node and His bundle in early fetal development (as with congenital structural heart disease), complete congenital heart block may also result from damage to the conducting system after it has been normally formed (as with SSA or SSB antibody-mediated damage to cardiac cells). Complete AV block arises in the fetus from blockage at the AV junction with, by definition, complete dissociation of the atria and the ventricles. The ventricular rate is usually between 40 and 60 bpm, and fetal hemodynamic compensation, presumably secondary to an increase in stroke volume, is frequently observed (Fig. 4.36). Complete AV block confers a guarded prognosis for the newborn. As many as 50% of infants with complete heart block have associated congenital cardiac malformations.[26] Even in the absence of significant underlying congenital heart disease, a pacemaker may need to be placed very soon after delivery.[28] Mothers of infants with congenital heart block in the absence of congenital heart disease are at increased risk for connective tissue disease, particularly systemic lupus erythematosus (SLE), either subclinical or overt.[29] The maternal disease may be nonexistent, heralded by a serologic abnormality, or associated with the current or subsequent development of severe connective tissue disease. Evaluation of the mother once fetal congenital heart block is diagnosed is clearly indicated as only 50% of fetuses with bradycardia are born to women with a history of connective tissue disease.[30]

The presence of specific antibodies to the soluble tissue ribonucleoprotein antigen Ro (SSA) in the serum of mothers giving birth to infants with complete heart block has been described.[31] There is immunofluorescent evidence of maternal anti-Ro immunoglobulin in the cardiac tissue of infants with congenital heart block. This finding suggests a transplacental passage of this immunoglobulin with direct effects on the fetal cardiac conduction system.[32] This anti-Ro immunoglobulin can be measured in the serum of pregnant women with SLE, and if present, patients should be counseled regarding the risk of congenital heart block in the fetus. It is controversial whether close fetal cardiac evaluation should be performed prospectively during pregnancy when a mother has anti-Ro immunoglobulins, as there is not a known effective treatment available to prevent the development of congenital heart block.

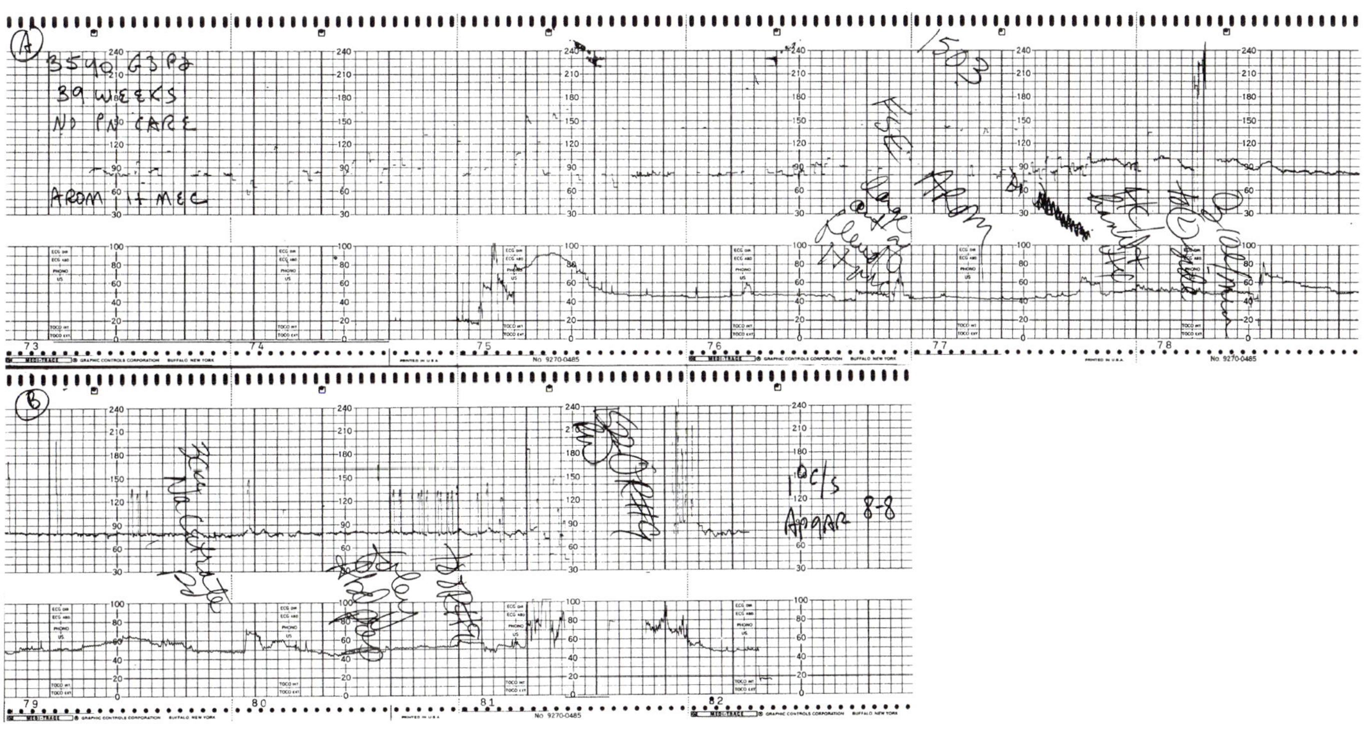

Figure 4.36. Example of emergency delivery for a patient presenting with a fetal heart rate of 80 bpm and no prenatal care. At delivery, the infant was discovered to have a congenital heart block. The mother was antinuclear antigen negative and asymptomatic for any connective tissue disease.

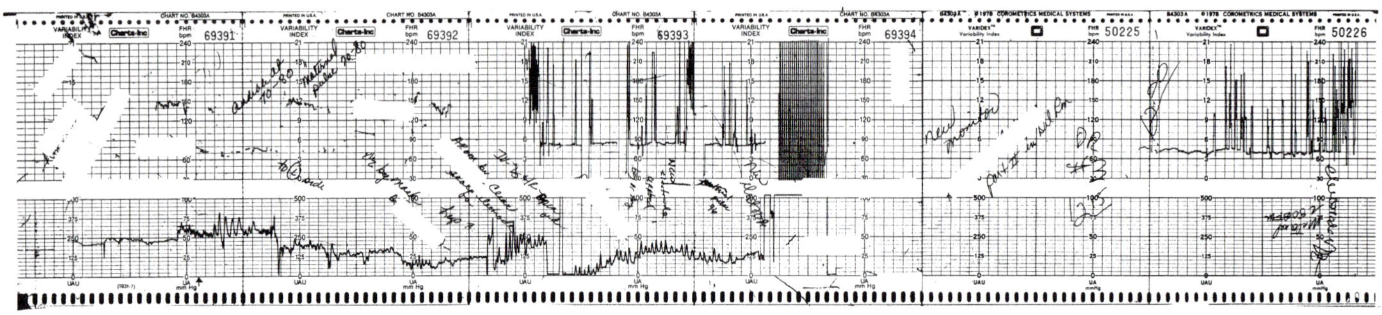

Figure 4.37. When complete heart block in the fetus is undiagnosed prior to entry into labor and delivery, it is not possible to determine the exact etiology of the abnormally slow fetal heart rate. The assumption that the heart rate was a prolonged fetal deceleration led to an emergent cesarean in this patient. At delivery, the infant was in no distress but maintained a heart rate of between 65 and 80 beats per minute. At discharge, he did not need a pacemaker, and the child continued to do well. The workup of the mother diagnosed serologic evidence for systemic lupus erythematosus, although she has remained asymptomatic.

Treatment of congenital heart block depends on the coexistence of major cardiac abnormalities and fetal and neonatal tolerance of the fixed low heart rate. As mentioned, temporary or permanent pacemakers may need to be placed following delivery. Complete fetal heart block resulting in nonimmune hydrops from heart failure in utero occurs in approximately 25% of cases and is associated with high mortality. The mother may be exposed to unnecessary surgical risks when the arrhythmia is unknown and confused with a preterminal bradycardia in the intrapartum period (Fig. 4.37). In a fetus with a complete heart block diagnosed before labor, the use of frequent intrapartum fetal pH determinations or continuous pulse oximetry of the fetus can result in a successful vaginal delivery. Our experience, however, has been that patients with fetal congenital heart block without congenital heart abnormalities incompatible with life are usually delivered via cesarean because of the difficulty in assessing fetal well-being intrapartum. When intermittent, it is possible to allow these patients a trial of labor (Fig. 4.38).

Many forms of fetal therapy have been suggested in cases of complete fetal heart block.[33] The treatment most often recommended is maternal administration of steroids, such as dexamethasone, in an effort to limit fetal inflammatory response to the transplacentally acquired maternal autoantibodies. Such treatment is associated with frequent and potentially severe maternal effects, and there is no evidence that the antibody-mediated damage of the fetal conduction system is reversible. Other therapies include intravenous gamma globulin (IVIG) and maternal plasmapheresis, but these therapies are not proven in the prevention or reversal of fetal heart block. Various medications to increase the FHR have also been reported (ie, ritodrine, terbutaline, and isoproterenol) with variable responses and no proven benefit. At the time of this writing, the STOP BLOQ study is enrolling pregnant people with anti-Ro immunoglobulins in an interventional clinical trial to determine whether PR interval screening and treatment of second-degree fetal AV block with dexamethasone or IVIG may prevent the development of complete AV block (ClinicalTrials.gov identifier NCT 04474223).

Direct pacing of the fetal heart in cases of complete heart block with nonimmune hydrops has also been reported. Carpenter reported the first case of percutaneous transthoracic fetal heart pacing with successful capture but fetal death within 3 hours.[34] More recently, Harrison performed open fetal surgery with placement of an epicardial pacing wire and pulse generator.[35] Once again, fetal death occurred quickly despite successful pacing.

Close monitoring of the fetus diagnosed with complete heart block is recommended. This includes both maternal perceptions of fetal movement and the use of real-time ultrasound to identify early development of cardiac decompensation. Such assessment includes observing early hydropic changes, ventricular size and function, and AV valve insufficiency. The exact role of either medical or surgical therapies for the treatment of fetal heart block remains unclear. The mortality rate for newborns with complete heart block is approximately 25%. After the neonatal period, survival is close to 90%

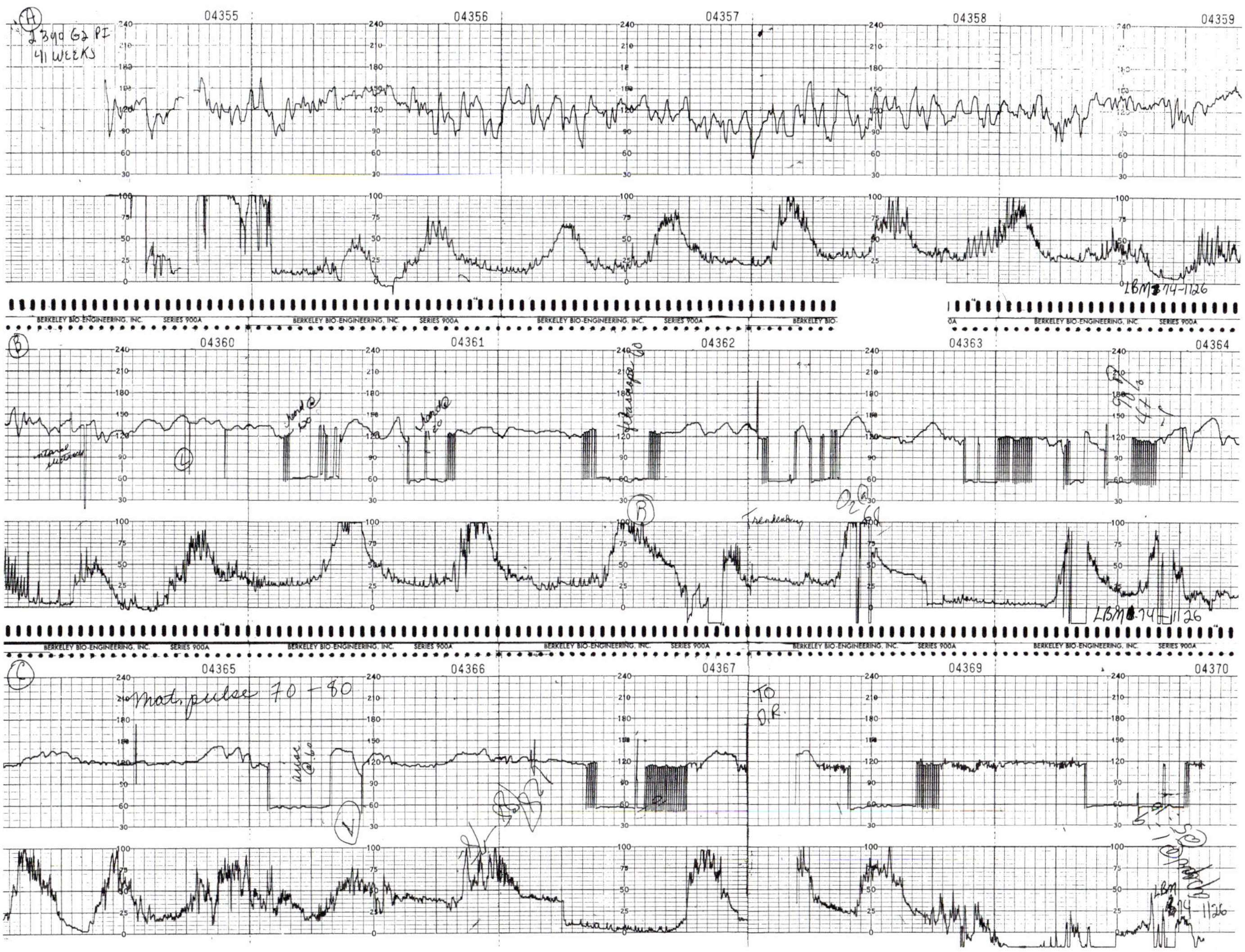

Figure 4.38. An interesting case of fetal heart block. Note that the **first panel**, recorded with a Doppler system containing excessive logic, shows an erratic pattern. The **middle and lower panels** are from a direct fetal scalp electrocardiograph (ECG). There are intermittent abrupt drops to 60 beats per minute (bpm) from the 120-bpm baseline. Where it says "heard at 120 bpm," the nurse was using a Doppler listening device and counting the atrial rate. With the third episode of 60 bpm, the nurse listened with a fetoscope (phone) and the rate of 60 bpm agreed with the ECG of 60 bpm, indicating the ventricular rate. Thus, a diagnosis of an intermittent 2-to-1 heart block was made.

with most deaths related to pacemaker failure.[36] The newborn with complete heart block in the absence of congenital heart disease frequently has neonatal lupus erythematosus often manifested by a distinctive skin rash caused by antibody deposition on basal keratinocytes.[30] Additional manifestations include anemia, thrombocytopenia, hepatosplenomegaly, hepatitis, myasthenia, or myopathy. This constellation of findings may appear to a greater or lesser degree and will disappear by 6 months of age.

Monitoring Fetal Arrhythmias

Accurate diagnosis of fetal arrhythmias is very difficult, if not impossible, using the FHR monitor alone. Monitors may have the logic system in operation at all times on the external mode and, therefore, heart rates above 200 bpm will often not even record. Figure 4.39 shows an expanded view of the recording of a fetal arrhythmia when the premature beat prompts a sudden rise and the following pause prompts a sudden drop in the

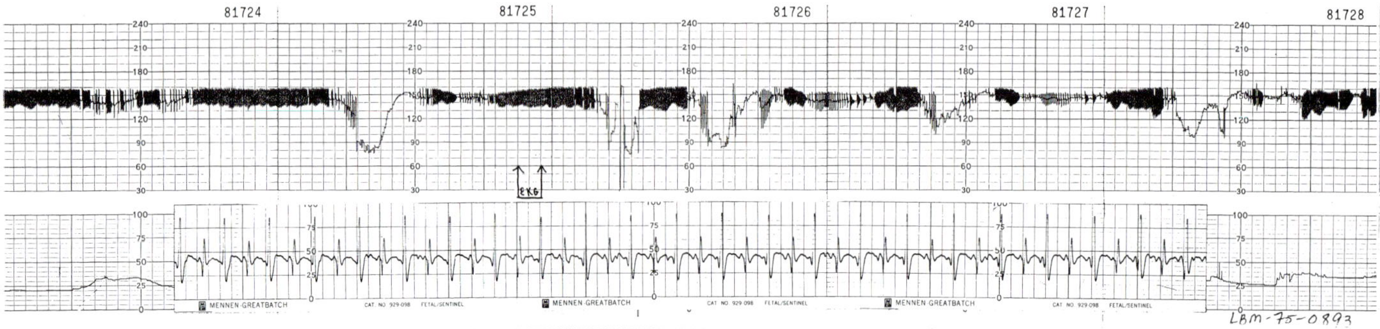

Figure 4.39. This tracing shows the fetal heart rate (FHR) pattern **above** and the simultaneous fetal electrocardiograph (ECG) **below**. The large vertical excursions on the FHR scale are caused by fetal arrhythmia, which is shown on the fetal ECG tracing to be owing to premature multifocal atrial contractions. Note the biphasic P waves.

rate, resulting in the characteristic vertical lines associated with the instantaneous FHR recording of fetal arrhythmias. Because electrical noise or maternal electrocardiograph (ECG) artifact can precipitate the same pattern, it is important to examine the raw fetal ECG tracing on the scope to differentiate between arrhythmia and artifact. Other examples of fetal arrhythmias and premature ventricle contractions are displayed in Figures 4.40–4.42. Congenital heart block is shown in Figure 4.43 in a patient with antepartum diagnosis early in the third trimester.

Although when very frequent, continuous monitoring of FHR may be difficult, and the clinical significance of these arrhythmias should be appreciated. Premature atrial and ventricular contractions usually have no clinical significance. Although there has been some association with other congenital abnormalities in the cardiac and other organ systems, this occurs infrequently. PACs and PVCs are not to be considered signs of fetal hypoxia and do not carry any significance as far as intervention. We do not recommend a fetal echocardiograph for patients with an antepartum finding of FHR irregularity consistent with PACs or PVCs. However, frequent assessment of FHR to rule out evolution to SVT is recommended. Sometimes, a terminal FHR pattern will show some PACs or PVCs,[37] but the significance of the pattern comes from the periodic and baseline FHR characteristics. Transient fetal cardiac standstill should be similarly managed. Position change, examination to rule out cord prolapse or rapid descent, and elevation of the presenting part are suggested maneuvers.[38] Figure 4.44 displays an example of transient fetal cardiac asystole mediated by vagal stimulations during a variable deceleration.

One will occasionally see a tracing with all downward deflections. This may be because of dropped beats

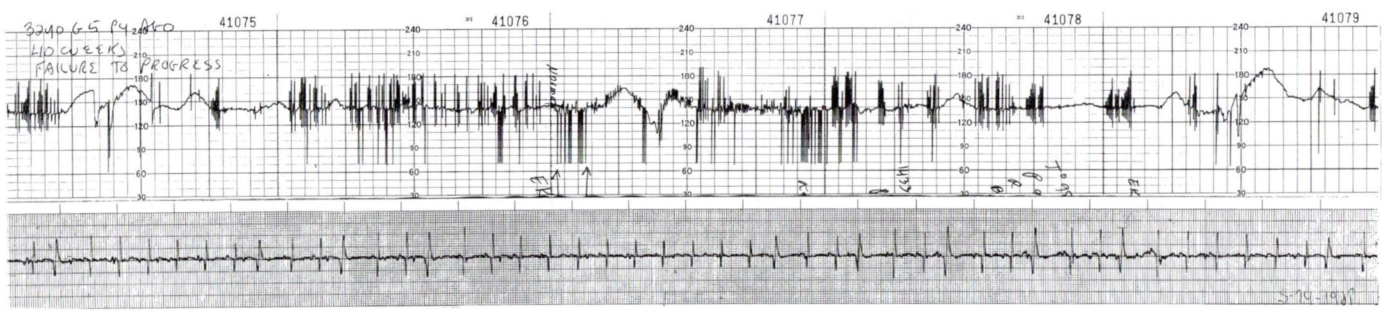

Figure 4.40. This tracing shows the fetal heart rate (FHR) patterns **above** and the simultaneous fetal echocardiograph (ECG) **below**. The large vertical excursions on the FHR scale are caused by fetal arrhythmia, which is shown on the fetal ECG tracing to be owing to premature ventricular contractions. Note the changing configuration of the fetal QRS complexes with each premature beat.

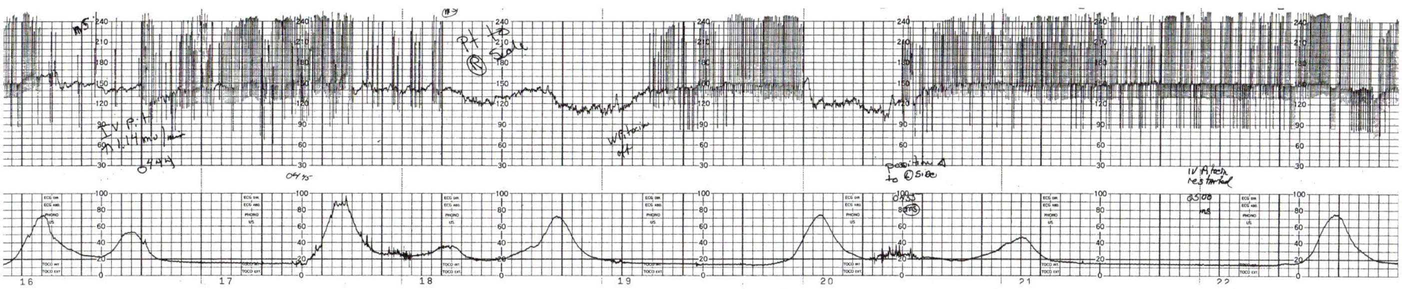

Figure 4.41. This tracing is an example of frequent multifocal premature ventricular contractions. Note the brief appearance of normal sinus rhythm following contractions.

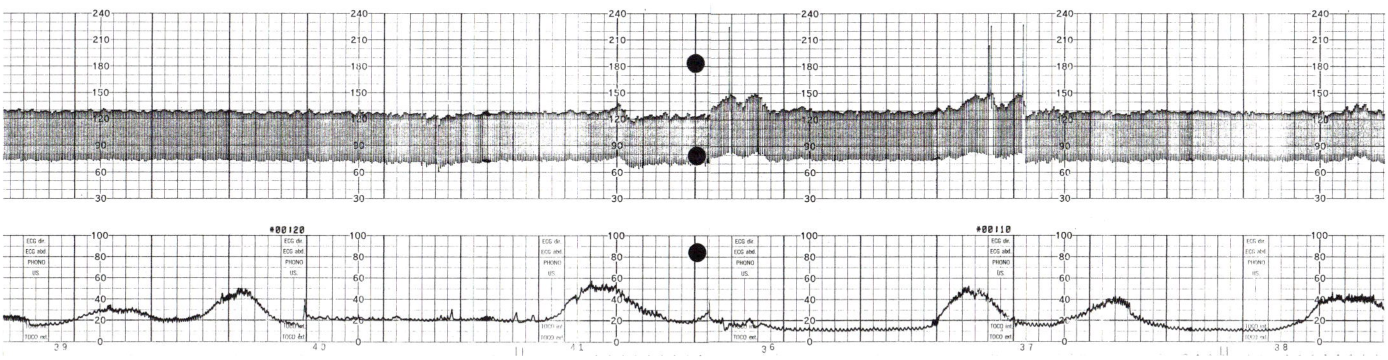

Figure 4.42. This is an example of frequent unifocal premature ventricular contractions. This was noted to be a bigeminy on neonatal electrocardiography.

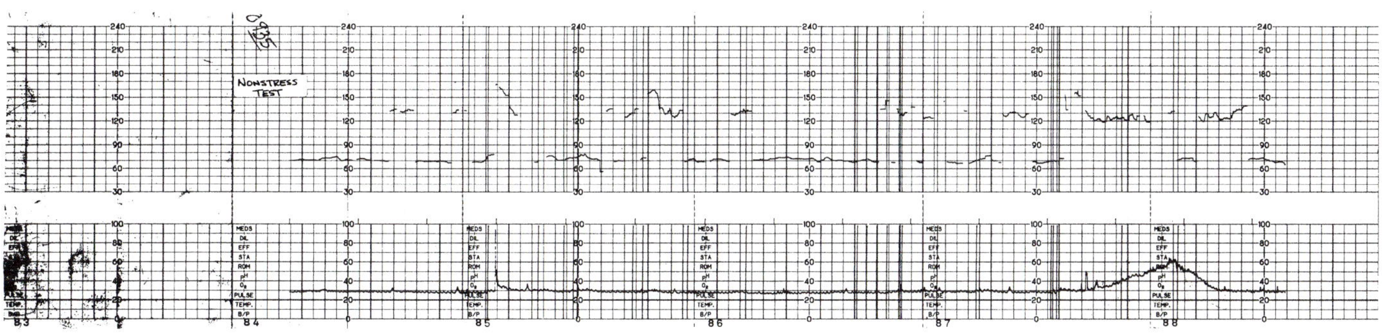

Figure 4.43. This is an example of intermittent congenital heart block detected during routine auscultation at the time of a prenatal visit. A nonstress test revealed areas of reactivity as well as a prolonged period of heart block. Ultrasound failed to reveal any structural cardiac defects or signs of cardiac failure. The patient was observed closely with no evidence of fetal deterioration. She was admitted in active labor at 35 weeks and delivered vaginally a normally grown, apparently healthy newborn. On postpartum day 3, because of frequent prolonged episodes of bradycardia and hypoxia, a pacemaker was placed in the neonate with excellent response. The workup of the mother was negative for any evidence of connective tissue disease.

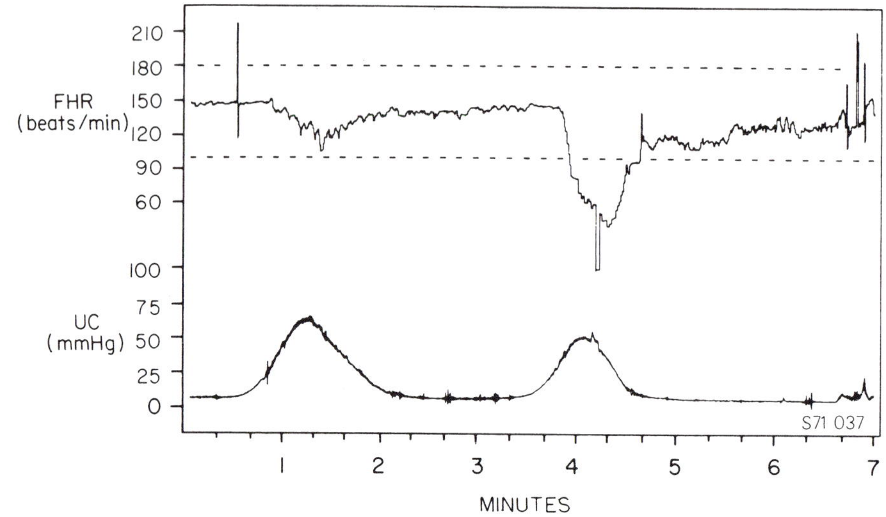

Figure 4.44. An example of a fetal heart rate (FHR)/uterine contraction (UC) tracing containing an episode of transient fetal cardiac arrest. At the 4-minute mark, during the course of severe variable deceleration, there was a transient fall of FHR to the zero level. Concomitant examination of the fetal electrocardiograph tracing proved the episode of transient fetal cardiac arrest. (From Yeh S, Zanini B, Petrie RH, Hon EH. Intrapartum fetal cardiac arrest: a preliminary observation. *Obstet Gynecol.* 1977;50(5):571-577, with permission.)

(Figs. 4.45 and 4.46), a very low amplitude signal, or premature beats where the interval is too short to be counted (<250 milliseconds) and causes only the compensatory pause to be shown. In rare cases, PVCs occur every other beat, creating the bigeminal rhythm noted in Figure 4.42.

The key to interpreting artifacts and arrhythmias is an understanding of fetal monitor instrumentation. The correct diagnosis and appropriate management can only be achieved with the careful application of technologic advances in the assessment of the fetal heart.

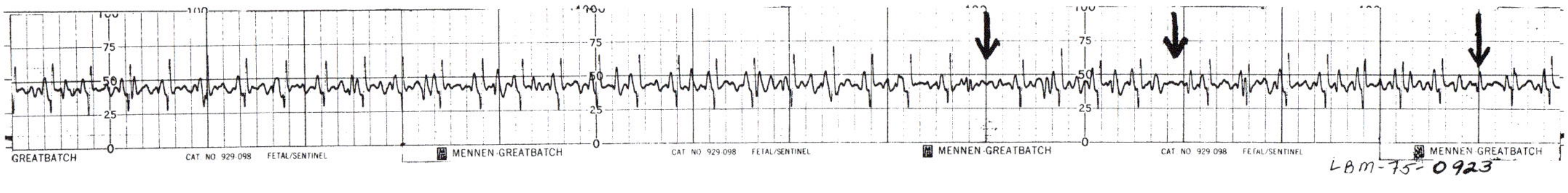

Figure 4.45. This tracing shows a series of downward deflections of the fetal heart rate in the **upper tracing**; the **lower tracing** of the simultaneous fetal electrocardiograph shows absent QRS complexes or dropped beats.

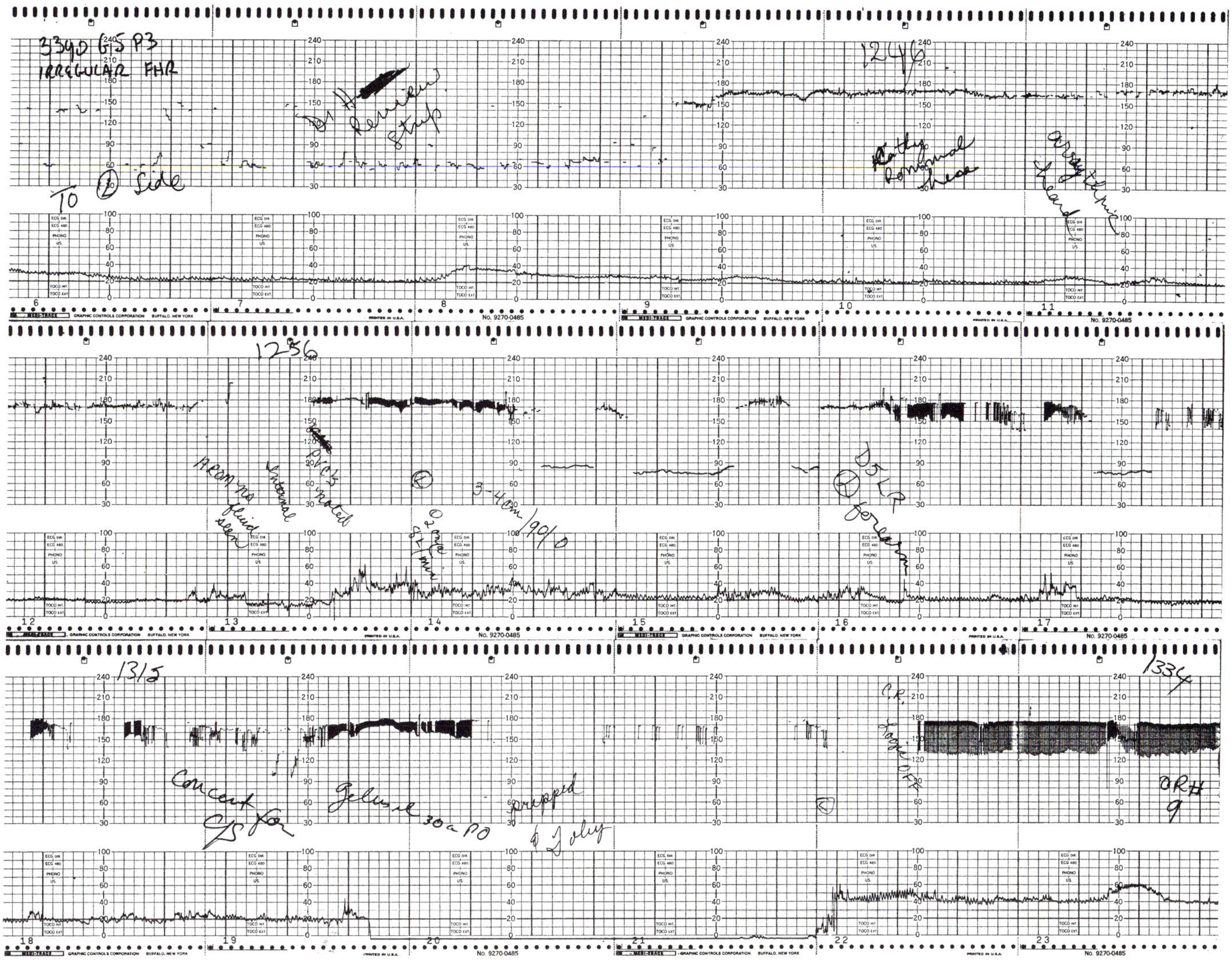

Figure 4.46. Intrapartum fetal arrhythmia evaluation. In the **middle panel**, an external monitor is recording a fetal heart rate of 80 to 90 bpm, most likely representing compensatory pauses of PVCs. In the **third panel**, when the logic is on, the monitor does not record because of the frequent premature beats with "abnormal" R-R intervals.

REFERENCES

1. Goodlin RC, Cheatham JP. Electronic fetal monitor paced by maternal implanted pacemaker. *Am J Obstet Gynecol.* 1985; 153(5):570-571.
2. Westgren M, Ingemarsson I. Maternal pacemaker activity mimicking fetal heart during labor. *Z Geburtshilfe Perinatal.* 1980;184(6):443-444.
3. Schneiderman CI, Waxman B, Goodman CJ Jr. Maternal-fetal electrocardiogram conduction with intrapartum death. *Am J Obstet Gynecol.* 1972;113(8):1130-1133.
4. Lackritz R, Schiff I, Gibson M, Safon L. Decelerations on fetal electrocardiography with fetal demise. *Obstet Gynecol.* 1978;51(3):367-368.
5. Nageotte MP, Freeman AG, Freeman RK, Dorchester W. Short term variability assessment from abdominal electrocardiogram during the antepartum period. *Am J Obstet Gynecol.* 1983; 145(5):566-569.
6. Fukushima T, Flores CA, Hon EH, Davidson EC Jr. Limitations of autocorrelation in fetal heart rate monitoring. *Am J Obstet Gynecol.* 1985;153(6):685-692.
7. Amato J. Fetal heart rate monitoring. *Am J Obstet Gynecol.* 1983;147:967-969.
8. Cremer M. Über die direkte Ableitung der Aktionsströme des menschlichen Herzens vom Oesophagus und über das Elektrokardiogramm des Fötus. *Munch Med Wochenschr.* 1906;53:811-813.
9. Larks SD, Dasgupta K. Fetal electrocardiography, with special reference to early pregnancy. *Am Heart J.* 1958;56(5):701-714.

10. Hon EH, Hess OW. The clinical value of fetal electrocardiography. *Am J Obstet Gynecol.* 1960;79(5):1012-1023.
11. Oldenburg JT, Macklin M. Changes in the conduction of the fetal electrocardiogram to the maternal abdominal surface during gestation. *Am J Obstet Gynecol.* 1977;129(4):425-433.
12. Jijón Knupp R, Andrews WW, Tita ATN. The future of electronic fetal monitoring. *Best Pract Res Clin Obstet Gynaecol.* 2020;67:44-52.
13. Monson M, Heuser C, Einerson BD, et al. Evaluation of an external fetal electrocardiogram monitoring system: a randomized controlled trial. *Am J Obstet Gynecol.* 2020;223(2):244.e1-244.e12.
14. Devoe LD, Gardner P, Dear C, Searle N. Monitoring intrauterine pressure during active labor: a prospective comparison of two methods. *J Reprod Med.* 1989;34(10):811-814.
15. Sherman DJ, Frenkel E, Kurzweil Y, Padua A, Arieli S, Bahar M. Characteristics of maternal heart rate patterns during labor and delivery. *Obstet Gynecol.* 2002;99(4):542-547.
16. Neilson DR Jr, Freeman RK, Mangan S. Signal ambiguity resulting in unexpected outcome with external fetal heart rate monitoring. *Am J Obstet Gynecol.* 2008;198(6):717-724.
17. Platt L, Manning F, Craigan G, Guttenburg M, Turkel SB. Antenatal detection of fetal A-V dissociation utilizing real time B-mode ultrasound. *Obstet Gynecol.* 1979;53(3 Suppl):59S-61S.
18. DeVore G, Siassi B, Platt L. Fetal echocardiography. III. The diagnosis of cardiac arrhythmias using teal time directed M-mode ultrasound. *Am J Obstet Gynecol.* 1983;146(7):792-799.
19. Ron M, Adoni A, Hochner-Celnikier D, Palti Z. The significance of baseline tachycardia in the post-term fetus. *Int J Gynaecol Obstet.* 1980;18(1):76-77.
20. Shenker L. Fetal cardiac arrhythmias. *Obstet Gynecol Surv.* 1979;34(8):561-572.
21. Heovall G. Congenital paroxysmal tachycardia: a report of three cases. *Acta Paediatr Scand.* 1973;62(5):550-552.
22. Klein A, Holzman I, Austin E. Fetal tachycardia to the development of hydrops-attempted pharmacologic cardioversion: case report. *Am J Obstet Gynecol.* 1979;134(3):347-348.
23. Kleinman CS, Copel JA. Electrophysiological principles and fetal antiarrhythmic therapy. *Ultrasound Obstet Gynecol.* 1991; 1(4):286-297.
24. Kleinman CS, Copel JA, Weinstein EM, Santulli TV Jr, Hobbins JC. In utero diagnosis and treatment of supraventricular tachycardia. *Semin Perinatol.* 1985;9(2):113-129.
25. Kleinman CS, Hobbins JC, Joffe CC. Echocardiographic studies of the human fetus: prenatal diagnosis of congenital heart disease and cardiac dysrhythmias. *Pediatrics.* 1980;65(6): 1059-1066.
26. Komaromy B, Gaal J, Lampe L. Fetal arrhythmia during pregnancy and labor. *Br J Obstet Gynaecol.* 1977;84(7):492-496.
27. Chan T, Potter RT, Liu L. Congenital intraventricular trifascicular block. *Am J Dis Child.* 1973;125(1):82-87.
28. Griffiths PS. Congenital heart block. *Circulation.* 1971;43:615.
29. Berube S, Lister G, Towes W, Creasy RK, Heymann MA. Congenital heart block and maternal systemic lupus erythematosus. *Am J Obstet Gynecol.* 1978;130(5):595-596.
30. McCauliffe DP. Neonatal lupus erythematosus: a transplacentally acquired autoimmune disorder. *Semin Dermatol.* 1995; 14(1):47-53.
31. Scott JS, Maddison PH, Taylor PV, Esscher E, Scott O, Skinner RP. Connective tissue disease, antibodies to ribonucleoprotein and congenital heart block. *N Engl J Med.* 1983;309(4):209-212.
32. Litsey S, Noonan J, O'Connor W, Cottrill CM, Mitchell B. Maternal connective tissue disease and congenital heart block: demonstration of immunoglobulin cardiac tissue. *N Engl J Med.* 1985;312(2):98-100.
33. Schmidt KG, Ulmer HF, Silverman NH. Perinatal outcomes of fetal complete AV block: a multi-centered experience. *J Am Coll Cardiol.* 1991;17(6):1360-1366.
34. Carpenter RJ, Strasburger JF, Gorsen A Jr. Fetal ventricular pacing for hydrops secondary to complete AV block. *J Am Coll Cardiol.* 1986;8(6):1434-1436.
35. Harrison MR. Fetal surgery. *Western J Med.* 1993;159(3):341-349.
36. Vetter VL, Rashkind H. CHB and connective tissue disease. *N Engl J Med.* 1983;309:236-238.
37. Cetrulo C, Schifrin BS. Fetal heart rate patterns preceding death in utero. *Obstet Gynecol.* 1976;48(5):521-527.
38. Kates RB, Schifrin BS. Fetal cardiac asystole during labor. *Obstet Gynecol.* 1986;67(4):549-555.

CHAPTER 5

Uterine Contraction Monitoring

Antonina Frolova

Electronic fetal monitoring comprises two main components: fetal heart rate (FHR) tracing and uterine contraction tracing.[1] The timing of FHR decelerations in relation to uterine contractions is crucial for FHR pattern interpretation and classification. Thus, accurate and interpretable uterine activity recording is essential. Uterine contraction monitoring serves the additional purpose of monitoring labor progress and can assist healthcare providers in making decisions regarding labor management interventions.

Although labor adequacy is defined by the progress of cervical dilation and fetal descent rather than contraction patterns, uterine contraction patterns can offer guidance in cases of abnormal labor progress. They can help determine the administration of uterotonics and decisions regarding the mode of delivery. Excessive uterine activity may also cause inadequate placental perfusion, resulting in fetal hypoxia and acidosis. Therefore, in the setting of labor induction or augmentation, the clinician must be aware of uterine activity, as overstimulation could lead to fetal compromise.

PHYSIOLOGY OF UTERINE CONTRACTIONS

Uterine contractions serve as the primary mechanism for the expulsion of intrauterine contents. For the majority of pregnancy, the uterine tissue remains in a quiescent state and resists contraction in the presence of increasing stretch caused by fetal growth. The transition into the contractile states, characterized by the presence of regular rhythmical contractions, may be insidious or abrupt, and the exact control of this transition is still unknown. The uterine smooth muscle or myometrium generates spontaneous action potentials through membrane depolarization, which in turn results in the opening of the voltage-gated L-type calcium channels and an increase in intracellular calcium (Ca^{2+}) (Fig. 5.1). Ca^{2+} can also be released from internal stores (sarcoplasmic reticulum) upon activation of the phospholipase C pathway. The Ca^{2+} binds calmodulin, activating myosin light chain kinase, which phosphorylates myosin. The phosphorylated myosin interacts with actin, resulting in cross-bridge cycling and contraction of the myocyte. Individual myometrial cells are interconnected through gap junctions, which increase in number before the onset of labor.[2] This increased connectivity enables the propagation of action potentials and the recruitment of more myocytes, resulting in stronger contractions within the uterus.

Uterine activity is often initially described or quantified in terms of contraction frequency, which is expressed as the number of contractions per unit of time (typically 10 minutes). This parameter is crucial and is believed to play a significant role in both fetal well-being and labor progress. According to the National Institute of Child Health and Human Development, and in agreement with the American College of Obstetrics and Gynecology (ACOG), ≤5 contractions in 10 minutes, averaged over a 30-minute window is considered normal, whereas >5 contractions per 10 minutes is abnormal and referred to as tachysystole.[1] Although the report does not define other characteristics of contractions as normal or abnormal, it acknowledges their importance. Contraction strength or intensity often refers to the peak intrauterine pressure or amplitude (the difference between peak and resting intrauterine pressure) (Fig. 5.2). Contraction duration is the time

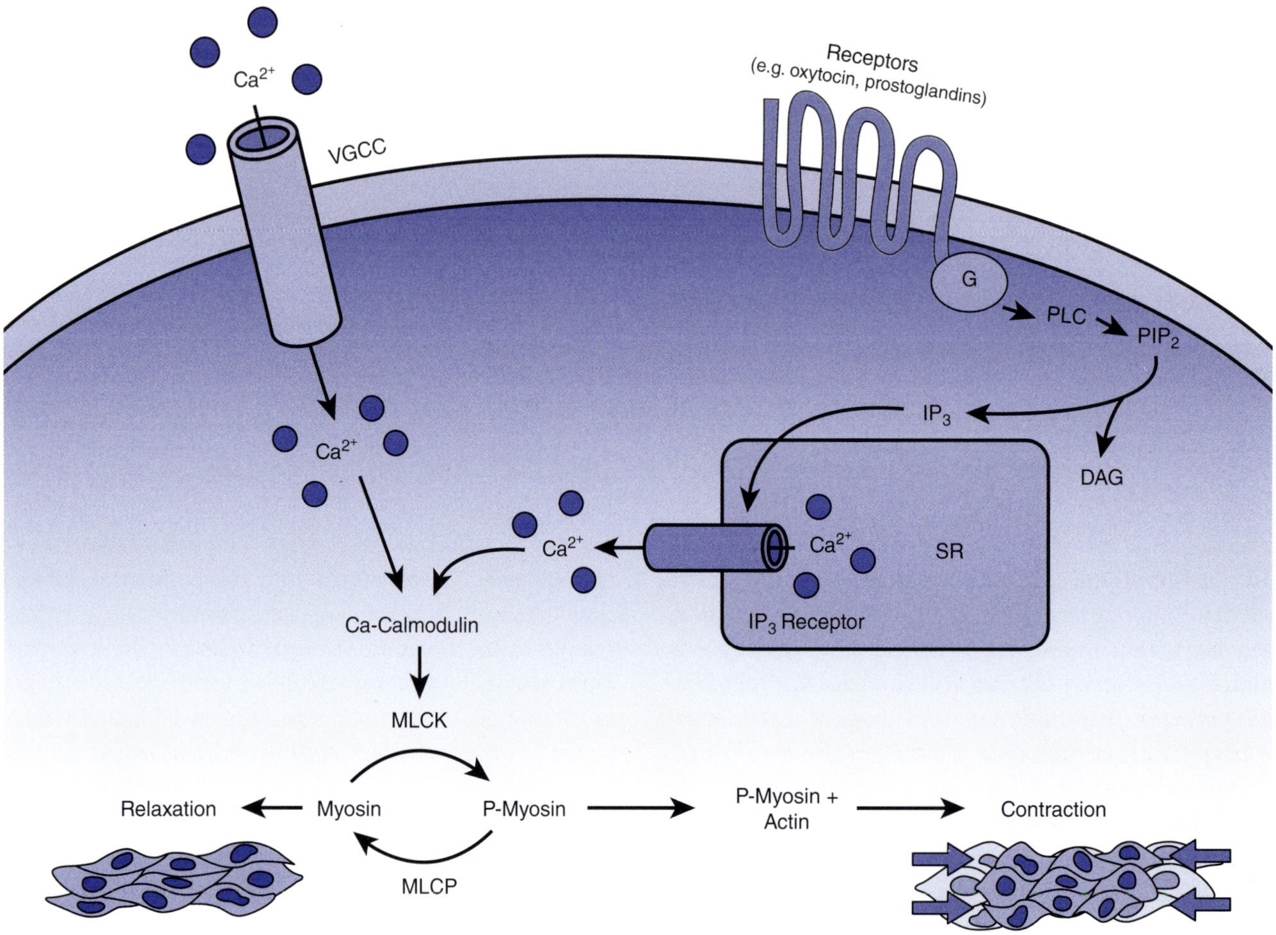

Figure 5.1. Schematic of excitation-contraction coupling in myometrial smooth muscle cells. MLCK, myosin light chain kinase; MLCP, myosin light chain phosphatase; PLC, phospholipase C; SR, sarcoplasmic reticulum; VGCC, voltage-gated calcium channel.

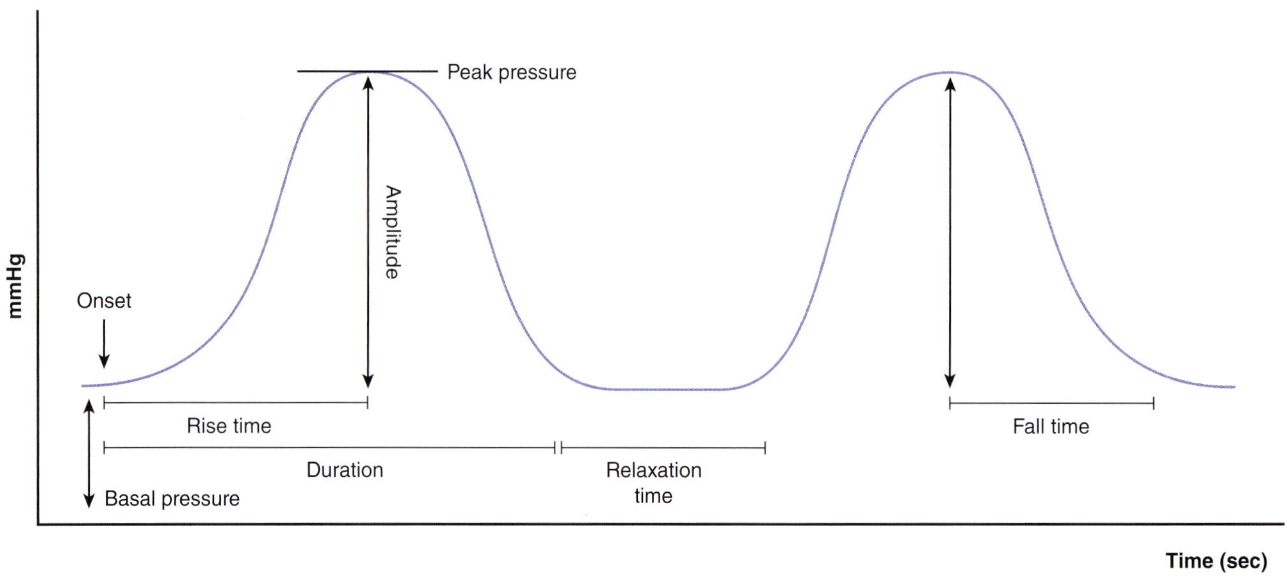

Figure 5.2. Quantifiable characteristics of uterine activity.

(measured in seconds) between the onset and end of a contraction. Contraction shape can be described by skewness and quantified by the time to reach peak pressure (Rise, R), the time from peak to return to baseline (Fall, F), and the F:R ratio. Additionally, resting tone refers to the intrauterine pressure between contractions, and relaxation time is the duration between the end of one contraction and the initiation of the next. Different methods of assessing uterine activity vary in their ability to accurately quantify all characteristics of contractions.

METHODS OF MONITORING UTERINE ACTIVITY

Patient Perception and Manual Uterine Palpation

One of the simplest methods for monitoring uterine activity is through maternal perception. This is typically felt as pain, which requires an average contraction intensity of 15 mm Hg.[3] However, individual contraction perception is highly variable and can be influenced by parity, weight, and gestational age.[4,5]

Manual palpation has long been used as a traditional method to assess uterine activity, with a lower threshold for detection of about 10 mm Hg. However, this method is also influenced by maternal weight and abdominal wall thickness. Although contractions can be detected earlier with external palpation, the absolute strength or intensity of a contraction can only be relatively assessed. One study assessed the accuracy of manual palpation by trained labor and delivery staff (residents, physicians, and nurses) in predicting contraction strength compared to the gold standard of intrauterine pressure catheter (IUPC) measurements.[6] When rating contractions as "mild," "moderate," or "strong," providers were only accurate 49% of the time compared to predetermined intrauterine pressure cutoffs. Although there was some difference in sensitivity by staff experience, the most accurate group (maternal-fetal medicine physicians) was only accurate 58% of the time. Effects of targeted training or individual reproducibility were not assessed. However, palpation accuracy, as defined in this study, was not influenced by maternal body habitus, maternal positioning, gestational age, or oxytocin use.

Furthermore, manual palpation is time-consuming, requires constant evaluation, and provides no permanent record. The process can be tedious, and in most cases, intermittent manual palpation is performed for short intervals. Both maternal perception and manual palpation also underestimate the duration of contractions and overestimate the relaxation time as they do not perceive the early and late portions (Fig. 5.3). Despite their inherent technical limitations, both of these methods can effectively detect contractions, quantify their frequency, and have the advantages of being readily available, inexpensive, and noninvasive.

External Tocodynamometry

The introduction of mechanical devices for external monitoring of uterine contractions dates back to as early as 1896.[7] Most of the early devices measured changes in abdominal wall shape or motion of the abdominal wall to detect uterine activity. The modern tocodynamometers (often referred to as "toco") utilize a pressure transducer, usually a centrally positioned spring-loaded piston that can be secured to the abdominal wall with a strap (Fig. 5.5). When a uterine contraction occurs, the piston is depressed, and this signal is transduced and recorded as a contraction. The toco is usually positioned near the fundus and adjusted for optimal contraction recording. A sensitivity calibration device, either on the toco or the monitor itself, is adjusted to set the resting pressure at 15 to 20 mm Hg for optimal tracing. However, it is important to note that contraction strength is only relatively accurate and can vary significantly depending on factors such as maternal position, body habitus, and belt tightness. These factors also impact the sensitivity of the recording. Consequently, the duration of contractions may appear to vary, with higher sensitivity resulting in a longer apparent duration (Fig. 5.4). Using external toco can most accurately identify the frequency of contractions and cannot provide the absolute intrauterine pressure or contraction strength.[8] However, if the toco placement and other variables remain constant, relative changes in contraction duration and intensity can be observed within an individual.

One of the advantages of external tocodynamometry is its noninvasive nature. Therefore, it is suitable for monitoring patients with intact membranes, including those in the antepartum period and those experiencing premature labor, as well as intrapartum monitoring. Toco use also allows for continuous and objective recording of uterine activity without the need for provider presence. However, there are several disadvantages associated with this technique, in addition to the limitations with regard to contraction intensity and duration quantification. External monitors generally cause more discomfort for the patient and may limit mobility, with the best tracings often obtained

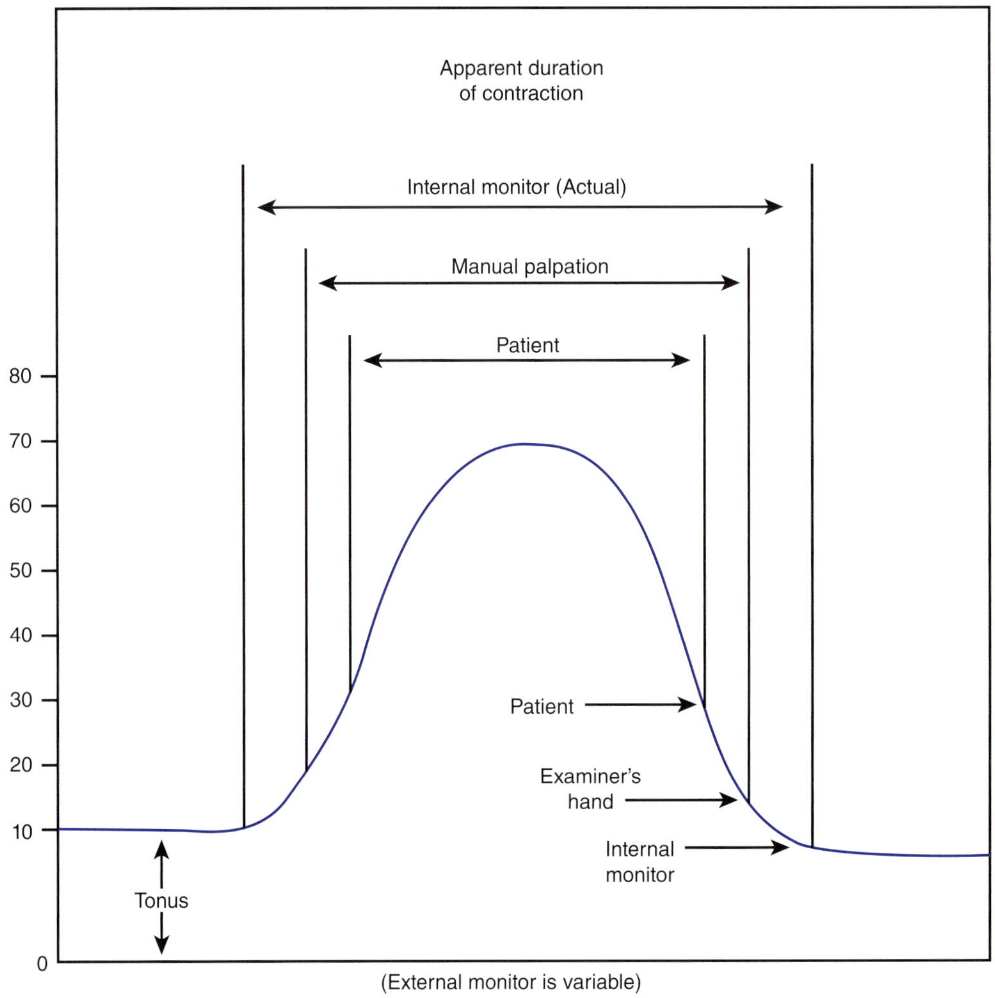

Figure 5.3. Relative sensitivity of various methods available for detection of uterine contractions.

when the patient is in a supine position. Some patients may produce poor or nonexistent tracings of uterine activity. Additionally, changes in maternal position can result in the loss of previously good contraction tracings, making the timing or recording of FHR decelerations challenging because of the loss of signal.

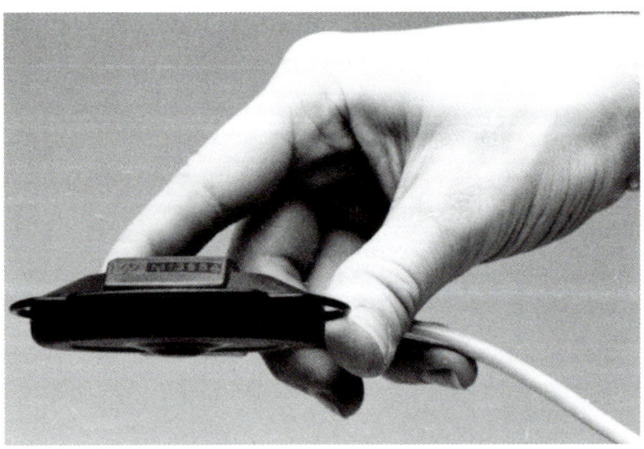

Figure 5.4. Tocodynamometer.

Internal Monitoring

Internal monitoring of uterine pressure is considered the "gold standard" and is perhaps the most accurate method of contraction monitoring available today. The history of intrauterine pressure recording dates back to 1872 when Friedrich Schatz first used a hydrostatic bag in the lower uterine segment after membrane rupture to measure pressure.[9] Since then, various techniques have been introduced to measure intrauterine pressure,[7] and currently, it is estimated that 15% to 20% of deliveries in the United States involve the use of an IUPC for labor management. There are two main types of commercially available IUPCs. The fluid-filled IUPC employs a catheter with a water column that transmits intrauterine pressure to an external transducer. However, this approach requires equilibration outside the uterus and frequent flushing, leading to potential errors and increased provider time spent troubleshooting. The other type of IUPC utilizes a catheter with a

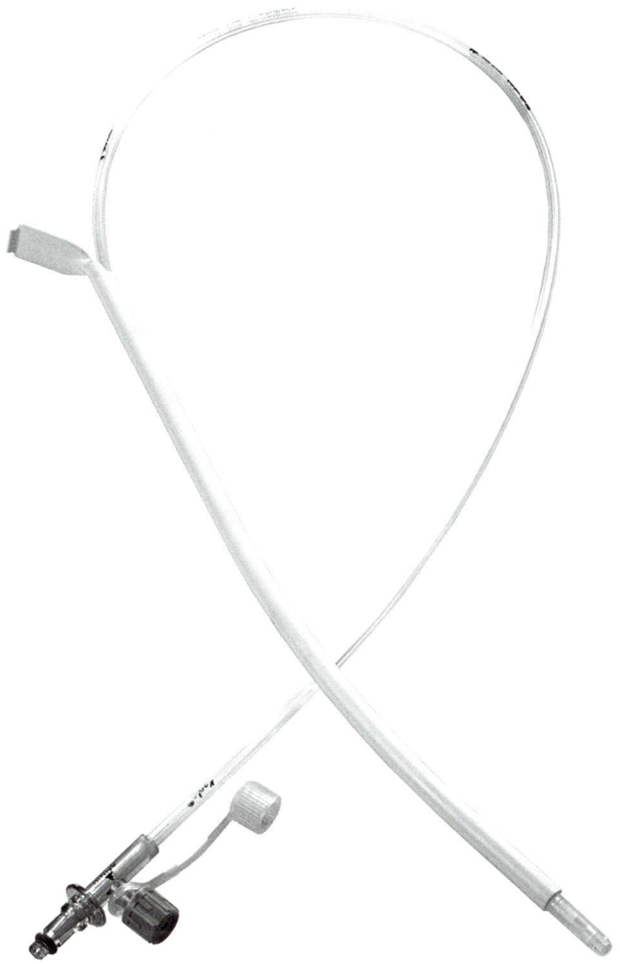

Figure 5.5. Internal pressure catheter with pressure sensor in tip (Reproduced with permission from Laborie Medical Technologies).

micro-pressure transducer or sensor at the tip, which is inserted into the amniotic cavity (Fig. 5.5). Multiple options for transducer- or sensor-tipped IUPCs exist, all of which demonstrate relatively similar efficacy in monitoring intrauterine pressure.[10]

The primary advantage of IUPCs over external tocodynamometry is the ability to precisely measure absolute intrauterine pressure or "strength" as well as baseline intrauterine pressure. IUPCs also provide more accurate assessment and recording of the frequency, duration, and relaxation time of uterine contractions (Fig. 5.4). Moreover, IUPCs offer greater patient comfort and are less influenced by maternal position or body habitus.

However, the use of IUPCs has certain limitations as it is an invasive procedure requiring membrane rupture before insertion. First, the use of IUPCs assumes that a contracting gravid uterus obeys the Pascal's law that states that pressure is equal throughout a closed fluid-filled system. In most cases, this holds true for the uterus, even after membrane rupture, as the fetal presenting part occludes the internal OS, maintaining a closed system. However, in situations where there are sealed-off pockets of fluid, especially with low amniotic fluid volume, there may be slight variations in pressure measurements.[11,12] A study by Arulkumaran et al examined 1429 contractions using two IUPCs placed in the same or different pockets and reported that 86% of contractions showed a ≤5 mm Hg difference, whereas 94% showed a ≤5 mm Hg difference in pressure.[11] Additionally, some studies have suggested a potential risk of maternal fever and infection associated with IUPC use.[13,14] However, these findings were subject to selection bias, and prospective randomized trials assessing IUPC use did not observe the same level of risk.[15-18] Rare occurrences of extramembranous placement, placental abruption, and uterine perforation have been reported following the insertion of an IUPC, emphasizing the importance of employing appropriate insertion techniques and acknowledging the invasive nature of this monitoring method.[19]

Electrohysterography

Electrohysterography (EHG), also known as transabdominal electromyography, utilizes electrodes placed on a patient's abdomen to measure and quantify the electrical potentials generated by the myometrium, rather than the physical forces of uterine contractions.[20] This is the newest commercially available method for contraction monitoring and much research is still underway to determine the utility and optimize the technology (electrode number, placement, etc). Nonetheless, preliminary findings suggest that EHG holds promise as a noninvasive alternative to external tocodynamometry, offering improvements in monitoring uterine activity. Maul et al showed a significant correlation between EHG and intrauterine pressure (Spearman's $r = 0.764$) and good predictive value for delivery within 48 hours (area under the curve 0.95).[21] Another study showed higher contraction detection by EHG versus external tocodynamometry when compared to IUPC data.[22] Moreover, EHG overcomes limitations associated with maternal body habitus or movement, making it a more reliable noninvasive monitoring method.[23,24] The available EHG devices use the same electrodes to monitor the fetal heart rate, maternal heart rate, and uterine activity, allowing for a lower number of monitors and greater patient satisfaction.

Despite its potential advantages, the use of EHG is currently limited by a lack of robust clinical experience and validation data. Specific populations, such as women with obesity and preterm gestations, require further investigation to understand the impact of relative tissue conductivity on EHG signals and its correlation with intrauterine pressure. Additionally, quantitative data on baseline intrauterine pressure is currently unavailable for EHG, a limitation shared with external tocodynamometry. Furthermore, EHG has been associated with a higher rate of "false positive" contraction detection, where electrical signals are present without a simultaneous increase in intrauterine pressure.[24] The implications of these contractions on labor progression remain unknown and could complicate the interpretation of fetal heart rate patterns.

QUANTITATION OF UTERINE ACTIVITY

For many reasons, it may be important to quantitate the amount of uterine activity per unit of time. The most practical reason would be to determine, in evaluating poor progress in labor, whether uterine contractions are sufficient. Because failure to progress is an indication for labor augmentation, adequate uterine activity must be defined. In 1959, Caldeyro-Barcia et al defined the Montevideo unit (MVU) as the product of the average contraction peak in mm Hg multiplied by the number of contractions in a 10-minute span.[25] Subsequent research demonstrated that in naturally progressing labor, uterine contraction pressures increase from approximately 100 MVUs in early labor to 250 MVUs at the end of the first stage.[3] This has been the quantitation measure most extensively used in research and clinical settings, although it does have the limitation of not including contraction duration or shape in its calculation. To address some of these limitations, El-Sahwi et al[26] defined the Alexandria unit as the MVU multiplied by the average contraction duration (in minutes). Other approaches, such as using the area under the curve with or without baseline tone (uterine activity integral,[27] uterine activity unit,[28] mean active pressure[29]; Fig. 5.6), have been proposed by different groups. As these are quite labor intensive, Miller et al[30] described a computerized approach for quantifying uterine activity by integrating the entire area under the curve (Fig. 5.6). Although these methods have been studied in a research setting, only the MVU has been adopted in clinical practice.

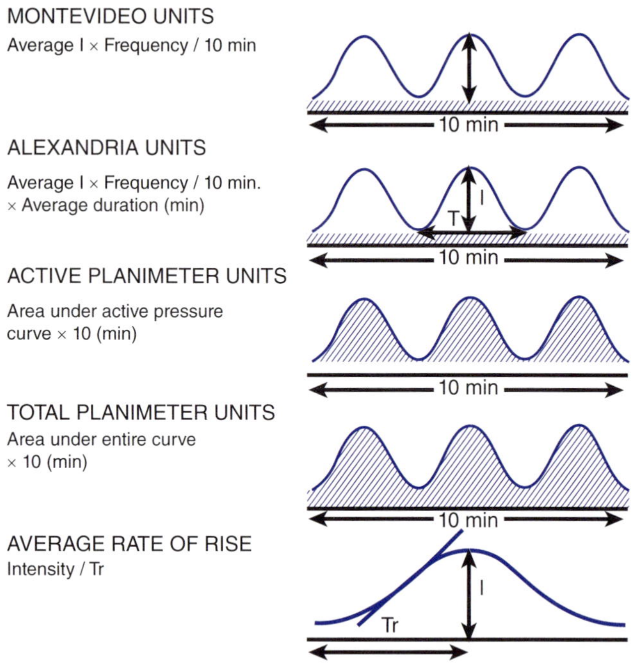

Figure 5.6. Available methods for quantitation of uterine activity. (Adapted from Miller FC, Yeh SY, Schifrin BS, Paul RH, Hon EH. Quantitation of uterine activity in 100 primiparous patients. *Am J Obstet Gynecol.* 1976;124(4):398-405.)

In 1989, Hauthe et al aimed to establish intrauterine pressure goals for oxytocin augmentation in cases of dysfunctional labor.[31] They reported that 91% of women undergoing labor induction and 75% of women undergoing labor augmentation achieved ≥200 MVUs, leading them to conclude that the arrest of labor should not be diagnosed until contractions of at least this strength are attained. Over the years, the threshold of 200 MVUs has become known as adequate uterine activity in labor, but this may be misleading. Some studies have shown no differences in MVU between women delivering vaginally or undergoing cesarean delivery because of labor arrest.[32] Additionally, almost half of the women with vaginal deliveries never reach MVUs of 200.[33] More recently, Mol et al did show that lower average MVUs are associated with increased risk of cesarean section, however, 44% of women delivering vaginally also had MVUs below 200.[34] Additionally, randomized trials comparing external tocodynamometry to universal IUPC use for contraction monitoring did not show a difference in cesarean delivery rates or other obstetric outcomes, suggesting no clinical advantage of quantitating intrauterine pressure in laboring women.[15-17] Therefore, the data regarding adequate MVUs remain inconclusive, and relying solely on contraction strength should be approached with caution during labor management.

ROLE OF UTERINE ACTIVITY MONITORING DURING LABOR

There are two main reasons for monitoring uterine activity during labor. The first is in order to assess fetal heart rate patterns, which cannot be accurately interpreted without adequate contraction recordings. The second is to monitor labor and uterotonic titration in the setting of abnormal labor progress. Data regarding the later indication are reviewed earlier.

Uterine contractions lead to the compression of uterine spiral arteries, resulting in the complete interruption of blood flow in the uterine arteries once intrauterine pressures reach ≥30 mm Hg.[35,36] This, in turn, results in an interruption of placental perfusion and intermittent fetal hypoxia. Klink et al showed that transcutaneous fetal scalp pO_2 (measured continuously) correlated with multiple contraction characteristics, but the strongest correlation was with the contraction frequency.[37] Subsequently, Peebles et al showed that contraction frequency was positively correlated with fetal cerebral oxyhemoglobin and negatively correlated with deoxyhemoglobin.[38] Stable fetal cerebral hemoglobin saturations were observed with intervals of 2 to 3 minutes between contractions, whereas shorter intervals resulted in decreased oxyhemoglobin-to-deoxyhemoglobin ratios. Hence, the time between contractions, known as the relaxation time, is likely crucial for adequate maternal-fetal gas exchange, fetal metabolic recovery, and maintenance of normal fetal acid-base balance. In cases of uterine tachysystole, where this recovery time is shortened, progressively lower fetal oxygen saturations and the accumulation of cord blood lactate are observed.[39,40] Bakker et al later demonstrated that fetal acidosis was associated with longer contraction durations, greater strength, and shorter relaxation time.[41] Recent data also indicate that baseline intrauterine pressure is linked to increased neonatal acidemia and lactate accumulation,[42] suggesting that both the relaxation time and the intrauterine pressure during this interval play a role in maintaining fetal oxygenation.

Despite the data linking fetal oxygenation and uterine activity, the evidence regarding uterine activity and neonatal morbidity is limited. Excessive uterine contractions can be inferred if fetal heart rate changes are observed in conjunction with uterine contractions and resolve upon cessation of contractions. Fetal compromise may manifest as reduced fetal heart rate variability, late decelerations, or prolonged decelerations. The fetus does possess several compensatory mechanisms that enable it to tolerate labor. During a contraction, fetal preload increases, and blood flow through the middle cerebral artery also increases, allowing for enhanced cerebral perfusion.[43,44] However, in compromised fetuses (such as those with fetal growth restriction, preeclampsia, etc), these compensatory mechanisms may be insufficient to counteract the hypoxic insults of uterine contractions. Whether there are long-term fetal effects attributed to uterine activity in the absence of fetal heart rate changes remains to be determined. Therefore, it is crucial to interpret fetal heart rate and uterine activity tracings together.

FACTORS AFFECTING UTERINE CONTRACTIONS

Several intrinsic and extrinsic factors can affect uterine contractility. These factors can manifest by decreasing or increasing contraction strength, frequency, or both. Labor is a common intrinsic factor that influences uterine activity. Caldeyro-Barcia et al, in their study of over 500 women, demonstrated that uterine activity progressively increases during spontaneous labor until the fetus is expelled.[3] The amplitude of contractions increases from an average of 30 mm Hg in early labor to 50 mm Hg in the later first stage and 50 to 80 mm Hg during the second stage. Similarly, the frequency of contractions increases from an average of 3 to 5 per 10 minutes. Maternal pushing efforts during labor can add 20 mm Hg or more to the recorded intensity of contractions, appearing as rapid, brief elevations of intrauterine pressure superimposed on the uterine contraction. The same group also found that maternal position can affect uterine contractility, with higher amplitude and lower frequency contractions observed in the lateral position compared to the supine position. Stretch, being a strong stimulus for muscle contractility, explains why polyhydramnios can influence uterine activity. In a uterus overdistended by polyhydramnios, the baseline tone increases while the amplitude of contractions decreases.[45] The effects are reversed with the removal of fluid in a dose-dependent manner. Some additional pathologic states that have been shown to alter uterine contractility are placental abruption, chorioamnionitis, and multiparity.

TABLE 5.1 Drugs affecting uterine contractions

Stimulating drugs
Acetylcholine
Ergonovine
Estrogen
Norepinephrine
Oxytocin
Propranolol
Prostaglandins
Quinine
Sparteine sulfate
Vasopressin
Inhibiting drugs
β-Sympathomimetics
Ritodrine, Orciprenaline, Isoxsuprine, Salbutamol, Fenoterol, etc
Calcium channel blockers
Nitroglycerin
Atosiban
Halothane
Magnesium sulfate
Progesterone
Prostaglandin synthetase inhibitors

Uterine activity can be affected by a number of medications and drugs (Table 5.1). The most commonly used uterotonic agent in labor management is oxytocin. Oxytocin binds to its receptor, a member of the G-protein coupled receptor superfamily, on the myometrial cell surface, subsequently activating the phospholipase C pathway and resulting in the release of intracellular Ca^{2+} stores from the sarcoplasmic reticulum (Fig. 5.1). Oxytocin increases the frequency, intensity, and synchrony of contractions. At lower doses, oxytocin-induced uterine contractions resemble physiological contractions; however, at higher doses, it can lead to tachysystole or tetanic uterine contractions.[25] The individual therapeutic dose of the drug varies widely, and dose titration is guided by cervical dilation and labor progress as the adequacy of contractions has not been established. The rate of titration has been a subject of great debate; however, Son et al have demonstrated that faster titration of oxytocin during augmentation results in shorter labor durations without any negative impacts on perinatal outcomes.[46] In this double-blind randomized trial, the maximum oxytocin doses ranged between 2 and 90 mU/min, highlighting once again the variability in individual response to this uterotonic.[47]

As oxytocin is quickly cleared from maternal circulation, a homolog with a longer half-life, carbetocin, has been developed for postpartum hemorrhage prevention. On the other hand, oxytocin receptor antagonists (eg, atosiban) have been developed for inhibition of preterm contractions and are approved for use in several countries.

Prostaglandins (PGs) are synthesized by the fetal membranes and decidua during labor, and synthetic forms have been developed for induction and postpartum hemorrhage management. Although all PGs are derived from their common precursor, arachidonic acid, each type has specific receptors and effects in the myometrium. The two major stimulating PGs are prostaglandin F2 alpha (PGF2α) and prostaglandin E (PGE). Upon activation of its receptor, PF, PGF2α triggers a signaling cascade similar to oxytocin, resulting in an increase in intracellular Ca^{2+}. PGEs can activate one of four receptors (EP1-4), of which EP1 and EP3 have pro-contractile effects in the myometrium. EP1 receptors activate a similar signaling pathway as oxytocin and PGF2α. However, EP3 receptors inhibit cAMP production and the activation of protein kinase A (PKA), both of which have pro-relaxation properties in the myometrium.

Medications that decrease uterine contractility should be considered in the context of preterm labor or fetal distress in labor caused by excessive uterine contractility. β2-adrenergic receptor (β2-AR) agonists exploit the pro-relaxation effects of cAMP and PKA in the myometrium. However, β2-ARs also have various roles in the cardiovascular system, limiting their use to short-term acute settings such as fetal distress during labor. Cyclooxygenase inhibitors exert their effects by inhibiting PG production and potentially affecting Ca^{2+} entry into the myometrial cell. Calcium channel inhibitors are another family of drugs that have been used for the inhibition of preterm contractions and the most commonly used Nifedipine blocks voltage-gated calcium channels (VGCCs). Magnesium competes with Ca^{2+} and thus inhibits Ca^{2+} entry into the myometrial cells. In vitro studies have shown that magnesium inhibits myometrial contractility, but its efficacy as a tocolytic in clinical settings has not been demonstrated.

Other drugs known to affect uterine contractility are listed in Table 5.1. Although they are not used in labor management because of their side effect profiles and unfavorable contractile characteristics, it is important to be aware of them when they are used for other maternal indications, as they may lead to unexpected labor and fetal compromise.

SUMMARY

The study of fetal monitoring is incomplete without detailed knowledge of uterine activity and its effects on fetal oxygenation and heart rate. Most significant periodic changes in the FHR occur at or after the time of the uterine contraction. The intent of this chapter has been to describe the details of contraction monitoring, the physiologic mechanisms of labor, and our current knowledge of the relationship between uterine activity and obstetric outcomes so that the reader might better be able to integrate this knowledge and understand the physiologic and pathophysiologic basis of fetal monitoring.

REFERENCES

1. Macones GA, Hankins GD, Spong CY, Hauth J, Moore T. The 2008 National Institute of Child Health and Human Development workshop report on electronic fetal monitoring: update on definitions, interpretation, and research guidelines. *J Obstet Gynecol Neonatal Nurs.* 2008;37(5):510-515. doi: 10.1111/j.1552-6909.2008.00284.x.
2. Garfield RE, Thilander G, Blennerhassett MG, Sakai N. Are gap junctions necessary for cell-to-cell coupling of smooth muscle?: an update. *Can J Physiol Pharmacol.* 1992;70(4):481-490. doi: 10.1139/y92-063.
3. Caldeyro-Barcia R, Poseiro JJ. Physiology of the uterine contraction. *Clin Obstet Gynaecol.* 1960;3:386-410. doi: 10.1097/00003081-196006000-00011.
4. Cottrill HM, Barton JR, O'Brien JM, Rhea DL, Milligan DA. Factors influencing maternal perception of uterine contractions. *Am J Obstet Gynecol.* 2004;190(5):1455-1457. doi: 10.1016/j.ajog.2004.02.024.
5. Newman RB, Campbell BA, Stramm SL. Objective tocodynamometry identifies labor onset earlier than subjective maternal perception. *Obstet Gynecol.* 1990;76(6):1089-1092.
6. Arrabal PP, Nagey DA. Is manual palpation of uterine contractions accurate? *Am J Obstet Gynecol.* 1996;174(1 Pt 1):217-219. doi: 10.1016/s0002-9378(96)70397-6.
7. Smith RP. A brief history of intrauterine pressure measurement. *Acta Obstet Gynecol Scand Suppl.* 1984;129:1-24. doi: 10.3109/00016348409157018.
8. Miles AM, Monga M, Richeson KS. Correlation of external and internal monitoring of uterine activity in a cohort of term patients. *Am J Perinatol.* 2001;18(3):137-140. doi: 10.1055/s-2001-14522.
9. Schatz F. Beiträge zur physiologischen Geburtskunde. *Arch. Gynecol Obstet.* 2005;4(1):34-111. doi: 10.3109/00016348409157018.
10. Dowdle MA. Comparison of two intrauterine pressure catheters during labor. *J Reprod Med.* 2003;48(7):501-505.
11. Arulkumaran S, Yang M, Tien CY, Ratnam SS. Reliability of intrauterine pressure measurements. *Obstet Gynecol.* 1991; 78(5 Pt 1):800-802.
12. Knoke JD, Tsao LL, Neuman MR, Roux JF. The accuracy of measurements of intrauterine pressure during labor: a statistical analysis. *Comput Biomed Res.* 1976;9(2):177-186. doi: 10.1016/0010-4809(76)90041-0.
13. Gee SE, Ma'ayeh M, Ward C, Buhimschi C, Klebanoff M, Rood K. Intrauterine pressure catheter use is associated with an increased risk of postcesarean surgical site infections. *Am J Perinatol.* 2020;37(6):557-561. doi: 10.1055/s-0039-1700861.
14. Harper LM, Shanks AL, Tuuli MG, Roehl KA, Cahill AG. The risks and benefits of internal monitors in laboring patients. *Am J Obstet Gynecol.* 2013;209(1):38.e1-38.e6. doi: 10.1016/j.ajog.2013.04.001.
15. Bakker JJ, Verhoeven CJ, Janssen PF, et al. Outcomes after internal versus external tocodynamometry for monitoring labor. *N Engl J Med.* 2010;362(4):306-313. doi: 10.1056/NEJMoa0902748.
16. Chia YT, Arulkumaran S, Soon SB, Norshida S, Ratnam SS. Induction of labour: does internal tocography result in better obstetric outcome than external tocography. *Aust N Z J Obstet Gynaecol.* 1993;33(2):159-161. doi: 10.1111/j.1479-828x.1993.tb02382.x.
17. Chua S, Kurup A, Arulkumaran S, Ratnam SS. Augmentation of labor: does internal tocography result in better obstetric outcome than external tocography? *Obstet Gynecol.* 1990; 76(2):164-167.
18. Halem KV, Bakker JJ, Verhoeven CJ, et al. Does use of an intrauterine catheter during labor increase risk of infection? *J Matern Fetal Neonatal Med.* 2012;25(4):415-418. doi: 10.3109/14767058.2011.582905.
19. Wilmink FA, Wilms FF, Heydanus R, Mol BW, Papatsonis DN. Fetal complications after placement of an intrauterine pressure catheter: a report of two cases and review of the literature. *J Matern Fetal Neonatal Med.* 2008;21(12):880-883. doi: 10.1080/14767050802220508.
20. Devedeux D, Marque C, Mansour S, Germain G, Duchene J. Uterine electromyography: a critical review. *Am J Obstet Gynecol.* 1993;169(6):1636-1653. doi: 10.1016/0002-9378(93)90456-s.
21. Maul H, Maner WL, Olson G, Saade GR, Garfield RE. Non-invasive transabdominal uterine electromyography correlates with the strength of intrauterine pressure and is predictive of labor and delivery. *J Matern Fetal Neonatal Med.* 2004;15(5): 297-301. doi: 10.1080/14767050410001695301.
22. Euliano TY, Nguyen MT, Darmanjian S, et al. Monitoring uterine activity during labor: a comparison of 3 methods. *Am J Obstet Gynecol.* 2013;208(1):66.e1-66.e6. doi: 10.1016/j.ajog.2012.10.873.
23. Euliano TY, Nguyen MT, Marossero D, Edwards RK. Monitoring contractions in obese parturients: electrohysterography compared with traditional monitoring. *Obstet Gynecol.* 2007;109(5): 1136-1140. doi: 10.1097/01.AOG.0000258799.24496.93.
24. Vlemminx MWC, Thijssen KMJ, Bajlekov GI, Dieleman JP, Van Der Hout-Van Der Jagt MB, Oei SG. Could electrohysterography be the solution for external uterine monitoring in obese women? *J Perinatol.* 2018;38(5):580-586. doi: 10.1038/s41372-018-0065-3.

25. Caldeyro-Barcia R, Poseiro JJ. Oxytocin and contractility of the pregnant human uterus. *Ann N Y Acad Sci.* 1959;75: 813-830. doi: 10.1111/j.1749-6632.1959.tb44593.x.
26. el-Sahwi S, Gaafar AA, Toppozada HK. A new unit for evaluation of uterine activity. *Am J Obstet Gynecol.* 1967;98(7):900-903. doi: 10.1016/0002-9378(67)90074-9.
27. Steer PJ. Monitoring in labour. *Br J Hosp Med.* 1977;17(3): 219-225.
28. Hon EH, Paul RH. Quantitation of uterine activity. *Obstet Gynecol.* 1973;42(3):368-370.
29. Phillips GF, Calder AA. Units for the evaluation of uterine contractility. *Br J Obstet Gynaecol.* 1987;94(3):236-241. doi: 10.1111/j.1471-0528.1987.tb02360.x.
30. Miller FC, Yeh SY, Schifrin BS, Paul RH, Hon EH. Quantitation of uterine activity in 100 primiparous patients. *Am J Obstet Gynecol.* 1976;124(4):398-405. doi: 10.1016/0002-9378(76)90100-9.
31. Hauth JC, Hankins GD, Gilstrap LC, 3rd, Strickland DM, Vance P. Uterine contraction pressures with oxytocin induction/augmentation. *Obstet Gynecol.* 1986;68(3):305-309. doi: 10.1097/00006250-198609000-00003.
32. Hauth JC, Hankins GD, Gilstrap LC, 3rd. Uterine contraction pressures achieved in parturients with active phase arrest. *Obstet Gynecol.* 1991;78(3 Pt 1):344-347.
33. Rouse DJ, Owen J, Savage KG, Hauth JC. Active phase labor arrest: revisiting the 2-hour minimum. *Obstet Gynecol.* 2001; 98(4):550-554. doi: 10.1016/s0029-7844(01)01516-2.
34. Mol BW, Logtenberg SL, Verhoeven CJ, et al. Does measurement of intrauterine pressure have predictive value during oxytocin-augmented labor? *J Matern Fetal Neonatal Med.* 2016;29(20):3239-3242. doi: 10.3109/14767058.2015.1123243.
35. Brotanek V, Hendricks CH, Yoshida T. Changes in uterine blood flow during uterine contractions. *Am J Obstet Gynecol.* 1969;103(8):1108-1116. doi: 10.1016/0002-9378(69)90515-8.
36. Fleischer A, Anyaegbunam AA, Schulman H, Farmakides G, Randolph G. Uterine and umbilical artery velocimetry during normal labor. *Am J Obstet Gynecol.* 1987;157(1):40-43. doi: 10.1016/s0002-9378(87)80342-3.
37. Klink F, Grosspietzsch R, Klitzing LV, Oberheuser F. Uterine contraction intervals and transcutaneous levels of fetal oxygen pressure. *Obstet Gynecol.* 1981;57(4):437-440.
38. Peebles DM, Spencer JA, Edwards AD, et al. Relation between frequency of uterine contractions and human fetal cerebral oxygen saturation studied during labour by near infrared spectroscopy. *Br J Obstet Gynaecol.* 1994;101(1):44-48. doi: 10.1111/j.1471-0528.1994.tb13008.x.
39. Palanisamy A, Lopez J, Frolova A, Macones G, Cahill AG. Association between uterine tachysystole during the last hour of labor and cord blood lactate in parturients at term gestation. *Am J Perinatol.* 2019;36(11):1171-1178. doi: 10.1055/s-0038-1676492.
40. Johnson N, van Oudgaarden E, Montague I, McNamara H. The effect of oxytocin-induced hyperstimulation on fetal oxygen. *Br J Obstet Gynaecol.* 1994;101(9):805-807. doi: 10.1111/j.1471-0528.1994.tb11951.x.
41. Bakker PC, Kurver PH, Kuik DJ, Van Geijn HP. Elevated uterine activity increases the risk of fetal acidosis at birth. *Am J Obstet Gynecol.* 2007;196(4):313.e1-313.e6. doi: 10.1016/j.ajog.2006.11.035.
42. Rimsza RR, Raghuraman N, Carter EB, Kelly JC, Cahill AG, Frolova AI. Association between elevated intrauterine resting tone during labor and neonatal morbidity. *Am J Perinatol.* 2023. doi: 10.1055/a-2022-9588.
43. Takahashi Y, Iwagaki S, Nakagawa Y, Kawabata I, Tamaya T. Uterine contractions increase fetal heart preload. *Ultrasound Obstet Gynecol.* 2003;22(1):53-56. doi: 10.1002/uog.142.
44. Li H, Gudmundsson S, Olofsson P. Acute centralization of blood flow in compromised human fetuses evoked by uterine contractions. *Early Hum Dev.* 2006;82(11):747-752. doi: 10.1016/j.earlhumdev.2006.03.011.
45. Caldeyro-Barcia R, Pose SV, Alvarez H. Uterine contractility in polyhydramnios and the effects of withdrawal of the excess of amniotic fluid. *Am J Obstet Gynecol.* 1957;73(6):1238-1254. doi: 10.1016/0002-9378(57)90267-3.
46. Son M, Roy A, Stetson BT, et al. High-dose compared with standard-dose oxytocin regimens to augment labor in nulliparous women: a randomized controlled trial. *Obstet Gynecol.* 2021;137(6):991-998. doi: 10.1097/AOG.0000000000004399.
47. Son M, Roy A, Grobman WA, et al. Maximum dose rate of intrapartum oxytocin infusion and associated obstetric and perinatal outcomes. *Obstet Gynecol.* 2023;141(2):379-386. doi: 10.1097/AOG.0000000000005058.

CHAPTER 6

Standard Nomenclature

Anna Graseck

Quantifying various parameters of fetal well-being by means of mathematical and statistical computations of the fetal heart rate (FHR) is difficult. This is because the interpretation of FHR tracings is both a study of pattern recognition and a process of evaluating multiple clinical and heart rate variables in determining the status of fetal oxygenation. Previous chapters have dealt with the basic understanding of the physiology and technology of electronic FHR monitoring. This chapter is devoted to the standard nomenclature used in the United States to describe the FHR and uterine contractions.

Initial efforts to arrive at universal nomenclature and criteria for various FHR patterns were challenging. In 1997, a workshop convened by the National Institute of Child Health and Human Development (NICHD) published a document in an attempt to create more consistent and uniform terminology and guidelines for interpreting FHR patterns.[1] At that meeting, the participants found there were only two situations where there was universal agreement with respect to the significance of FHR patterns. The first was the pattern with normal baseline rate and variability and no periodic decelerations. It was agreed that such patterns were consistent with normal oxygenation and there were no requirements for intervention with respect to fetal well-being. The second patterns that were agreed to by the group as being consistent with hypoxia sufficient to cause death or damage were those patterns with repetitive late or variable decelerations or bradycardia all of which were accompanied by absent FHR variability. Any patterns between these two extremes could not gain general agreement from the group with respect to significance or management.[1]

In 2008, the Eunice Kennedy Shriver National Institute of NICHD partnered with the American College of Obstetricians and Gynecologists and the Society for Maternal-Fetal Medicine to sponsor a workshop focused on electronic FHR monitoring.[2] This workshop gathered a diverse group of investigators with expertise and interest in the field to accomplish three goals: (a) to review and update the definitions for FHR pattern categorization from the prior workshop, (b) to assess existing classification systems for interpreting specific FHR patterns and make recommendations about a system for use in the United States, and (c) to make recommendations for research priorities for electronic fetal monitoring (EFM). A complete clinical understanding of EFM necessitates discussion of uterine contractions, baseline FHR rate and variability, presence of accelerations, periodic or episodic decelerations, and the changes in these characteristics over time. A number of assumptions and factors common to FHR interpretation in the United States are central to the proposed system of nomenclature and interpretation. Two such assumptions are of particular importance. First, the definitions are primarily developed for visual interpretation of FHR patterns but should be adaptable to computerized systems of interpretation. Second, the definitions should be applied to intrapartum patterns but also be applicable to antepartum observations.

CLASSIFICATION OF FETAL HEART RATE TRACINGS

A variety of systems for EFM interpretation have been used in the United States and worldwide. Based on a careful review of the available options, a three-tiered system for the categorization of FHR patterns was recommended by the NICHD working group (see box). It is important to recognize that FHR tracing patterns provide information only on the current acid-base status of the fetus. Categorization of the FHR tracing evaluates the fetus at that point in time; tracing patterns can and will change. An FHR tracing may move back and forth between the categories depending on the clinical situation and management strategies used.

Category I FHR Tracings Are Normal

Category I FHR tracings are strongly predictive of normal fetal acid-base status at the time of observation. Category I FHR tracings may be monitored in a routine manner, and no specific action is required.

NICHD 2008 terminology three-tier FHR interpretation system
Category I: Normal FHR pattern
Baseline rate 110-160 bpm
Baseline FHR variability: moderate (5-25 bpm)
Late and variable decelerations absent
Early decelerations present or absent
Accelerations present or absent
Category II: Equivocal FHR patterns
Baseline rate and variability
Baseline rate: Bradycardia (<110 bpm) not accompanied by absent variability
Tachycardia (>160 bpm)
Variability minimal (= or <5 bpm but present)
Variability absent without recurrent decelerations
Marked baseline variability (>25 bpm)
Periodic changes
Absence of induced accelerations after fetal stimulation
Recurrent variable decelerations accompanied by minimal or moderate baseline variability
Prolonged deceleration >2 min but <10 min
Recurrent late decelerations with moderate baseline variability
Variable decelerations with other characteristics such as slow return to baseline or overshoot
Category III: Abnormal FHR patterns
Absent FHR variability *and* of the following:
Recurrent late decelerations
Recurrent variable decelerations
Bradycardia
Sinusoidal pattern

bpm, Beats per minute.

Category II FHR Tracings Are Indeterminate

Category II FHR tracings are not predictive of abnormal fetal acid-base status, yet presently there is not adequate evidence to classify these as category I or category III. Category II FHR tracings require evaluation and continued surveillance and reevaluation, taking into account the entire associated clinical circumstances. In some circumstances, either ancillary tests to ensure fetal well-being or intrauterine resuscitative measures may be used with category II tracings.

Category III FHR Tracings Are Abnormal

Category III tracings are associated with abnormal fetal acid-base status at the time of observation. Category III FHR tracings require prompt evaluation. Depending on the clinical situation, efforts to expeditiously resolve the abnormal FHR pattern may include but are not limited to provision of maternal oxygen, change in maternal position, discontinuation of labor stimulation, treatment of maternal hypotension, and treatment of tachysystole with FHR changes. If a category III tracing does not resolve with these measures, delivery should be undertaken.

PATIENT IDENTIFICATION

Many modern monitoring systems have electronic storage of patient information and EFM tracings. These systems require patient data entry before starting the monitor on a new patient. However, many hospitals continue to store paper records for backup medical records, for teaching purposes, or because some information (eg, continuous fetal pulse oximetry data) may not be stored on the digital record. Therefore, it is important to appropriately label the paper record as well. Monitors should be identified numerically and tracings labeled accordingly. Should a technical problem occur, it can be traced to the correct monitor. Also, different monitors may have different logic and other technical characteristics, and when a facility has various brands, the clinician can better interpret the tracing by taking the make and model into consideration.

UTERINE CONTRACTIONS

Uterine contractions are quantified as the number of contractions present in a 10-minute window, averaged over a 30-minute period. Contraction frequency alone is a partial assessment of uterine activity. Other factors such as duration, intensity, and relaxation time between contractions are equally important in clinical practice.

Listed as follows is the terminology used to describe uterine activity:

- *Normal*: five contractions or less in 10 minutes, averaged over a 30-minute window
- *Tachysystole*: more than five contractions in 10 minutes, averaged over a 30-minute window

Characteristics of uterine contractions

- The terms hyperstimulation and hypercontractility are not defined and should be abandoned.
- Tachysystole should always be qualified as to the presence or absence of associated FHR decelerations.
- The term tachysystole applies to both spontaneous and stimulated labor. The clinical response to tachysystole may differ depending on whether contractions are spontaneous or stimulated.

BASELINE FETAL HEART RATE

The normal baseline FHR ranges from 110 to 160 beats per minute (bpm). The NICHD defined baseline FHR as the mean FHR during a 10-minute window. The mean is expressed in increments of 5 bpm. Changes of shorter duration are called "periodic changes." Although it is appropriate to attempt to create a defined duration of a periodic change, for which a more sustained rate becomes a baseline change, this is often inconsistent with what is the obvious physiologic explanation for a prolonged periodic change. For example, a profound hypotensive episode that results in a prolonged deceleration will ultimately return to the original baseline when the insult is reversed. Thus the deceleration may have lasted longer than 10 minutes and, according to the previous NICHD definition, would now be called a bradycardia, but it was truly not a baseline change. Similarly, a fetus that is unusually active may have an acceleration that lasts considerably longer than 10 minutes but returns to the original baseline when the fetus returns to a more quiet state.

TABLE 6.1 Causes of fetal tachycardia
Fetal hypoxia
Maternal fever
Parasympatholytic drugs
Atropine
Hydroxyzine hydrochloride (Atarax or Vistaril)
Phenothiazines
Maternal hyperthyroidism
Fetal anemia
Fetal sepsis
Fetal heart failure
Chorioamnionitis
Fetal cardiac tachyarrhythmia
β-Sympathomimetic drugs

Fetal Tachycardia

Fetal tachycardia is defined as a baseline heart rate in excess of 160 bpm. Factors associated with or causing tachycardia are listed in Table 6.1. Because tachycardias represent increased sympathetic and/or decreased parasympathetic autonomic tone, they are generally associated with a loss of variability (Fig. 6.1). Most fetal tachycardias

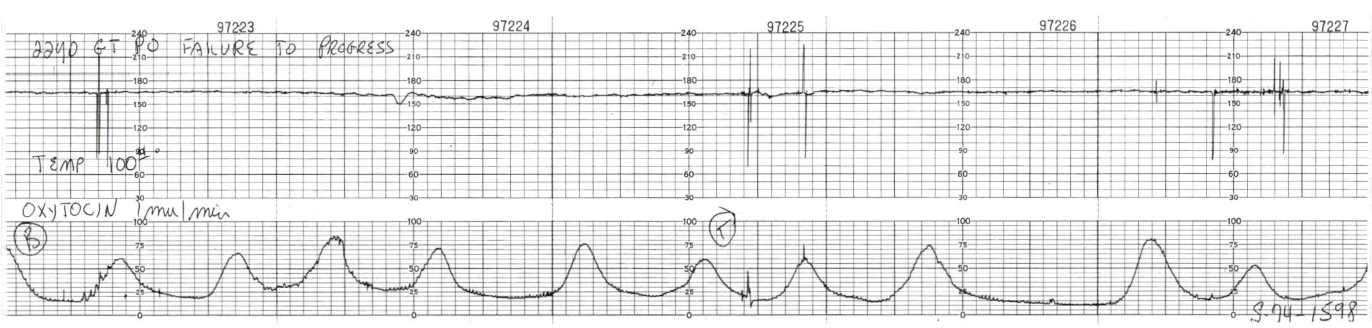

Figure 6.1. Fetal tachycardia. The fetal heart rate 165 beats per minute. This tachycardia is associated with maternal fever (note temperature [100.4°F]). Also, note the associated loss of variability. The absence of associated decelerations and the presence of an explanation (fever) make hypoxia an unlikely cause.

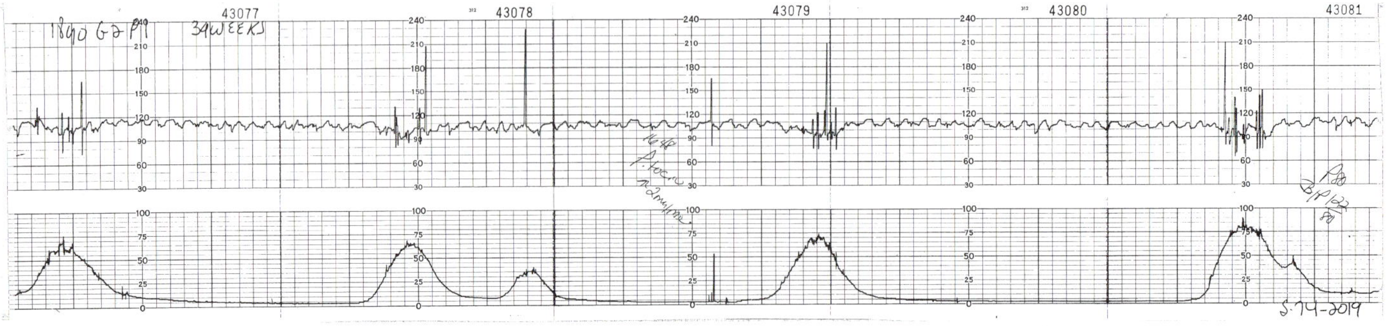

Figure 6.2. Fetal bradycardia. The fetal heart rate is 110 beats per minute. There is normal variability present by direct internal scalp electrode monitoring. Four hours later, the patient delivered a 3025-g baby with Apgar scores of 9 at 1 minute and 10 at 5 minutes. Mother and baby did well.

do not reflect a hypoxic fetus, particularly when present in a term gestation. In a preterm fetus or when seen in a term pregnancy without an obvious explanation (eg, maternal fever), close evaluation is critical.

Fetal Bradycardia

Bradycardia is a baseline FHR of <110 bpm. Bradycardia, within the range of 80 to 110 bpm with moderate variability, generally indicates good oxygenation without acidemia (Fig. 6.2). Slowing of the baseline heart rate is most likely in response to an increased vagal tone.[3] Fetal bradycardia that is first noted at the initiation of monitoring may be difficult to distinguish from a prolonged deceleration. Generally, prolonged decelerations are associated with loss of variability and their rate fluctuates up and down rather than remaining consistent unless rates below 70 bpm are seen.

Actual baseline FHRs of <70 bpm are generally seen without variability and may represent congenital heart block (Fig. 6.3). Persistent bradycardia from complete atrioventricular dissociation should alert the clinician to the possible diagnosis of maternal connective tissue disease, most often systemic lupus erythematosus, which results in fetal heart block and bradycardia consequent to transplacental passage of maternal antibodies that have an affinity for fetal cardiac conduction fibers[4] (see Chapter 4). Structural cardiac defects and cytomegalovirus infections are also potential etiologies of congenital heart block. To reliably establish that fetal cardiac activity is present and that the persistent bradycardia is caused by fetal heart block, confirmation with real-time ultrasound is necessary. Ultrasound allows for a further advantage in that cardiac structure can be carefully evaluated as well (see Chapter 7). However, ultrasound is really only an option in the antepartum period because it may not be possible to take the time required to make this evaluation in labor where either a bradycardia or prolonged deceleration may require urgent operative intervention.

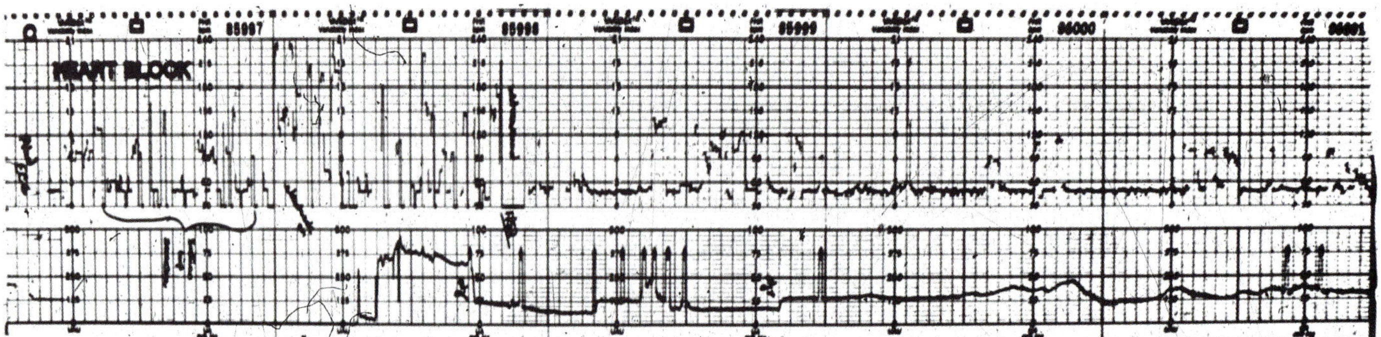

Figure 6.3. Fetal bradycardia caused by complete heart block. Note the rate of 50 beats per minute with a lack of variability.

When the diagnosis of complete fetal heart block is made antenatally, the problem then becomes how to monitor the fetus in labor because the normal alterations in FHR in response to hypoxemia and other central nervous system (CNS) input cannot be transmitted to the ventricles. Thus, in this situation, the FHR cannot be used as a way to monitor for fetal hypoxemia and to rule out acidemia. Intermittent scalp pH is theoretically an option, but it is not routinely available in the United States. Additionally, the need for repeating the test every 30 minutes makes this option unrealistic except in very rapid labor. Although no longer available in the United States, fetal pulse oximetry would be a logical option, and limited data suggest that this is a safe and effective way of monitoring patients whose fetal arrhythmia prevents adequate FHR monitoring.[5] Because of these limitations, an elective cesarean section is usually performed, simply because there is no other way to monitor the fetus.

Bradycardia with moderate variability may occur in the second stage and is not indicative of abnormal fetal acid-base status. Other, rarer causes of fetal bradycardia are maternal hypothermia, prolonged hypoglycemia, beta-blocker therapy, and fetal panhypopituitarism with brain-stem injury.[6] Persistent bradycardia requires careful evaluation to ensure that it is not the maternal heart rate being recorded in the presence of fetal demise or secondary to signal ambiguity. Real-time ultrasound can establish the correct diagnosis and thus avoid unnecessary and potentially dangerous therapy in the presence of an already dead fetus. Maternal heart rate can also be recorded from the Doppler transducer and in the rare situation where the fetus is dead, the MHR may be recorded from a fetal scalp electrode (see Chapter 4).

Variability

In the 2008 NICHD update on nomenclature, FHR variability was classified as follows:

- Absent
- Minimal (1-5 bpm)
- Moderate (5-25 bpm)
- Increased (>25 bpm)

In determining the immediate fetal status, the most important single FHR characteristic is variability. Moderate variability (6-25 bpm peak to trough) is a reflection of intact neurologic modulation of the FHR and of intact or normal cardiac responsiveness. The two components are short-term and long-term variability (LTV) (Fig. 6.4). Short-term variability (STV) is the beat-to-beat irregularity caused by the normal variance in intervals between consecutive cardiac cycles. It is a consequence of the constant "push-pull" effect of sympathetic and parasympathetic nervous system input. LTV is the waviness of the FHR tracing, generally at a frequency of 3 to 5 cycles per minute. With older EFM systems, using external Doppler, FHR variability could not be accurately determined because Doppler monitoring can artifactually increase FHR variability owing to the imprecision of the signal. With contemporary Doppler signal processing systems, however, variability can be accurately assessed. Although there is utility in distinguishing between LTV and STV in research settings because the mathematical quantification of these two types is different, there is no current evidence that the distinction between the two has any clinical relevance. Perhaps the single exception to this is the sinusoidal tracing that is absent short term but uniformly increased LTV. Increased variability has been shown in animals to be a sign of mild hypoxia.[7] However, when

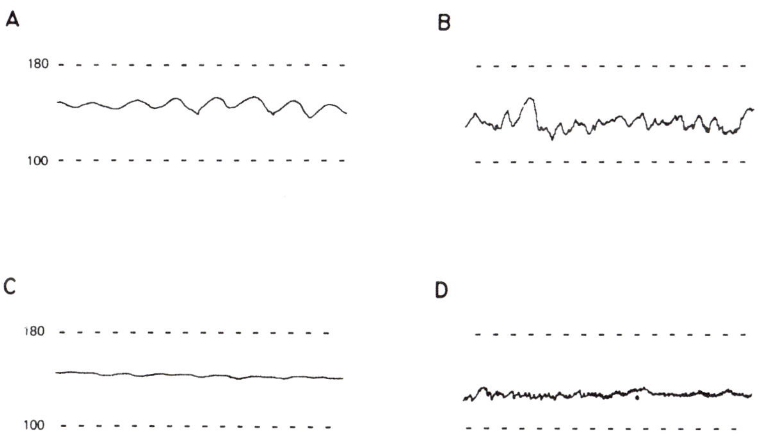

Figure 6.4. Long-term variability (LTV) is demonstrated in **(A and B)** and is absent in **(C and D)**. Short-term variability (STV) alone is shown in **(D)** and its concurrent presence with LTV is shown in **(B)**. Absence of both LTV and STV is seen in **(C)**. (From Zanini B, Paul RA, Huey JR. Intrapartum fetal heart rate: correlation with scalp pH in the preterm fetus. *Am J Obstet Gynecol.* 1980;136(1):43-47, with permission.)

TABLE 6.2 Causes of decreased FHR variability

Hypoxia/acidosis
Drugs CNS depressants Parasympatholytics
Fetal sleep cycles
Congenital anomalies
Extreme prematurity
Fetal tachycardia
Preexisting neurologic abnormality

CNS, central nervous system; FHR, fetal heart rate.

TABLE 6.3 Examples of drugs causing decreased fetal heart rate variability

Analgesics/narcotics Meperidine Heroin Morphine
Barbiturates Phenobarbital Secobarbital
Tranquilizers Diazepam
Phenothiazines Promethazine
Parasympatholytics Atropine
General anesthetics
Corticosteroids Betamethasone
Magnesium sulfate

FHR variability is moderate or increased, fetal pH is usually normal.

As gestation advances and the fetal autonomic nervous system matures, the baseline FHR decreases, and both STV and LTV increases. This is thought to reflect an increase in vagal control of cardiovascular reflexes. Decreased variability may be seen with prematurity, fetal sleep cycles, or anything that causes fetal CNS depression. Fetal hypoxemia with acidemia is the most worrisome cause; however, any condition that depresses the CNS can also decrease variability (Table 6.2). In labor, it is critical to carefully review the strip for the presence or absence of late, variable, or prolonged decelerations when decreased variability is seen. It is highly unlikely that minimal or absent variability reflects CNS depression caused by metabolic acidemia unless there are decelerations indicating ongoing hypoxemia. The exception to this rule may occur in the fetus who presents in labor with absent variability without decelerations, as one cannot rule out a hypoxic insult prior to the initiation of electronic monitoring. Especially in the absence of significant decelerations, other causes of CNS depression should be considered. Certain drugs may be responsible (Table 6.3), particularly drugs that depress the CNS (Fig. 6.5) and drugs with autonomic blocking effects. Parasympathetic blocking drugs decrease variability while increasing baseline heart rate. Sympatholytic drugs (eg, beta-adrenergic blockers) also decrease variability but decrease baseline heart rate.

Baseline heart rate variability is also associated with fetal wakefulness. When the fetus is sleeping, there may be decreased variability (Fig. 6.6). Usually the variability will spontaneously return to its previous level after a reasonable time, although the duration of fetal sleep states in labor is not as consistent as in the antepartum period. Stimulation of the fetus by manipulation of the uterus or noise may arouse the fetus and cause the variability to return or result in an FHR acceleration, both of which reliably predict the absence of abnormal fetal academia. The new onset of loss of variability in the absence of periodic FHR decelerations with contractions is not a sign of fetal hypoxia.

From an intrapartum monitoring perspective, the most ominous cause of decreased variability is fetal hypoxemia where FHR decelerations precede the loss of variability. In the presence of heart rate patterns such as persistent late decelerations, loss of variability is associated with a high incidence of fetal acidosis and low Apgar scores[8] (Fig. 6.7), particularly in the case of preterm infants.[9] A most difficult heart rate pattern to interpret is absent variability seen in the fetus with a normal baseline heart rate and no decelerations. This may represent a previous insult to the fetus that has since been corrected but has resulted in persistent neurologic damage. Also, this pattern may be seen in fetuses with significant congenital anomalies, especially in the central nervous and cardiac systems.[10] Extreme prematurity is associated with decreased variability and nonreactive FHR patterns. Finally, these patterns can be idiopathic and occur in a subsequently vigorous and healthy neonate. Table 6.2 lists the causes of decreased variability.

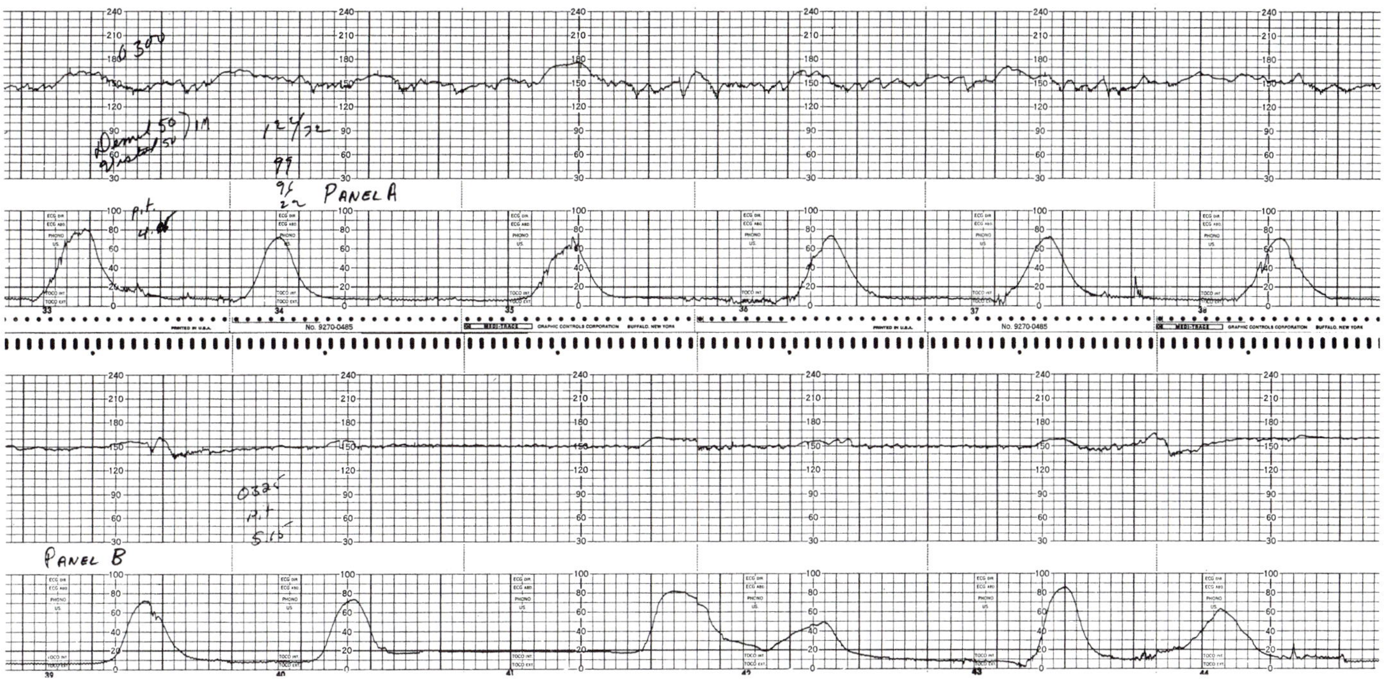

Figure 6.5. Narcotics are among the most frequent causes of decreased fetal heart rate variability in labor. In (**A**), Demerol and Vistaril are given intramuscularly. At the beginning of (**B**), about 20 minutes later, there is a noticeable decrease in variability without a change in baseline heart rate.

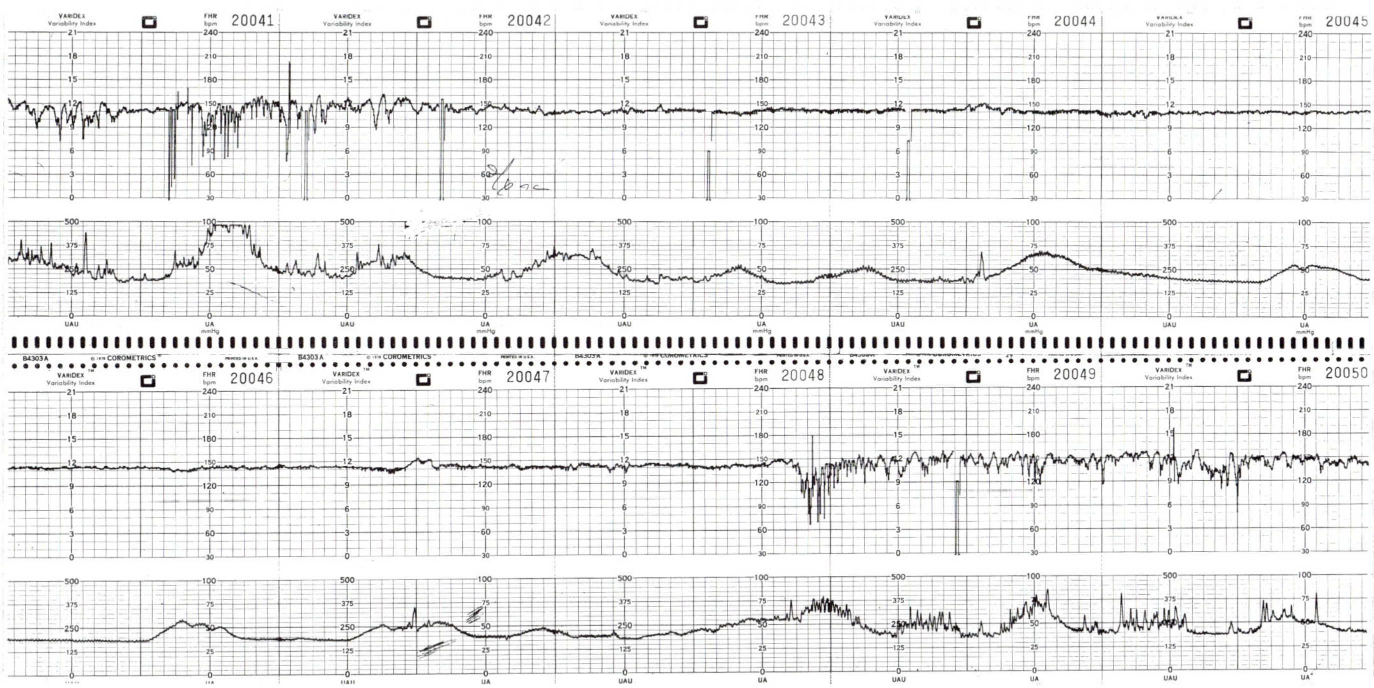

Figure 6.6. Spontaneous changes in variability occur normally in labor. Note the abrupt decrease in variability at **Panel 20042**, which again abruptly returns to normal at **Panel 20048**. This decreased variability lasted 20 to 30 minutes. There were no medications used. A vigorous normal baby was subsequently delivered.

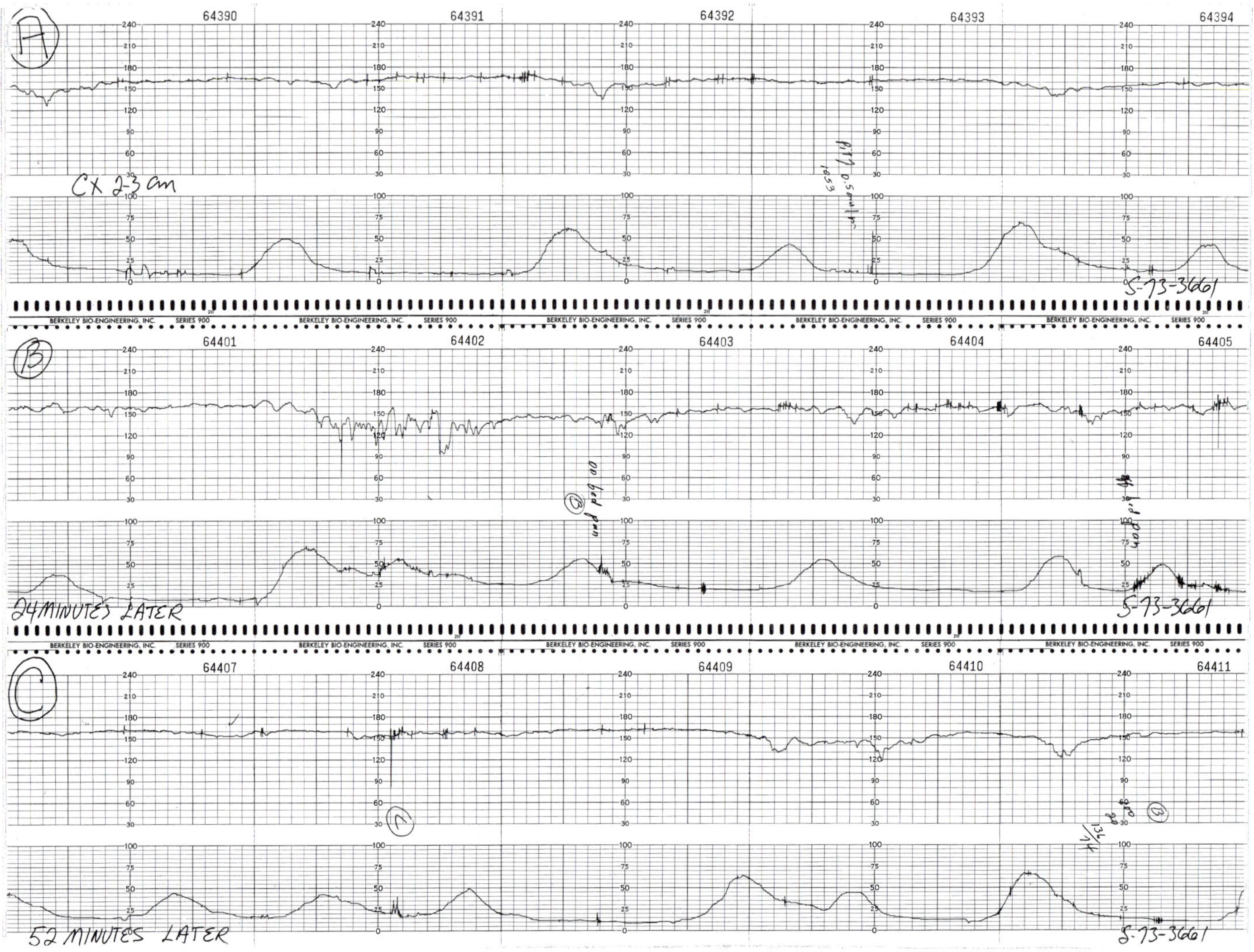

Figure 6.7. Persistent late decelerations are seen after most contractions. At **Panel 64407** and after, variability is notably decreased. There is an associated fetal tachycardia.

PERIODIC CHANGES

Tachycardia, bradycardia, and alterations in variability involve baseline FHR changes. Periodic changes are transient heart rate accelerations or decelerations that ultimately return to the original or a newly established baseline heart rate. Generally, these periodic changes occur in response to contractions and may also be seen with fetal movement.

Decelerations

There are four principal types of decelerations named according to shape and temporal relationship to contractions. These are early, late, variable, and prolonged decelerations (Table 6.4). Decelerations are defined as recurrent if they occur with at least one-half of the contractions (Table 6.4).

Early Decelerations

Early decelerations are uniformly shaped decelerations of gradual onset and gradual return to baseline (Fig. 6.8). They begin early in the uterine contraction cycle, have their nadir at the peak of the contraction, and return to baseline before completion of the contraction. Acceleration of the heart rate generally does not precede or follow early deceleration. An important characteristic of early deceleration is the minimal amplitude. The degree of FHR slowing is generally proportional to the strength of the contraction but rarely falls below 100 to 110 or 20 to 30 bpm below baseline. Early decelerations are thought to be caused by fetal

TABLE 6.4 Definitions of decelerations, NICHD 2008 terminology

Late deceleration Visually apparent usually symmetrical *gradual* decrease and return of the fetal heart rate (FHR) associated with a uterine contraction. A *gradual* FHR decrease is defined as from the onset to the FHR nadir of ≥30 seconds. The decrease in FHR is calculated from the onset to the nadir of the deceleration. The deceleration is delayed in timing with the nadir of the deceleration occurring after the peak of the contractions. In most cases, the onset of the nadir and recovery of the deceleration occurs after the beginning, peak, and ending of the contraction, respectively.
Early deceleration Visually apparent usually symmetrical *gradual* decrease and return of the FHR associated with a uterine contraction. A *gradual* FHR decrease is defined as one from the onset to the FHR nadir of ≥30 seconds. The decrease in FHR is calculated from the onset to the nadir of the deceleration. The nadir of the deceleration occurs at the same time as the peak of the contraction. In most cases, the onset, nadir, and recovery of the deceleration are coincident with the beginning, peak, and ending of the contraction respectively.
Variable deceleration A visually apparent *abrupt* decrease in FHR. An *abrupt* FHR decrease is defined as from the onset of the deceleration to the beginning of the FHR nadir of <30 seconds. The decrease in FHR is calculated from the onset to the nadir of the deceleration. The decrease in FHR is ≥15 beats per minute, lasting ≥15 seconds, and <2 minutes in duration. When variable decelerations are associated with uterine contractions, their onset, depth, and duration commonly vary with successive uterine contraction.

head compression, with altered cerebral blood flow precipitating cardiac slowing through a vagal reflex. Early deceleration is generally seen in the active phase of labor, between 4 and 7 cm of cervical dilation. It is not associated with tachycardia, loss of variability, or other heart rate changes. Early deceleration is an FHR pattern that is not associated with fetal hypoxia, acidosis, or low Apgar scores.

Late Decelerations

In shape and uniformity, late decelerations are similar to early decelerations, but the timing is delayed relative to the uterine contraction (Fig. 6.9). The onset of the deceleration is often seen 30 seconds or more after the onset of the contraction. The nadir of the deceleration occurs after the contraction peak, and usually, the return to baseline occurs after the contraction is over. In recognizing late decelerations, several important characteristics in addition to the timing are important. The descent and return are gradual and smooth. There are usually no accelerations seen preceding or following the deceleration. The FHR rarely falls more than 30 to 40 bpm below baseline and usually not by more than 10 to 20 bpm. Late decelerations are significant

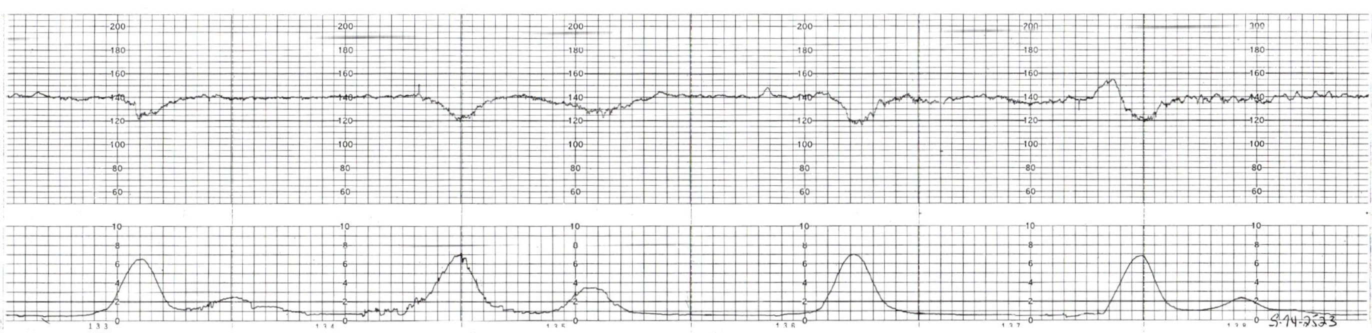

Figure 6.8. Early decelerations are seen with each contraction on this panel. They are uniform, mirror the contractions, and decelerate only 10 to 20 beats per minute.

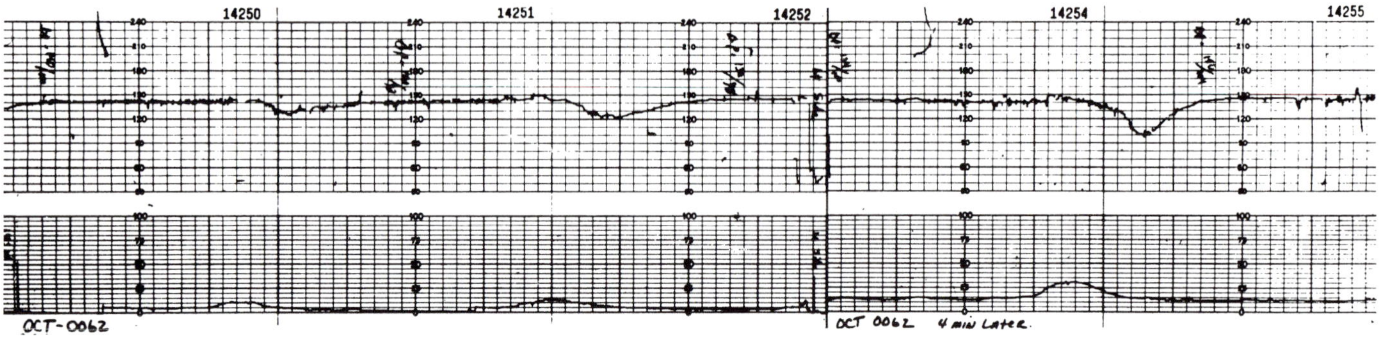

Figure 6.9. Late decelerations are seen after each of the three contractions. They are uniform, smooth, and drop only 20 to 30 beats per minute below baseline. There are no associated accelerations.

and concerning when they are persistent and not correctable. Variability is often increased during the deceleration. Late decelerations may occur before fetal metabolic acidemia develops and in this case, they are caused by vagal stimulation. After fetal metabolic acidosis develops, the late decelerations are caused by fetal myocardial depression (see Chapter 2). Although late decelerations may be associated with hypoxia, acidemia, and hypotension, only a decrease in fetal oxygen tension is essential for late decelerations to occur. The degree of this hypoxia and the appearance of late decelerations are related to many factors, including, on occasion, the strength and duration of the uterine contraction. There may be a correlation between the magnitude of late decelerations (amount of slowing) and the degree of hypoxia, but this is not always the case, as the most depressed fetuses may have only shallow late decelerations. Persistent late decelerations are significant and potentially ominous. The association of late decelerations with loss of variability and/or elevation of baseline FHR is of more significance than the decelerations alone and reflects fetal intolerance to the hypoxic stress of uterine contractions.

The cause of late decelerations is uteroplacental insufficiency (UPI) elicited by intervillous stasis occurring during uterine contractions, and the factors that lead to this hypoxia may be intrinsic or extrinsic to the placenta. Decreased uterine blood flow is a much more common cause of late deceleration than poor exchange from other causes. Causes of decreased flow include supine hypotension and decreased uterine artery perfusion secondary to epidural or spinal anesthesia. The most common cause of late deceleration is uterine hyperactivity or hypertonus, often as a result of excessive oxytocin stimulation. Late decelerations seen in association with vaginal bleeding and/or spontaneous uterine hyperactivity may be the result of premature placental separation (abruptio placentae) (Fig. 6.10). Several disease states, including chronic hypertension, postmaturity, intrauterine growth restriction, diabetes mellitus, hypertensive disorders of pregnancy, and collagen vascular disease, may compromise placental exchange.

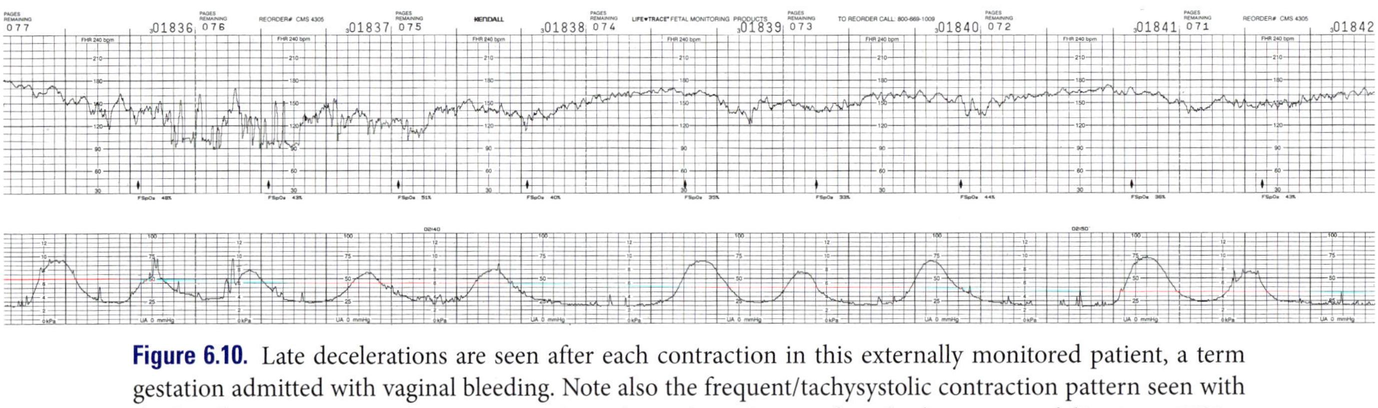

Figure 6.10. Late decelerations are seen after each contraction in this externally monitored patient, a term gestation admitted with vaginal bleeding. Note also the frequent/tachysystolic contraction pattern seen with the first five contractions. At cesarean section, a large abruption was found subsequent to delivering a 3500-g female with Apgar scores of 7 at 1 minute and 8 at 5 minutes.

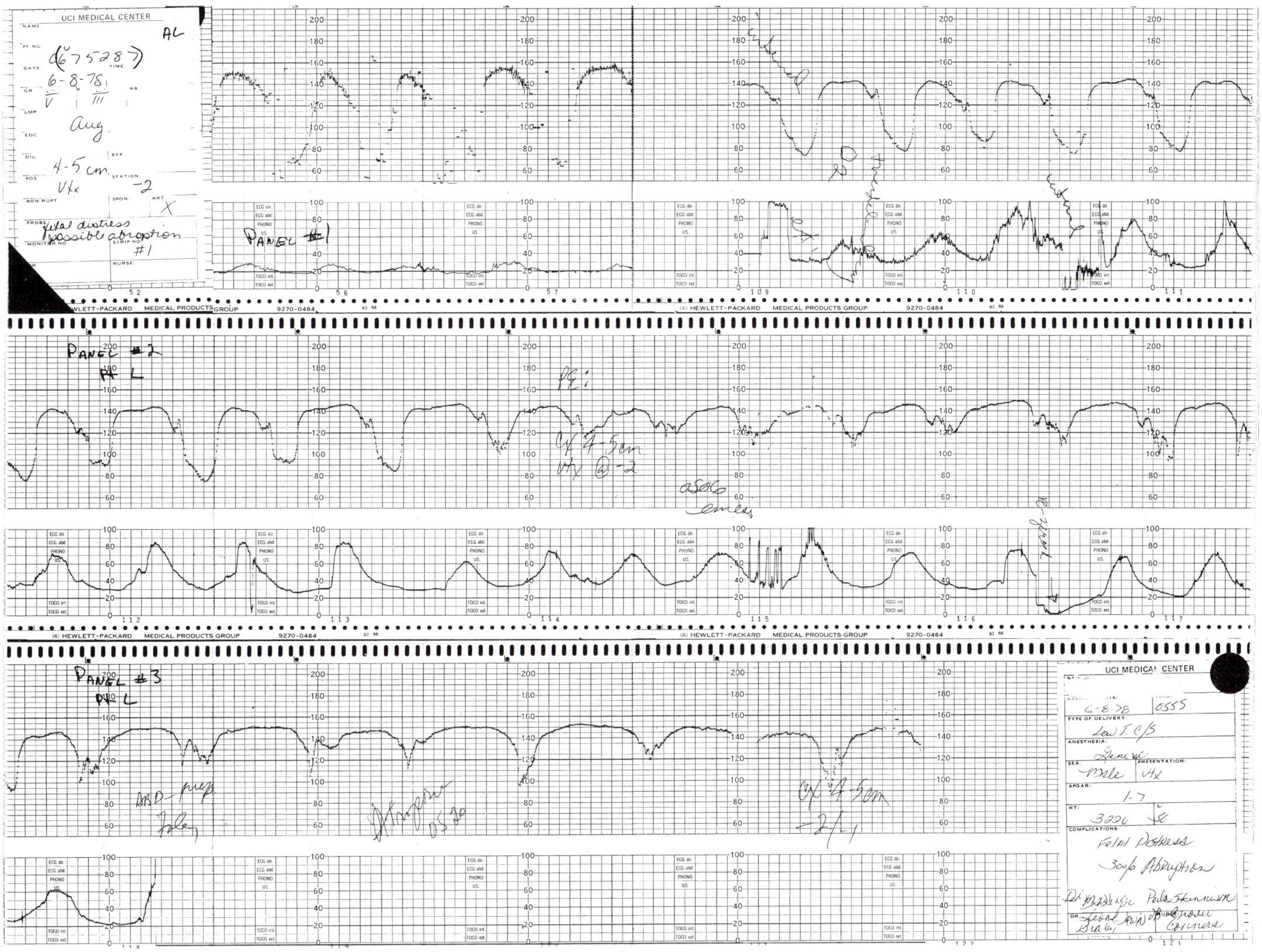

Figure 6.11. This is a gravida 5, para 3 admitted at term with contractions and minimal vaginal bleeding. On the internal monitor (second half of **Panel 1**), persistent late decelerations are noted that fail to respond to oxygen and position change. Variability is poor throughout and the baseline heart rate gradually increased from 140 to 155 beats per minute. In the presence of late decelerations, poor variability, and rising baseline rate are signs of fetal intolerance to hypoxia and developing acidosis. In this case, a female with Apgar scores of 1 at 1 minute and 7 at 5 minutes was delivered. The 30% abruption is the cause of the late decelerations.

The decreased intervillous blood flow associated with contractions (labor) may further aggravate this exchange and produce late decelerations. Because each contraction can produce hypoxic stress, the persistence of late deceleration may precipitate metabolic acidosis. Recurrent late decelerations are predictive of neonatal acidemia.[11] Additional causes of concern in the presence of recurrent late decelerations are loss of accelerations and the loss of variability (Fig. 6.11). Tachycardia may also occur with the development of fetal acidosis, although for unknown reasons, this is not as consistently seen as it is with progressively severe variable decelerations. Decreased variability and fetal tachycardia are important signs of developing acidosis, and their presence with persistent late decelerations correlates highly with neonatal depression.

Variable Decelerations

The most frequently seen FHR deceleration pattern in labor is variable decelerations. This aptly named pattern is variable in nearly all respects: shape, duration, intensity, and timing relative to uterine contractions. It is commonly the result of umbilical cord compression but can result from any interruption of umbilical blood flow that is acute and intermittent. Other causes of interruption of cord flow include cord stretch and

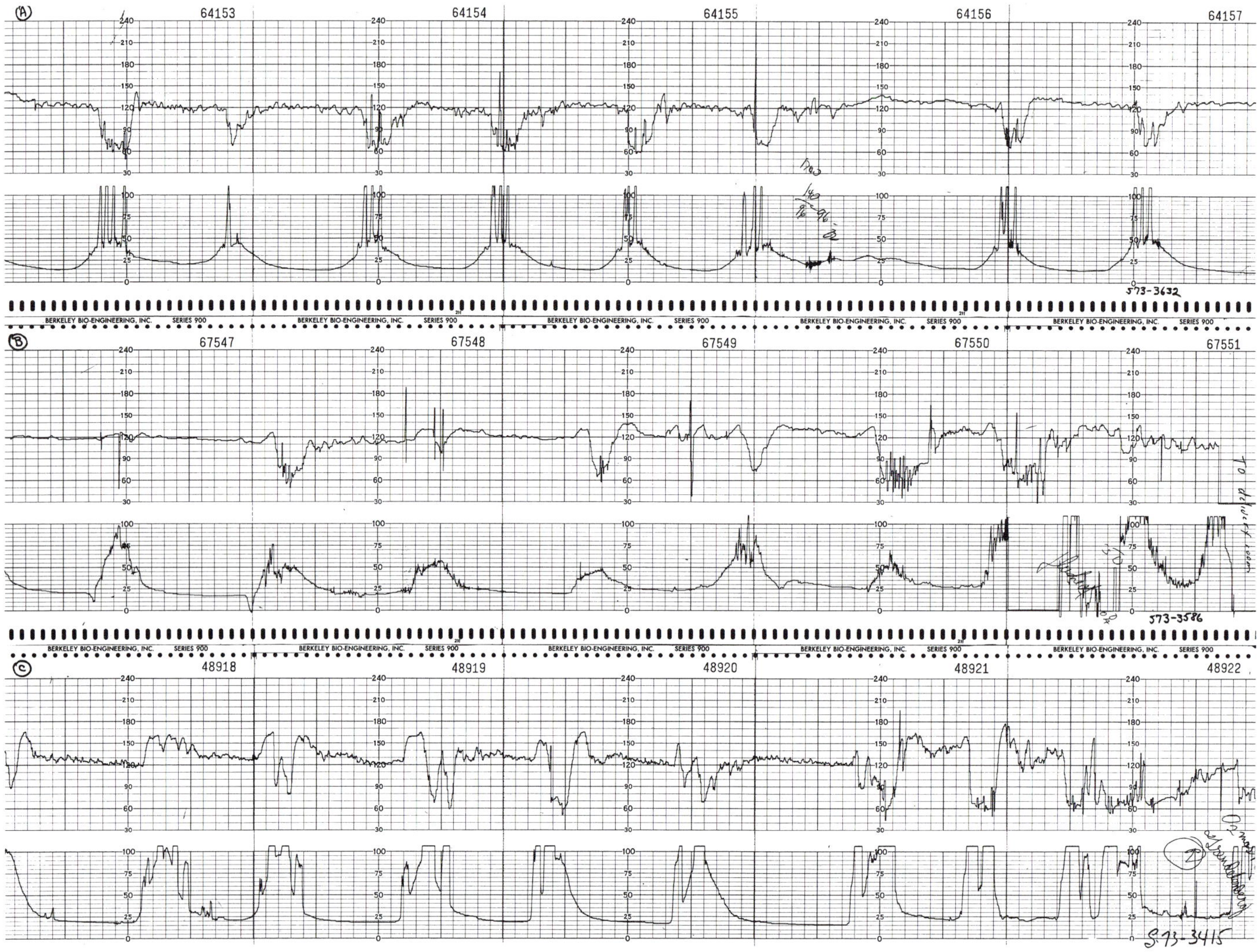

Figure 6.12. Typical variable decelerations are seen in this patient in the second stage of labor. Although all are occurring with contractions, they are variable in depth, duration, and shape. They are abrupt in onset and return to baseline. There are accelerations seen preceding and following most of these decelerations.

cold (eg, rapid infusion of room-temperature amnioinfusion). In addition, head compression may also produce or alter the shape, depth, and duration of variable decelerations. Because cord compression during labor occurs most often during uterine contractions, variable decelerations usually coincide with uterine contractions (Fig. 6.12). This is, however, an inconsistent occurrence, and such decelerations may be seen with one but not the subsequent contraction. Characteristically, these decelerations are very abrupt in both onset and return to baseline. Small abrupt accelerations of the FHR usually precede and/or follow these decelerations. Variable decelerations are also occasionally observed during antepartum monitoring with fetal movement. This is more common in preterm fetuses, perhaps because of a relative decrease in the amount of Wharton's jelly in the cord compared to at term.[12] There appears to be an association between the presence of variable decelerations on antepartum monitoring and both oligohydramnios and subsequent abnormal FHR tracings in labor. The degree of oligohydramnios correlates with the frequency of severe variable decelerations in labor.[13] Assessment of amniotic fluid volume should be considered in antepartum patients with frequent variable decelerations during FHR testing and in patients with variable decelerations occurring relatively early in labor.

It is useful to think of four potential groups of causes of variable decelerations, because these groups aid in understanding the pathophysiology, determining the best method(s) for correction, and predicting the most likely progression (Table 6.5). Variable

TABLE 6.5 Causes of variable decelerations and their relationships to labor

Oligohydramnios
Onset usually in the early active phase of labor or after membrane rupture
Descent
Onset usually at 8-10 cm of dilation
Often associated with nuchal cords
Aggravated by pushing efforts
Cord prolapsed
Sometime after the rupture of membranes
Associated with unengaged station or abnormal presentation
Unusual causes
True knots, short cords, limb entanglement occult prolapse, etc
Onset and progression variably related to labor

decelerations that begin early in the active phase of labor are often associated with and caused by oligohydramnios (Fig. 6.13). These will not likely respond to position change but may well be reversed or ameliorated by amnioinfusion if they progress to require intervention. Those developing during or just before the onset of the second stage of labor are most likely caused by umbilical cord stretch or compression. This time in labor coincides with an acceleration of descent of the fetal presenting part, and these decelerations are most commonly seen in association with cord encirclement about the fetal neck (nuchal cords). It is presumed that in such circumstances, the variable decelerations are caused by cord stretch as the fetus descends. Such events are so common that experienced labor and delivery nurses know that it is time to examine the patient because the new appearance of variable deceleration often heralds the onset of the second stage (Fig. 6.14). Rarely the appearance of variable decelerations can announce the presence of umbilical cord prolapse, and this is another important reason to examine the patient. The final category of causes of cord compression can be thought of as "unusual cords" including such things as short cords, true knots, cord entanglement about fetal small parts, and occult cord prolapse. The course of cord compression is most unpredictable in such circumstances.

The vast majority of variable decelerations are not associated with significant hypoxia, or acidosis. Thus the challenge of evaluating and managing these patterns depends on the ability to distinguish between patterns that do and do not require further evaluation and management. In terms of fetal compromise, any insult should vary directly with the duration and degree of cord compression. With persistent mild degrees of cord compression, mild respiratory acidosis may develop from carbon dioxide (CO_2) retention. However, if the placental function is adequate and contractions are not too frequent, this CO_2 retention should clear rapidly with reversal of the respiratory acidosis. Should cord compression be prolonged and/or repetitive, progressive fetal hypoxia and resultant metabolic acidosis may also develop. Neonatal acidemia correlates more strongly with variable decelerations when they are either repetitive or have an increasing deceleration area. The deceleration area is defined as the sum of the areas of deceleration under the baseline over a given period. Thus tracings with increased deceleration area reflect both the frequency of variable decelerations and increased depth and duration of the deceleration.[11,14]

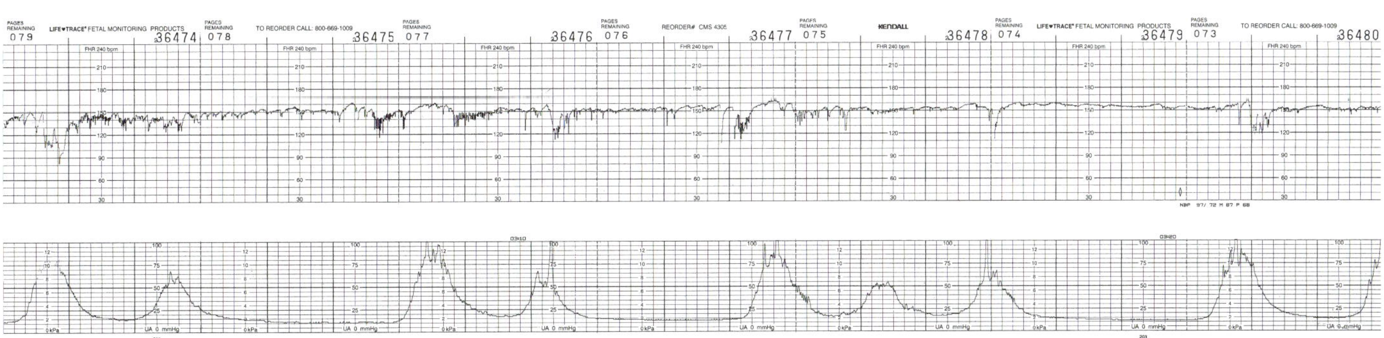

Figure 6.13. This nulliparous patient is at 41.5 weeks in early labor. Note the occasional mild variable decelerations. The amniotic fluid volume on ultrasound was noted to be markedly reduced. Subsequently, at the time of amniotomy, thick meconium was noted and amnioinfusion was started. Variable decelerations appearing in early labor are unusual, and oligohydramnios should always be considered as an etiology of cord compression.

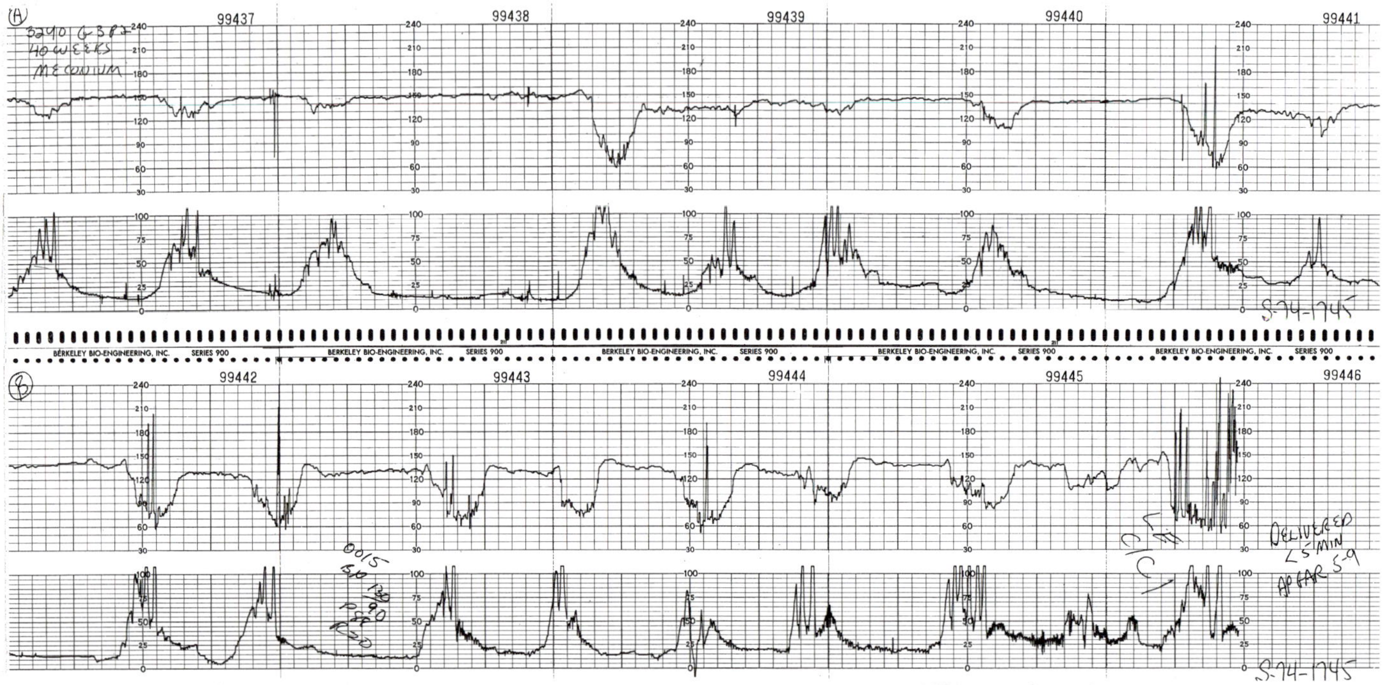

Figure 6.14. Variable decelerations here, as they often do, herald the onset of the second stage of labor in **Panel A**. Maternal pushing can be detected by the short spikes on top of the contractions. The reason for this is probably a nuchal cord that is stretched during the descent of the fetal vertex. Although the decelerations become larger and more regular, baseline heart rate and variability remain unchanged and do not signify hypoxia. A term-size infant with Apgar scores of 5 at 1 minute and 9 at 5 minutes was delivered <5 minutes after the monitor was removed and there was indeed a tight nuchal cord.

Deceleration area has been used in research studies to quantify variable decelerations but is not routinely calculated clinically. Other schematics have been suggested to characterize the severity of variable decelerations. Kubli et al[15] graded variable decelerations on the basis of the level and duration of decelerations, without considering other parameters. Mild variable decelerations have a duration of <30 seconds, regardless of level, or deceleration not below 70 to 80 bpm, regardless of duration (Fig. 6.15). Moderate variables have a level <80 bpm regardless of duration (Fig. 6.16). Severe variables are <70 bpm for >60 seconds (Fig. 6.17). Another heuristic is the "rule of 60s," positive if at least two of the following are true: duration at least 60 seconds, the lowest value is 60 bpm or lower, or depth from baseline is 60 or more bpm.[16] While using a different cut point, this correlates with the Kubli "severe" variable deceleration. It has the added benefit of including as

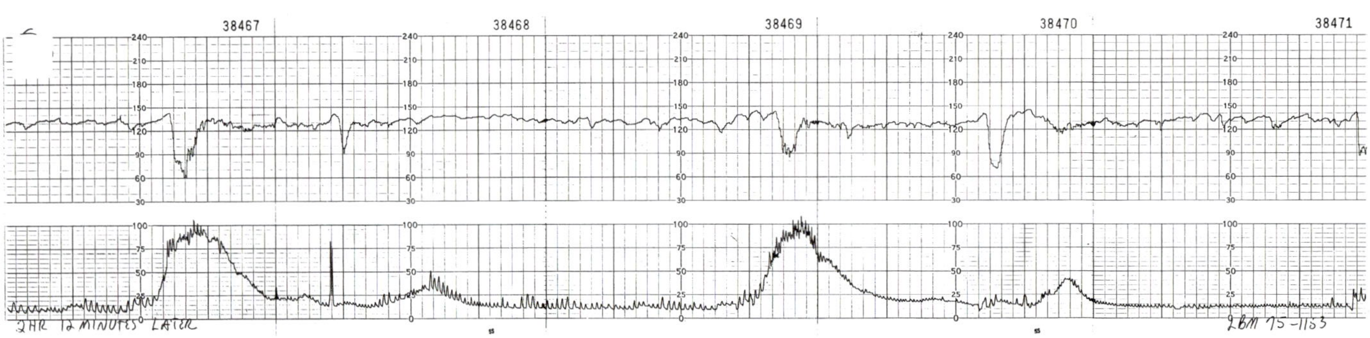

Figure 6.15. Mild variable decelerations are seen in this patient in early labor. They are occurring with contractions and probably with fetal movement. Baseline heart rate and variability are normal.

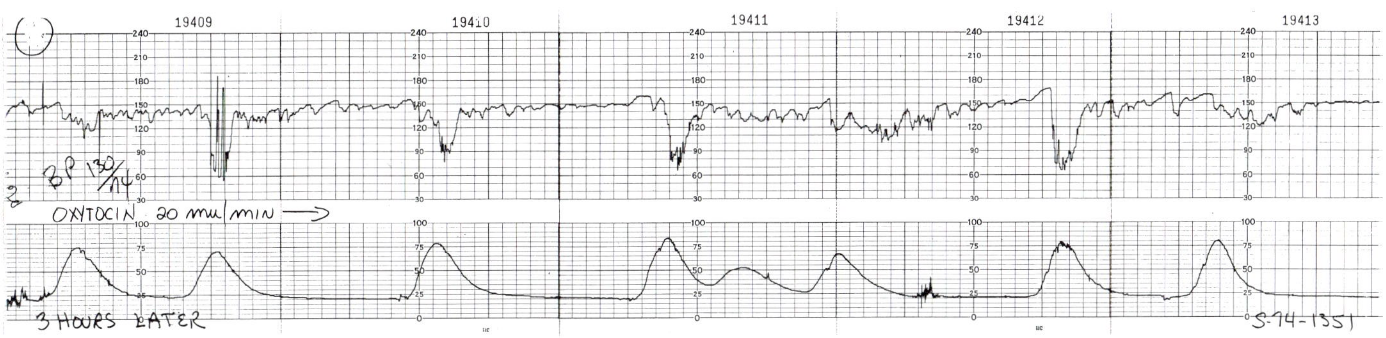

Figure 6.16. Moderate variable decelerations are seen in this panel. Baseline heart rate and variability are normal.

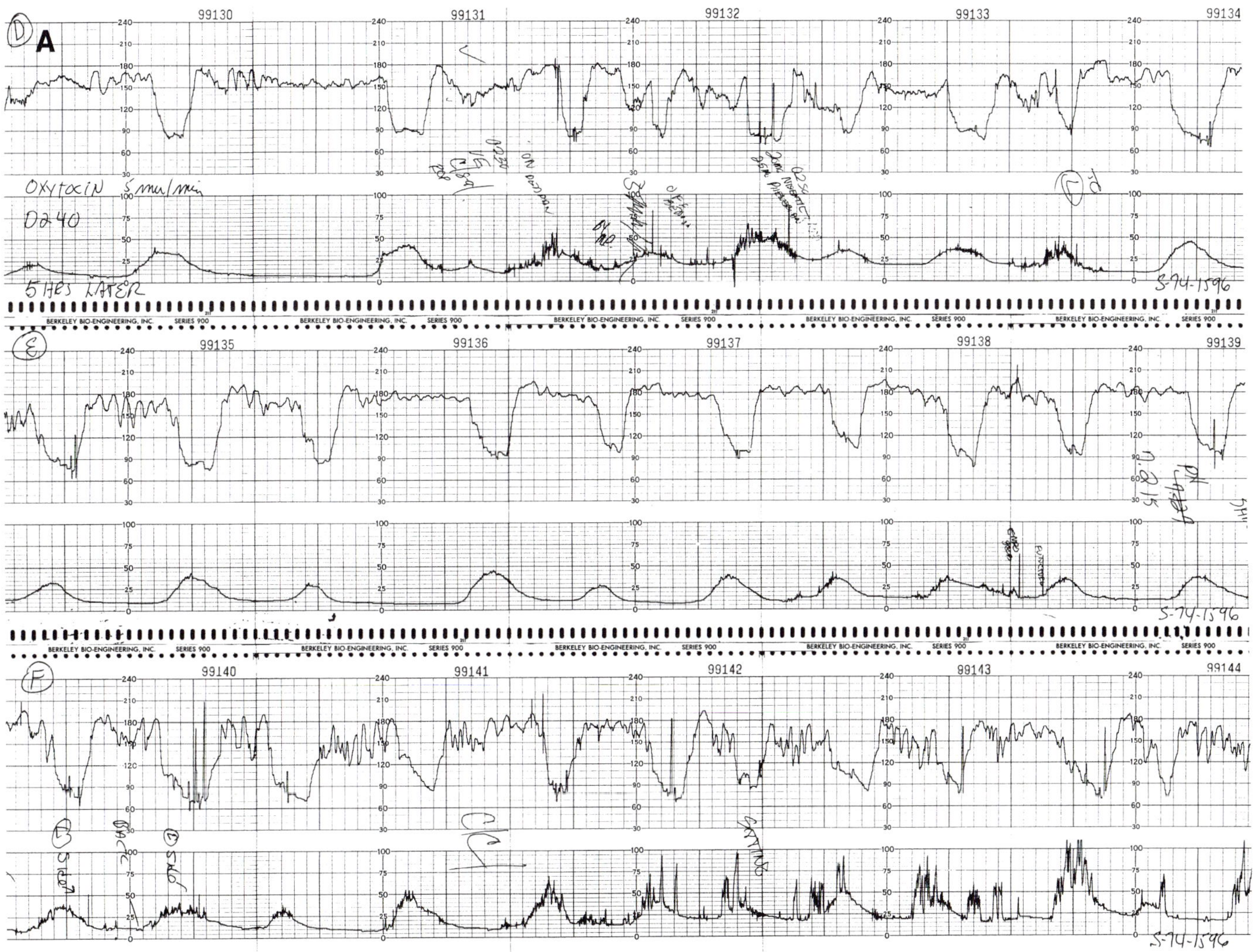

Figure 6.17. Severe variable decelerations are seen in a 14-year-old primigravida admitted at 43 weeks with meconium-stained amniotic fluid. Variable decelerations are seen throughout, becoming progressively deeper and more prolonged. Baseline heart rate is somewhat erratic from 140 to 180 beats per minute. Increased heart rate variability seen in G and H probably represents early hypoxia between contractions. A 2760-g infant with Apgar scores of 6 at 1 minute and 5 at 5 minutes was delivered. The low 5-minute Apgar score may have been caused by meconium in the airway and difficult ventilation. *(Continued)*

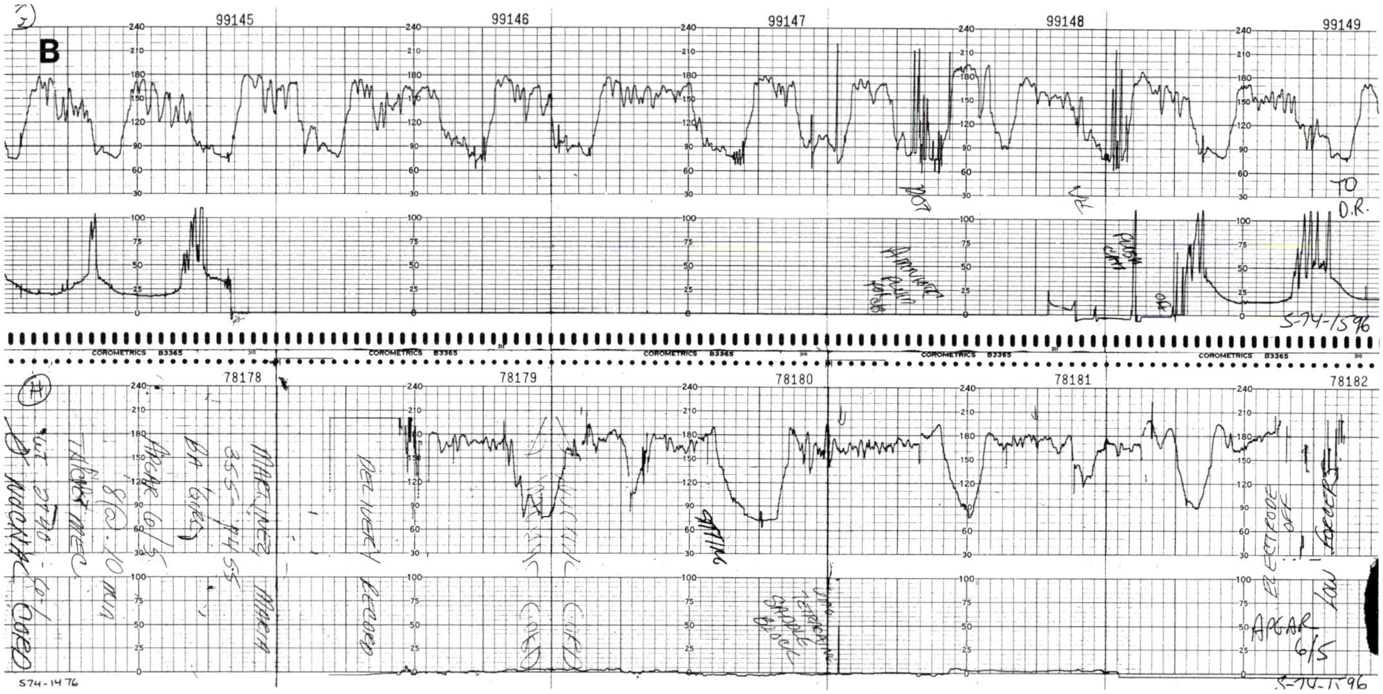

Figure 6.17. *(Continued)*

severe decelerations those that may occur in the setting of a tachycardia, for instance, a drop from a baseline level of 180 down to 80 or 90 bpm. Each of these systems of classifying variable decelerations emphasizes that increasing depth, frequency, and duration of variable decelerations increase the risk that fetal acidemia is present.

With variable decelerations, the depth and duration of the decelerations correlate to the degree of hypoxia when present, but are not always indicative of hypoxia, because they are initially caused by a baroreceptor reflex (Fig. 6.18). To evaluate how a given fetus is responding to or tolerating these variable decelerations, other parameters of the FHR tracing require evaluation. Loss of variability and baseline tachycardia suggest possible progressive neurologic depression from hypoxia and acidosis (Fig. 6.19). In the presence of variable decelerations that are persistent, deeper, and of greater duration, the development of these additional warning signs, in the absence of other causes such as drugs, is an important sign that the fetus is not tolerating the intermittent cord compression. The other sign of fetal intolerance to cord compression is a slow return of the variable deceleration pattern to baseline heart rate (Fig. 6.20). Usually, variable decelerations are very abrupt in both their descent and return to baseline. Should the return to baseline persistently become more gradual, the indication is that progressive hypoxia is developing. This slow return probably represents a component of late deceleration that would be consistent with developing fetal hypoxia. Sometimes, distinct variable decelerations are followed by distinct late decelerations when simultaneous cord compression and primary UPI occur (Fig. 6.21). With mild variable decelerations, especially without tachycardia or loss of variability, it is unlikely that the cord compression has caused the hypoxia and late decelerations. Therefore, a placental perfusion or exchange problem probably coexists with cord compression. Variable decelerations with slow return to baseline is one of the most confusing and difficult patterns to interpret and manage. These patterns may or may not be associated with fetal hypoxia. A study using fetal pulse oximetry demonstrated that when this pattern is preceded in its development by late or severe variable decelerations, then it is a sign of progressive hypoxia; but when slow return to baseline is associated with neither, then it is no more often associated with hypoxia than if the variable decelerations with which it occurs did not have a slow return to baseline.[17]

As variable decelerations become more severe and hypoxia is present or more severe, and especially as acidosis develops, additional FHR changes are common. The variable deceleration pattern will begin to

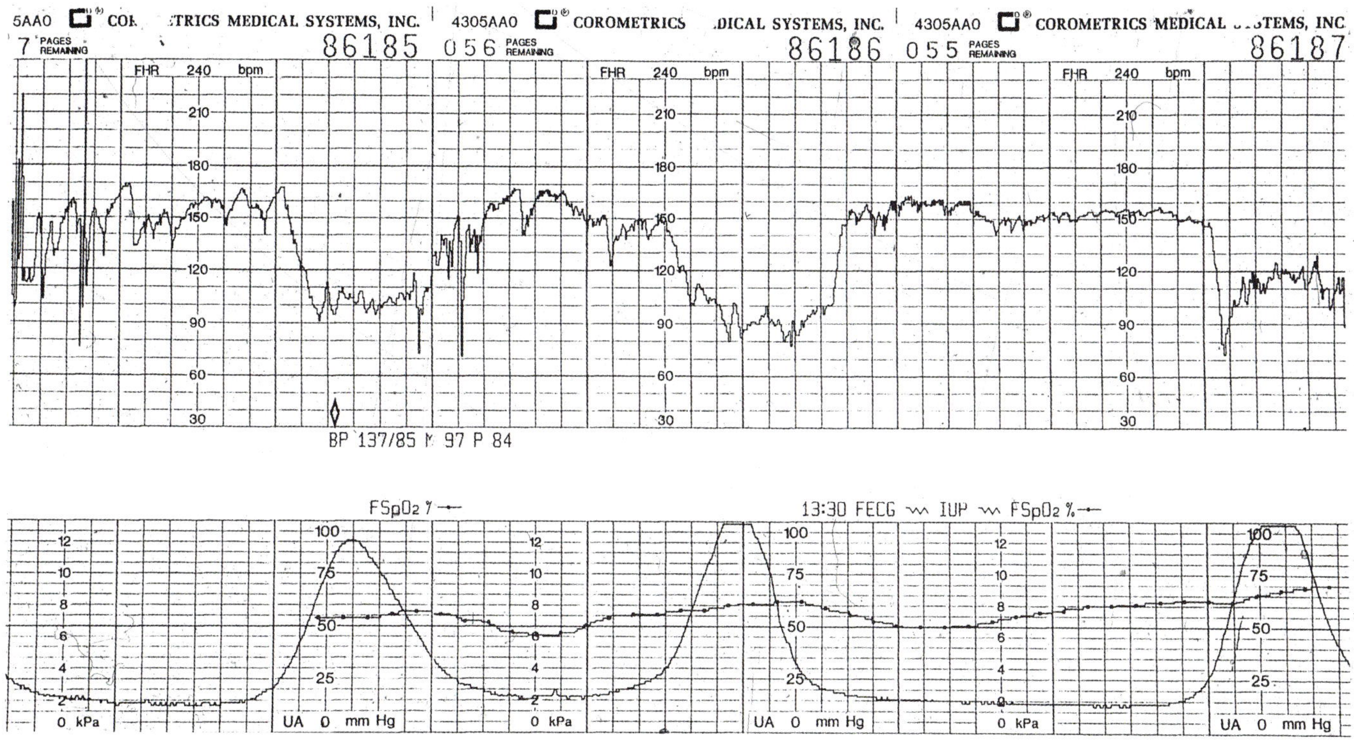

Figure 6.18. These deep variable decelerations dropping to 80 beats per minute and lasting up to 1 minute are seen in conjunction with a fetal pulse oximeter that shows normal fetal oxygen saturation values between 50% and 60%. Because the inciting stimulus of a variable deceleration is the increase in peripheral vascular resistance in the fetal circulation, and a slowing of the fetal heart rate that is the result of a baroreceptor reflex, even marked decelerations are often not associated with hypoxia.

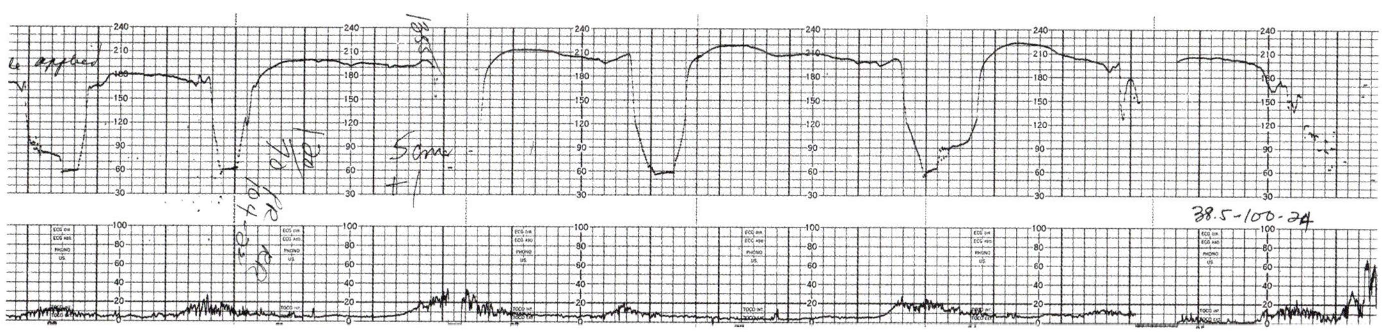

Figure 6.19. Severe ominous deceleration is seen with increasing heart rate to 210 beats per minute and virtually absent variability. A premature baby was delivered by cesarean section with Apgar scores of 1 at 1 minute and 2 at 5 minutes.

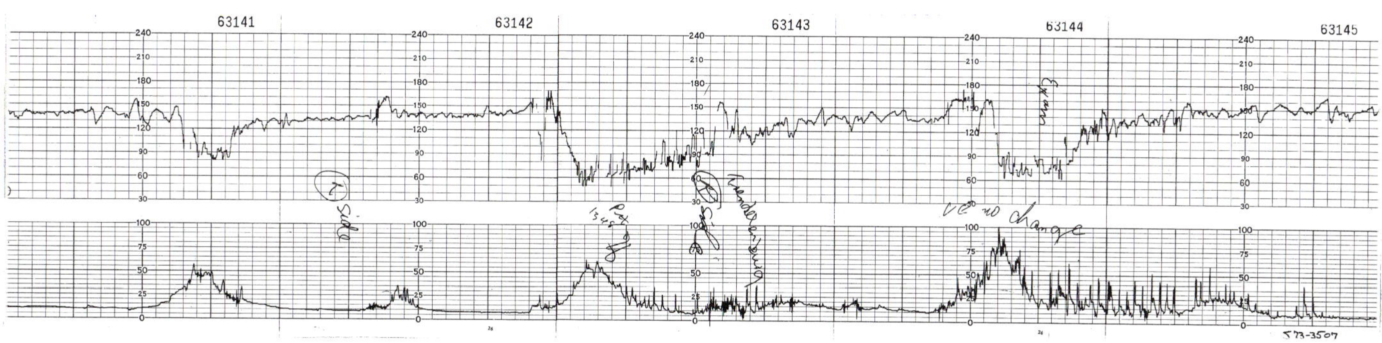

Figure 6.20. Severe decelerations are seen with a slow return to baseline. Baseline heart rate and variability are normal.

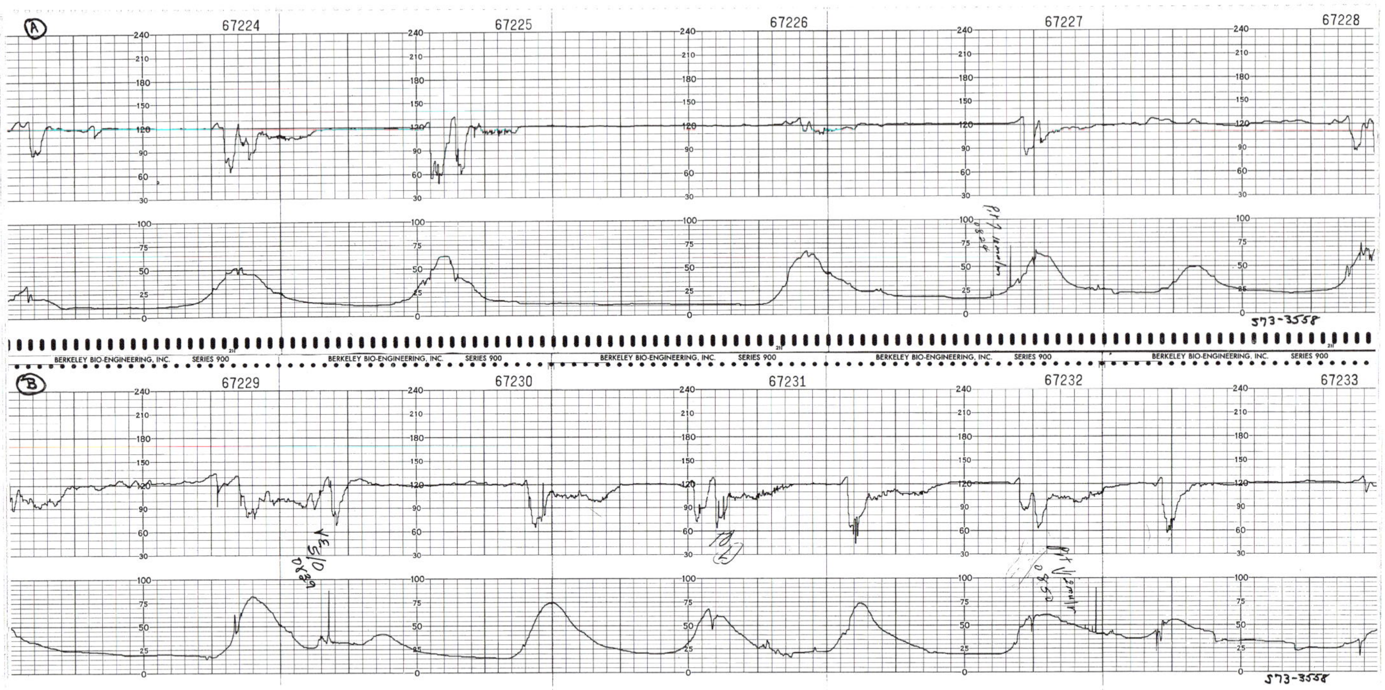

Figure 6.21. Mixed mild variable and late decelerations are seen with most contractions. With such mild variable decelerations, it is unlikely that progressive cord compression has caused the hypoxia, but a coexistent uteroplacental insufficiency probably exists. Poor variability suggests acidosis may also be present.

appear smoother and rounded or blunted (Fig. 6.22). This change can be partially reproduced with atropine or may be seen in a very premature fetus. In extreme situations, with severe and progressive variable deceleration, the contraction may be followed by a blunt acceleration described by Goodlin and Lowe[18] as "overshoot." This is a transient smooth acceleration lasting more than a minute and occurring after severe variable decelerations. There is no acceleration preceding the deceleration. The overshoot lacks abruptness, is without STV within the acceleration, and returns to baseline very gradually. This pattern is only seen with variable decelerations, usually with a flat baseline and with blunted changes as previously described.

Another finding that may occur when variable decelerations approach 50 to 60 bpm is transient cardiac asystole. Junctional rhythms are common if the FHR decreases below 70 bpm, with ventricular escape beats seen on occasion. Prolonged asystole is quite unusual and sudden death exceedingly rare. These do not seem to alter the likelihood that the decelerations correlate with hypoxia and acidosis over and above the appearance of the remainder of the pattern.

Rather than attempting to quantify variable decelerations and using this as some means to determine intrapartum management, we view variable decelerations as primarily reflex or as indicating developing fetal hypoxia. Reflex variable decelerations do not suggest fetal hypoxia and have the following components:

1. The deceleration lasts no more than 30 to 45 seconds.
2. There is a rapid return to baseline from the nadir of the deceleration.
3. Moderate variability of the baseline FHR is present.
4. The baseline rate is not increasing.

Variable decelerations that suggest developing fetal hypoxia are those that become deep and long lasting and have delayed return to baseline with or without overshoot. Decreasing baseline variability or an increasing baseline FHR are signs of developing fetal hypoxemia.[16]

In contrast to late decelerations, what makes variable decelerations so difficult to manage is their unpredictability. Because the second stage precedes delivery by only a relatively short time, and intervention is usually immediately possible should truly ominous patterns develop, more prolonged and deeper

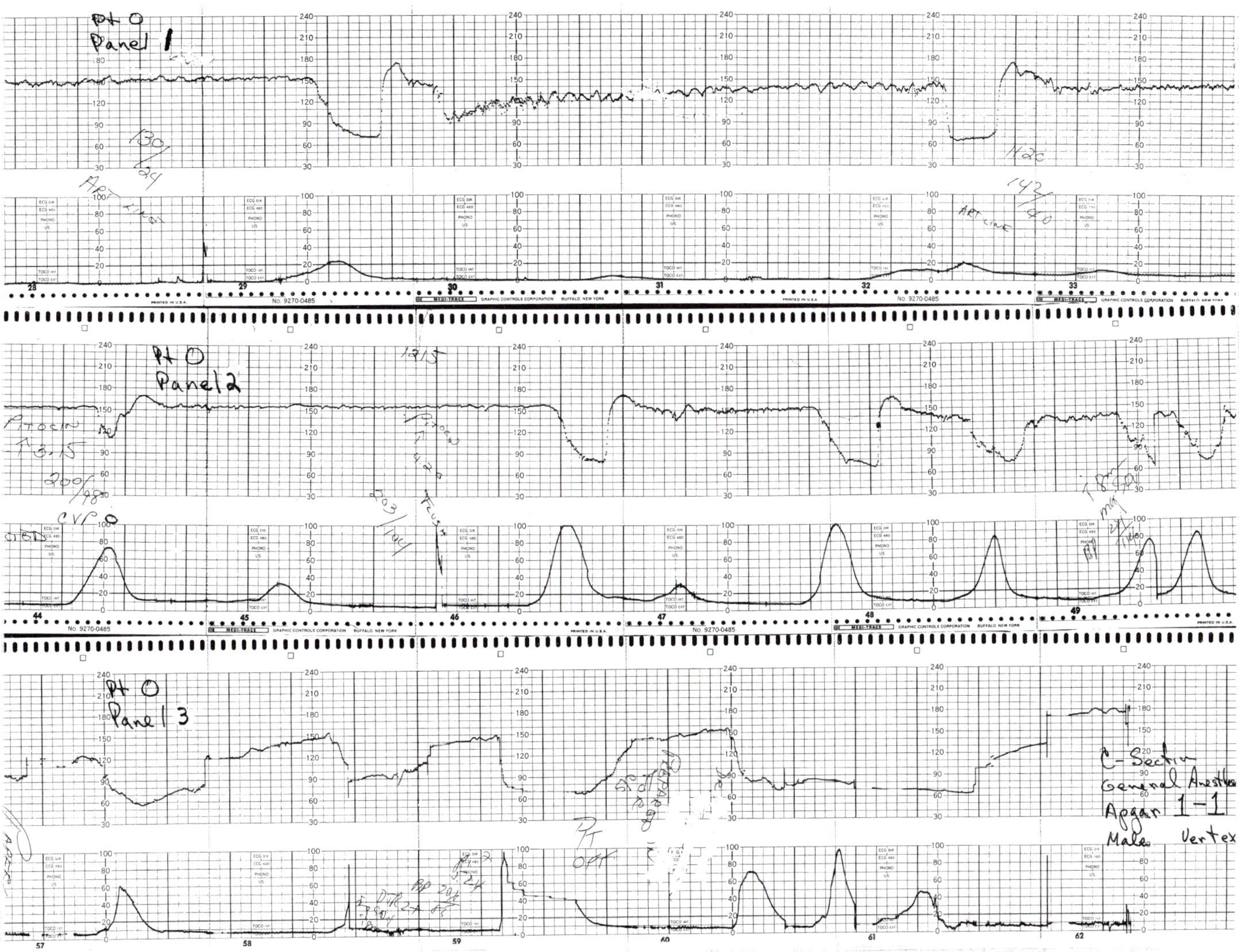

Figure 6.22. Severe variable decelerations are seen throughout these three panels. The blunted (rounded and not abrupt) accelerations seen following the decelerations are not the usual abrupt acceleration and may represent an overshoot. Variability is progressively lost and decelerations become ominously prolonged. Delivery in this 30-week severe preeclamptic was by cesarean section and a severely depressed neonate with Apgar scores of 1 at 1 minute and 1 at 5 minutes was delivered.

variable decelerations can be tolerated. This is true as long as the baseline heart rate is not rising and moderate variability is maintained (Fig. 6.14). Because cord compression is more frequent in the second stage and is likely to be more severe, having to deal with this issue in practice is a very common problem. To what extent head compression is involved in the production of these decelerations is not totally clear; however, the depth and progression of many of these decelerations do make it clear that cord compression is the main component, and referring to these second-stage decelerations as early deceleration is inappropriate. If loss of variability and an increasing baseline develop with the more severe second-stage variable decelerations, expeditious delivery definitely becomes warranted (Fig. 6.23).

Prolonged Decelerations

Prolonged decelerations are isolated decelerations lasting more than 2 minutes. A prolonged deceleration that then lasts more than 10 minutes becomes bradycardia. In either case, these are difficult to classify in terms of pathophysiology because they may be seen in a multitude of situations. As might be expected, cord compression can cause prolonged decelerations. This

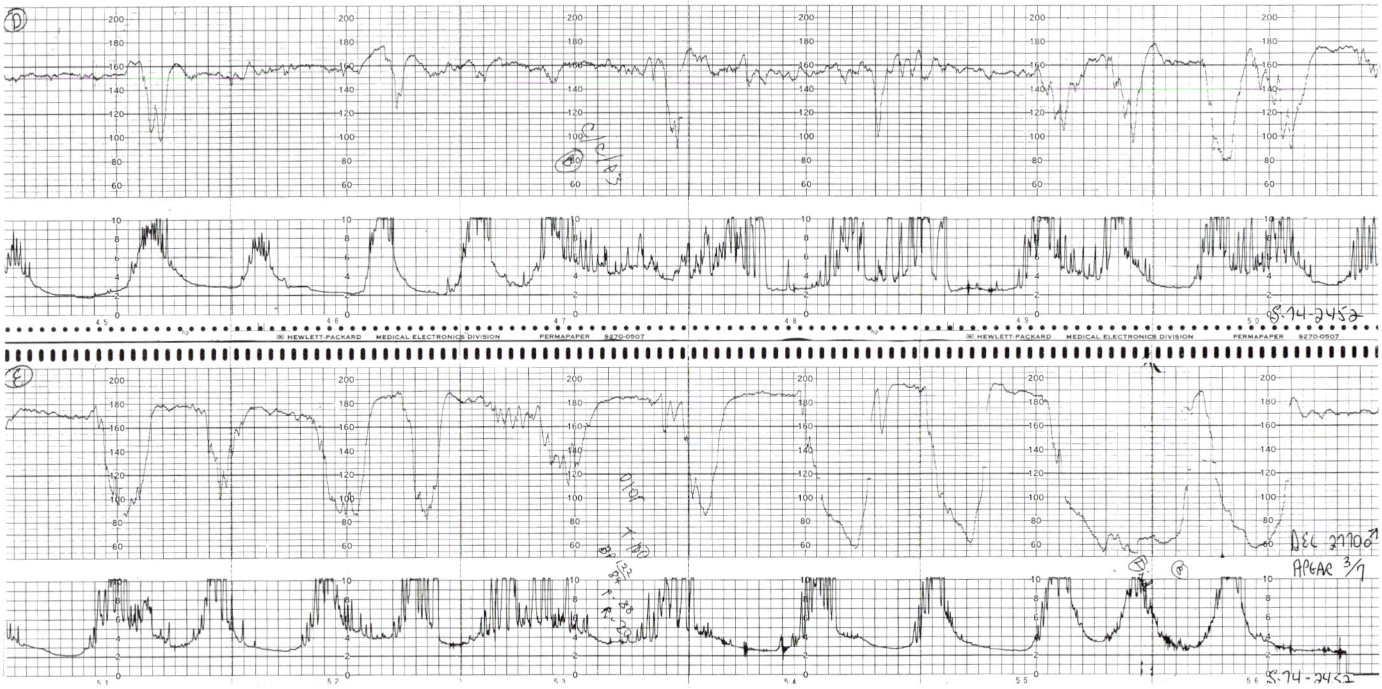

Figure 6.23. The patient is being monitored with an internal electrode and intrauterine catheter. There is a rapid progression of variable decelerations from mild to severe. The baseline heart rate rises from 150 beats per minute (bpm) at the beginning to 190 bpm. The heart rate variability is normal at the beginning of the tracing but is markedly decreased just before delivery. The patient was delivered by low forceps of a 2770-g male with Apgar scores of 3 at 1 minute and 7 at 5 minutes and a single loop of tight nuchal cord.

is generally seen either with the progression of severe variable deceleration or with sudden occult cord prolapse (Fig. 6.24) but may also occur solely as recurrent prolonged decelerations. Profound placental insufficiency may cause prolonged decelerations. This is most characteristically seen with hypotension from the supine position or following epidural or spinal anesthesia (Fig. 6.25).

Hypertonic or tetanic uterine contractions may precipitate UPI-induced prolonged decelerations (Fig. 6.26). Tetanic uterine contractions can be seen with oxytocin, breast hyperstimulation, abruptio placenta, or with uterine artery vasospasm. Cocaine ingestion has been implicated in the development of vasospasm and abruptio placenta. Maternal hypoxia causing such decelerations might be seen with seizures, respiratory depression secondary to a high-spinal anesthetic, or following an overdose of narcotics or magnesium sulfate. Frequently, prolonged decelerations of the FHR, especially when the duration is

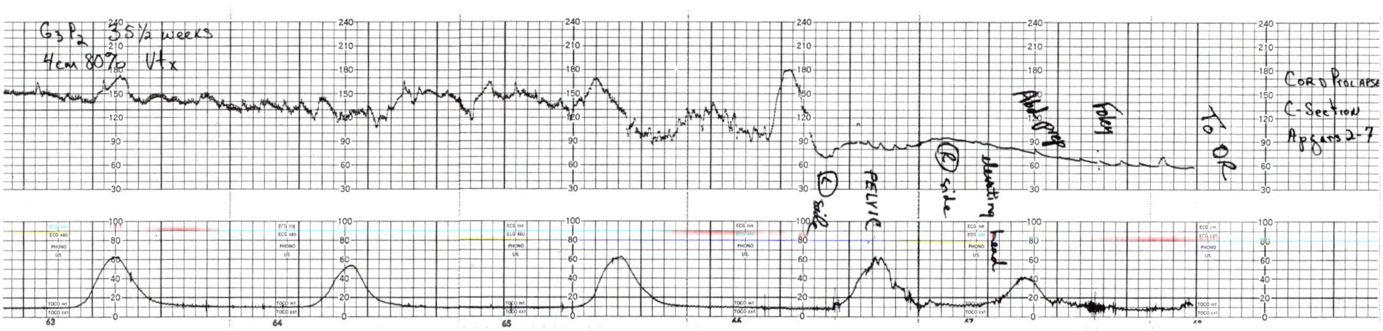

Figure 6.24. A sudden prolonged deceleration is seen in this patient in the early active phase of labor. An immediate pelvic examination revealed cord prolapse, and a cesarean section was performed.

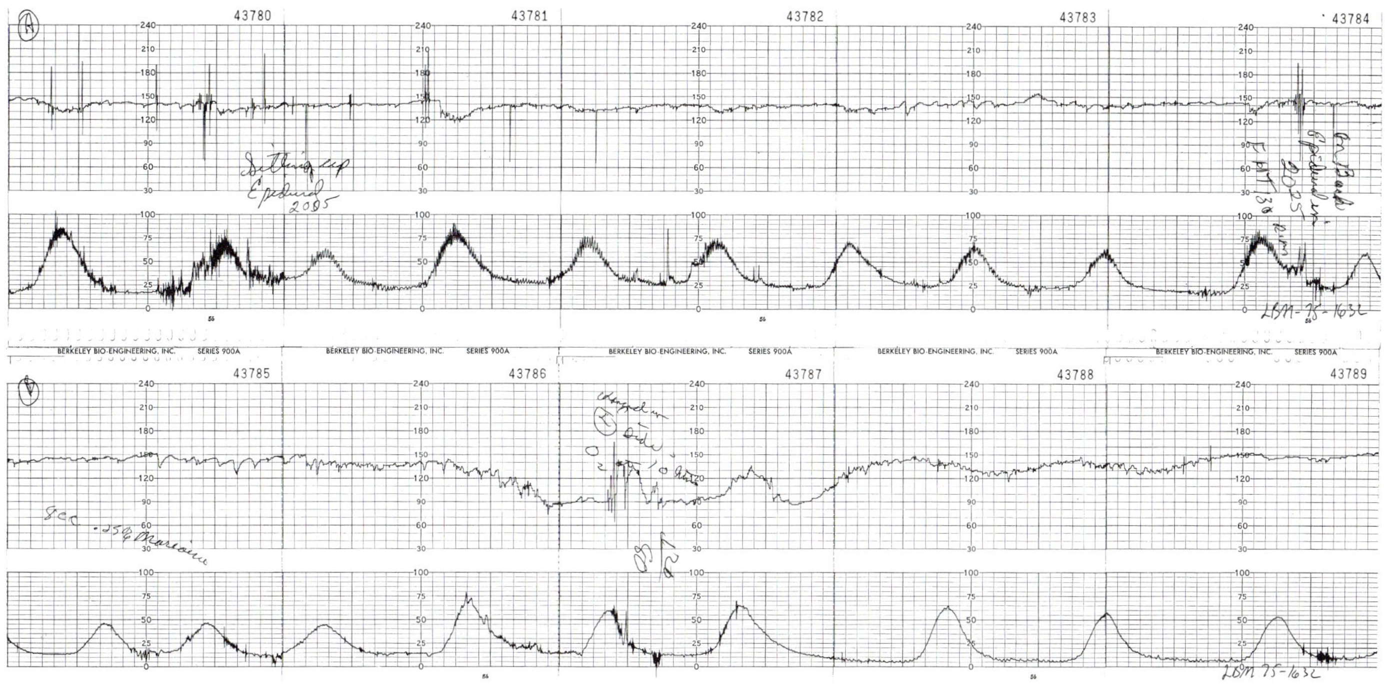

Figure 6.25. A prolonged deceleration is seen after injection of epidural anesthesia with Marcaine. This is followed by several late decelerations, often seen following such epidural-induced decelerations. The pattern subsequently returned to normal and a vigorous newborn was delivered vaginally.

more than 4 to 5 minutes, are associated with rebound tachycardia and loss of variability (Fig. 6.27). This may be because of the release of fetal epinephrine or may reflect some degree of fetal CNS depression or injury. If the original insult does not recur immediately, and the fetus was well-oxygenated before the insult, the placenta is very effective in resuscitating the fetus. Generally, allowing placental resuscitation is a better choice than operative intervention in these situations. The loss of variability and tachycardia are not necessarily prognostically ominous because the insult may no longer be present and the placenta can effectively restore the fetus to its normal well-oxygenated state. Occasionally, in addition to the loss of variability and tachycardia seen after such prolonged decelerations, there may be a period of late decelerations. These usually clear spontaneously with *in-utero* recovery of the fetus.

Prolonged decelerations may not always return to baseline. When seen following a protracted course of severe variable decelerations or a prolonged period of recurrent late decelerations, such a prolonged deceleration

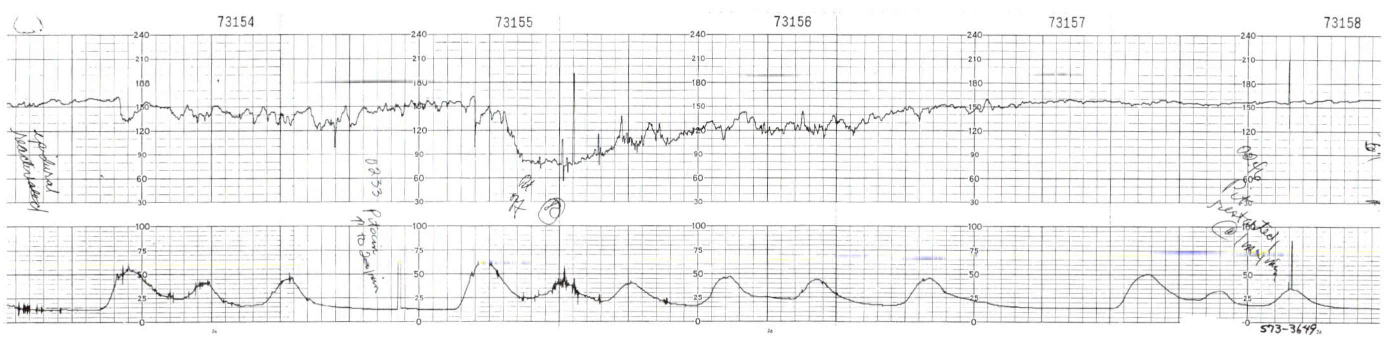

Figure 6.26. Here a prolonged deceleration is seen associated with excessive uterine activity secondary to oxytocin hyperstimulation. Again, a rebound tachycardia with decreased variability follows the prolonged deceleration. Pitocin was stopped and restarted at a lower rate and the heart rate subsequently returned to normal.

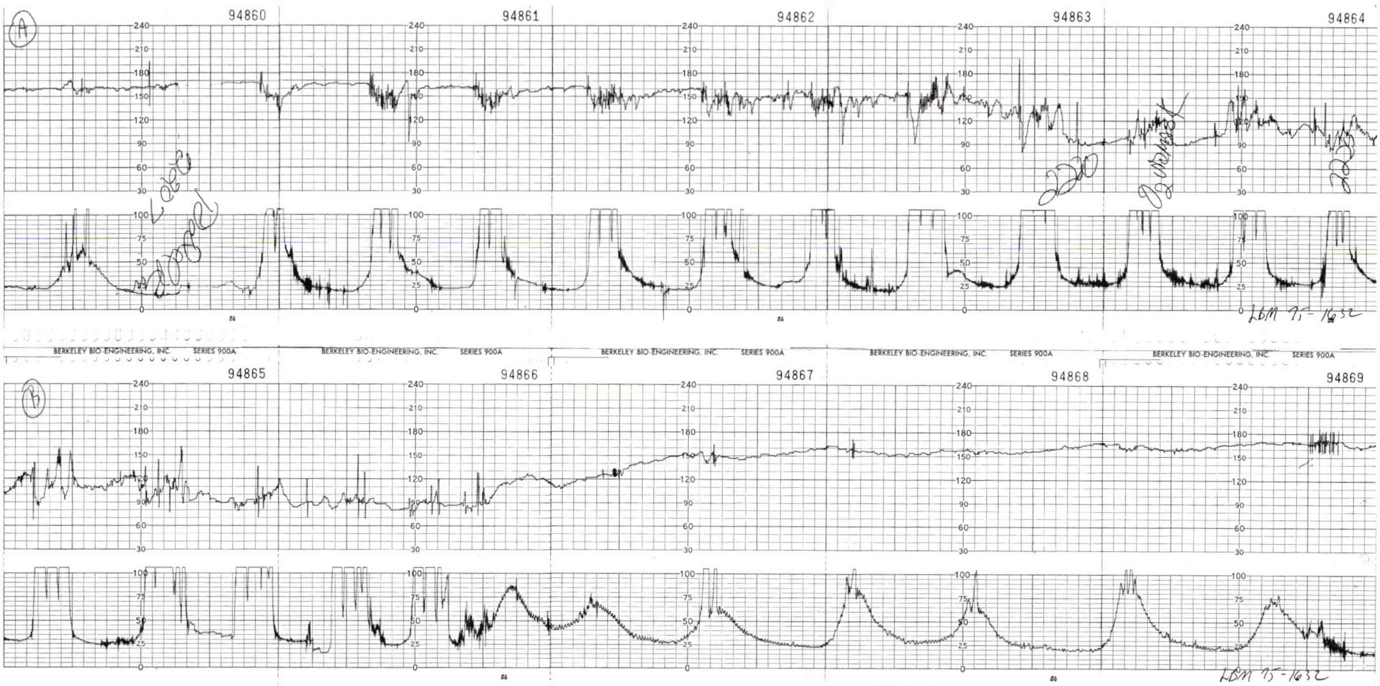

Figure 6.27. A prolonged deceleration from a baseline heart rate of 160 to 90 beats per minute (bpm) is seen lasting 12 minutes in the second stage of labor. An apparent cause is not present. Tachycardia to 170 bpm and decreased variability are seen after this deceleration. Also, some subtle late decelerations are probably present during this time. Again, the heart rate pattern returned to normal. No further significant decelerations recurred and a vaginal delivery of an Apgar 7 infant occurred approximately 15 minutes later.

may occur just before fetal death (Fig. 6.28). Recurrent prolonged decelerations without apparent etiology probably represent cord compression and are the most difficult of all patterns to manage. This is because one cannot prognosticate fetal tolerance based on previous performance of the FHR in labor or on such parameters of the FHR as variability. Such prolonged decelerations may just continue to recur, and prolonged cord compression may cause fetal death.

There are a few other, more benign, causes of prolonged declarations that merely represent an active fetal vagus nerve and not fetal hypoxia. Occasionally, such decelerations are associated with the pelvic examination (Fig. 6.29), application of scalp electrode, rapid descent of the fetus through the birth canal (Fig. 6.30), or with sustained maternal Valsalva maneuver (Fig. 6.31). Such decelerations generally do not last more than a few minutes and are not usually followed by tachycardia or loss of variability.

Accelerations

Because periodic changes are defined as transient changes above and below the baseline, accelerations are the counterpart of decelerations. The frequency and amplitude of acceleration increase with gestational age. At 32 weeks and beyond, acceleration is defined as an abrupt increase in FHR of 15 bpm lasting at least 15 seconds from the onset to return to baseline. Below 32 weeks, the threshold is 10 bpm with a 10-second duration, though controversy exists on how frequently these accelerations are absent in normal fetuses during the 24- to 28-week range.[12] Accelerations of the FHR occur most commonly in the antepartum period, in early labor, and in association with variable decelerations. There are at least two physiologic mechanisms responsible for accelerations. Accelerations associated with fetal movement or uterine contractions (Fig. 6.32) seem to have the same significance as FHR variability in that their presence represents fetal alertness or arousal states. The other cause of accelerations seems to be partial umbilical cord occlusion. If the low-pressure umbilical vein is compressed and the higher pressure umbilical artery remains patent, a period of decreased placental return and fetal hypotension results in baroreceptor response. The normal baroreceptor response to hypotension or decreased cardiac return is an increase in heart rate, with a resultant acceleration.

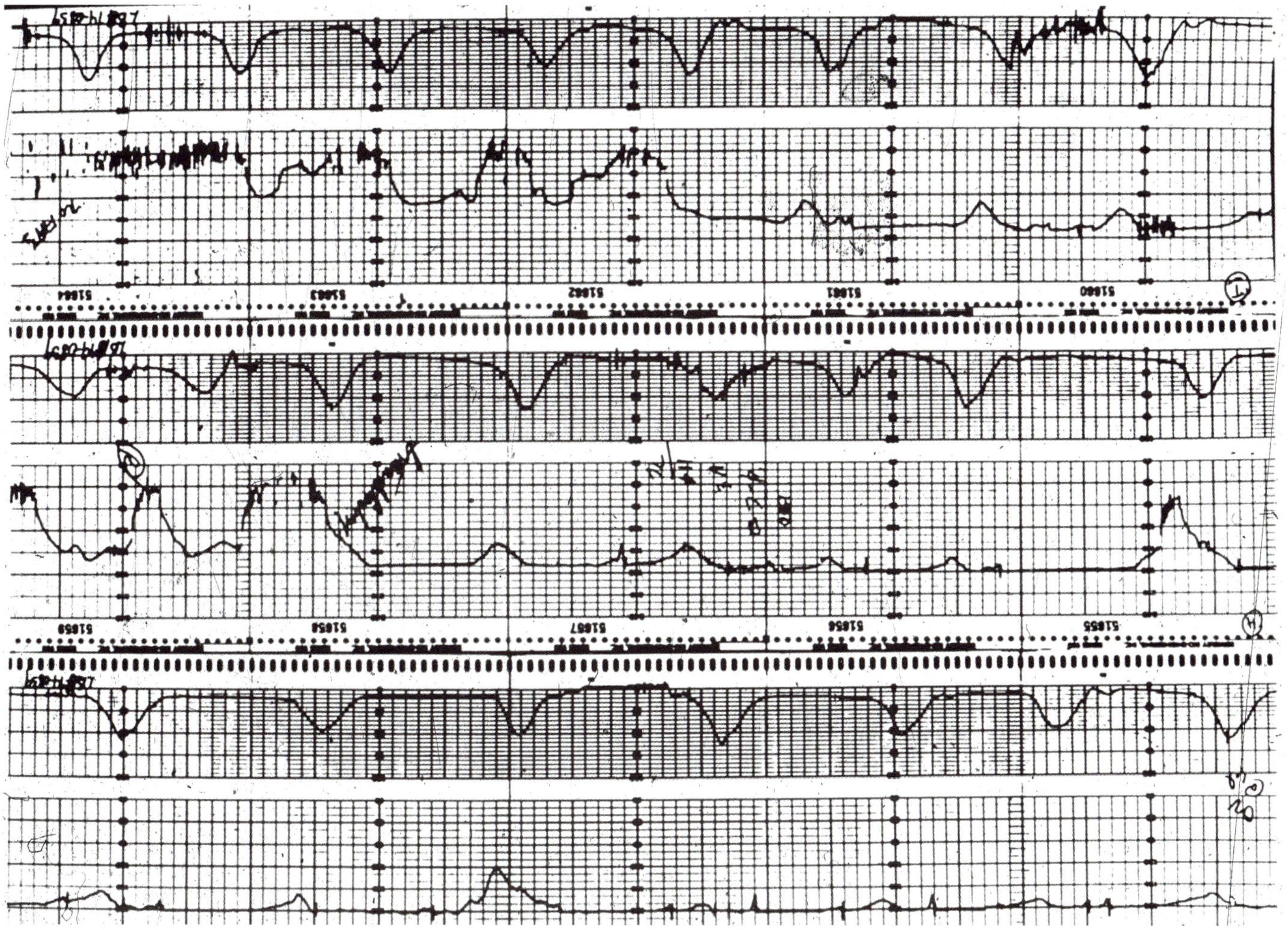

Figure 6.28. This fetus in labor is having recurrent late decelerations with absent variability and tachycardia. At the end of the strip, a terminal bradycardia is seen immediately preceding the demise of the fetus.

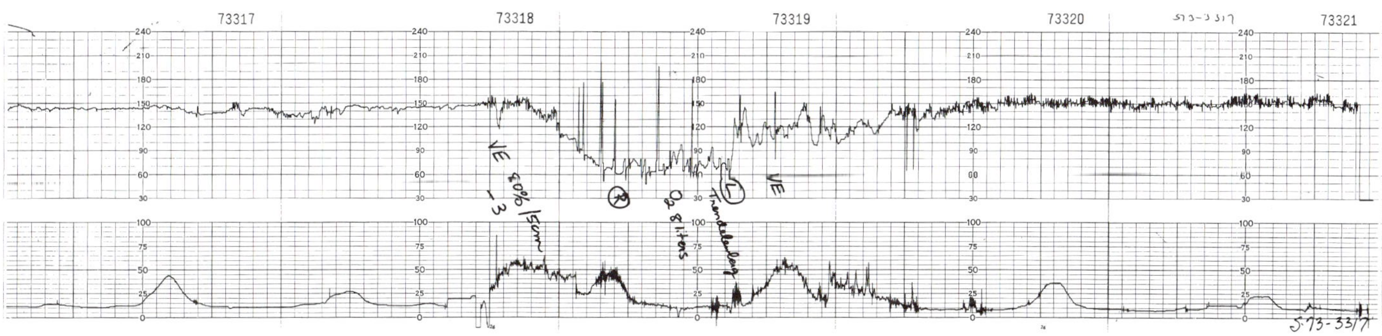

Figure 6.29. A prolonged deceleration is seen after a pelvic examination. Also, note the uterine hyperactivity commonly seen following a pelvic examination (Ferguson reflex?). This probably represents a fetus with an active vagal reflex.

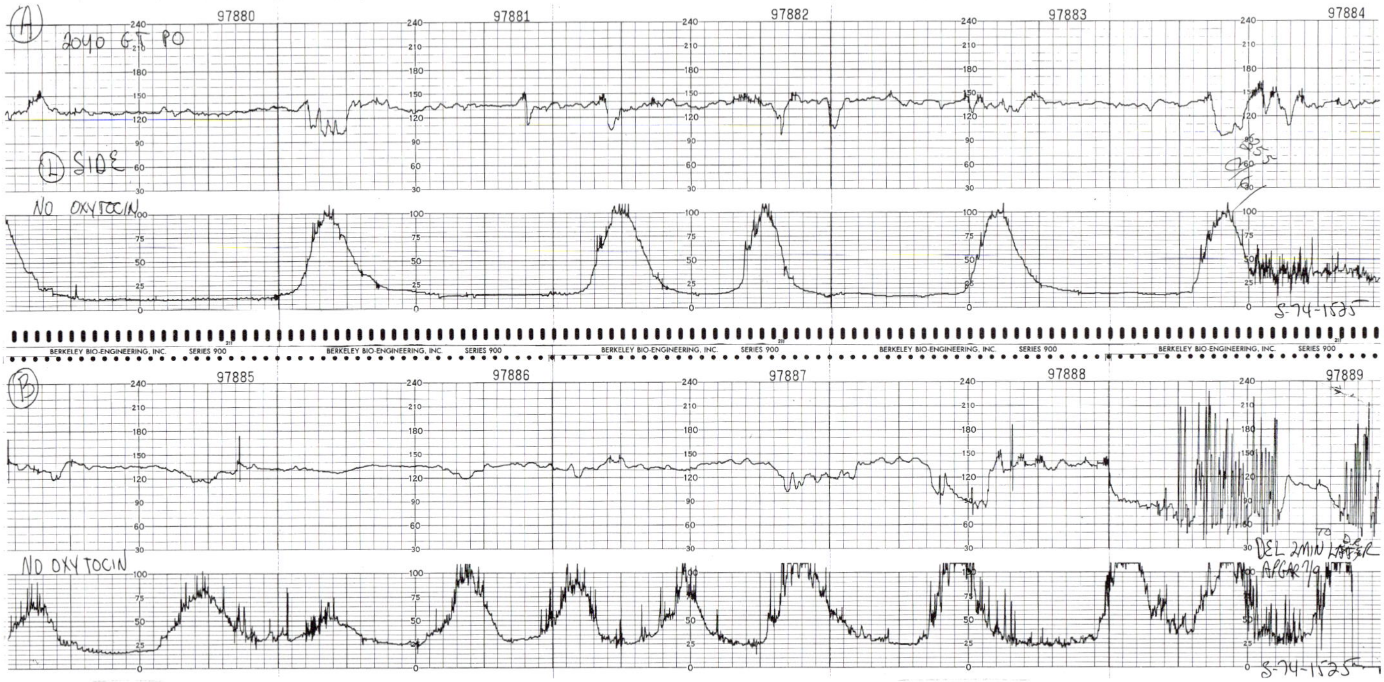

Figure 6.30. In this case, a prolonged deceleration is seen at the end of **Panel B**. This patient progressed rapidly from 6 cm at the end of **Panel A** to delivery 2 minutes after the end of **Panel B**. Such prolonged decelerations should incite the performance of a pelvic examination, not only to rule out cord prolapse, but as is often the case, to check for rapid descent as occurred here.

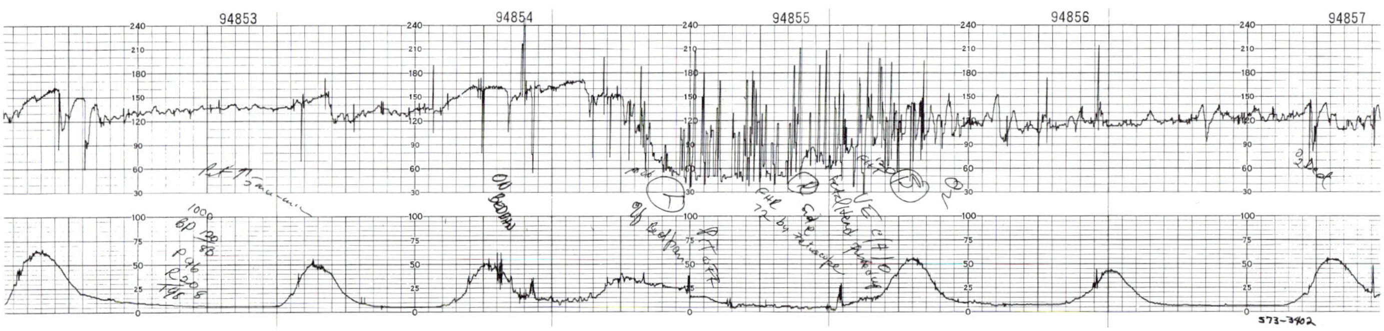

Figure 6.31. Here, a prolonged deceleration occurs while the patient is on a bedpan. Again, a fetal vagal reflex may cause decelerations with maternal Valsalva.

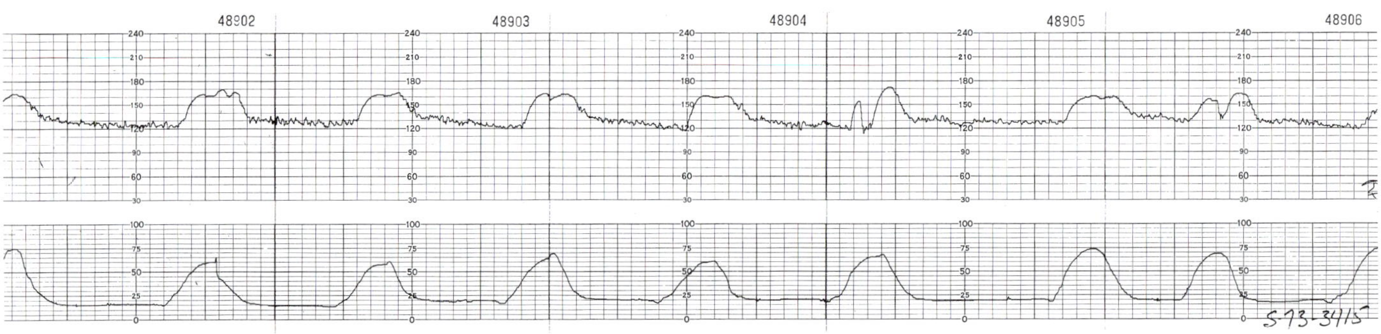

Figure 6.32. Accelerations of the fetal heart rate are seen with each contraction. Baseline heart rate and variability are normal. Such a pattern indicates a normal fetal pH.

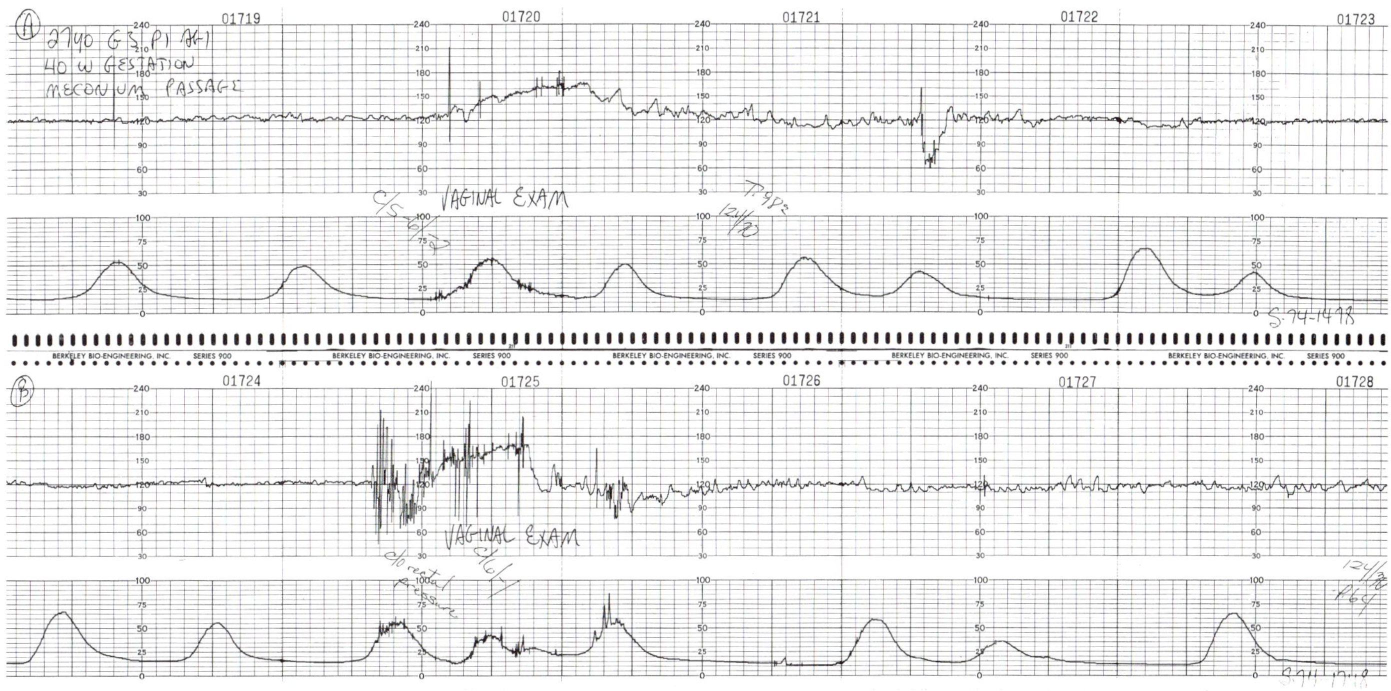

Figure 6.33. Just as a vaginal examination may precipitate prolonged deceleration (Fig. 6.30A), a vaginal examination may stimulate the fetal heart rate to accelerate as occurs in both panels.

The presence of FHR accelerations in the intrapartum period indicates the absence of acidosis. Hypoxia with a normal pH may or may not result in the loss of accelerations. These accelerations may occur with contractions, fetal movement, or without apparent stimulus. In addition, as with decelerations, accelerations may be seen in response to pelvic examination and stimulation of the fetal head (Fig. 6.33). Virtually all of these accelerations are associated with fetal movement. Indeed, as described in Chapter 8, accelerations with intrapartum pelvic examination or fetal scalp stimulation reflect normal fetal pH. This is the rationale for using spontaneous or stimulus-produced accelerations in the presence of FHR patterns with concerning decelerations and/or decreased variability to reassure the clinician that the baby is neither depressed nor acidotic. It cannot be emphasized enough, however, that the absence of FHR accelerations in the intrapartum period is not in and of itself alarming as long as variability is normal and there are no deceleration patterns indicative of possible fetal hypoxia. Thus in labor, fetuses are often inactive, and long periods with the absence of accelerations occur that do not, in and of themselves, constitute a concerning scenario. One other problem created by accelerations of the FHR is that, at times, it is difficult to be sure whether one is dealing with decelerations or with accelerations with return to baseline (Fig. 6.34). This is especially true in the beginning of the monitoring period when the baseline has not been established. This is an important practical problem because there may be cases of misinterpretation with intervention for fetal distress when, in reality, there were no decelerations but rather accelerations mistaken for baseline heart rate and return to baseline mistaken for decelerations. There are three clues to help avoid this difficulty. First, accelerations and decelerations are rounded at their peak, whereas the baseline tends to be flat. Second, with accelerations especially, there is usually a period preceding or following without periodic changes when the baseline may be more clearly determined. Third, accelerations are almost always associated with fetal movement that can be documented by patient symptoms, palpation, or ultrasound.

Unusual Patterns

Sinusoidal Pattern

Originally described in separate reports from Shenker[19] in 1973 and Kubli et al[20] in 1972, the sinusoidal FHR is a rare but distinct baseline pattern. Observed in antepartum, intrapartum, and neonatal FHR monitoring,

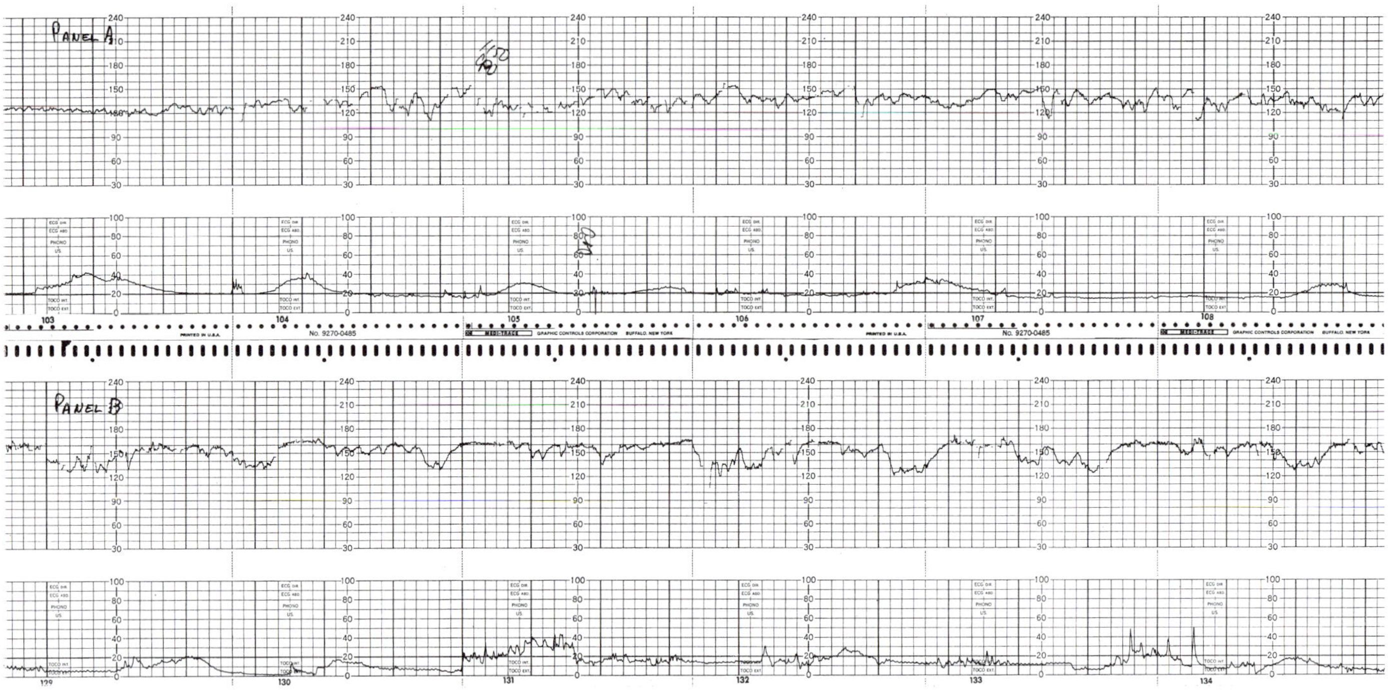

Figure 6.34. In **Panel B**, accelerations with a return to baseline could easily be confused for late decelerations. Looking back at **Panel A**, it can be seen that the real baseline heart rate is 120 to 130 beats per minute. Also, note that the return to baseline tends to be flat rather than rounded at the nadir as late decelerations would be.

this pattern is strongly associated with fetal hypoxemia, often resulting from severe fetal anemia (Fig. 6.35). This fetal anemia may result from Rh sensitization, fetal-maternal hemorrhage, or *in-utero* fetal hemorrhage and has an associated increased perinatal morbidity and mortality. The sinusoidal FHR pattern has been reported following the intrapartum administration of analgesics such as butorphanol (Stadol)[21] and meperidine (Demerol),[22] in association with chorioamnionitis.[23] In the absence of acidosis or anemia, sinusoidal heart rate following analgesic administration does not appear to have an ominous significance for the fetus, and the mechanism of this heart rate change is unclear. Many times, benign FHR patterns with increased LTV may be easily confused with sinusoidal patterns (Fig. 6.36).

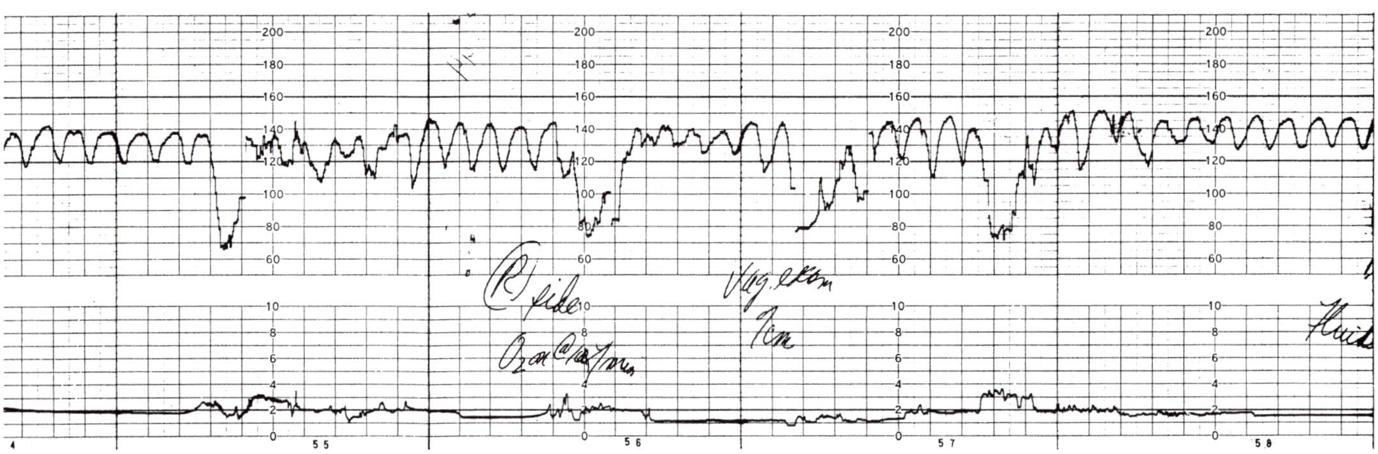

Figure 6.35. Intrapartum sinusoidal fetal heart rate pattern. There are also moderate variable decelerations present. (From Klavin M, Laver A, Boscola M. *Clinical Concepts of FHR Monitoring.* Hewlett-Packard Co., 1977:106, with permission.)

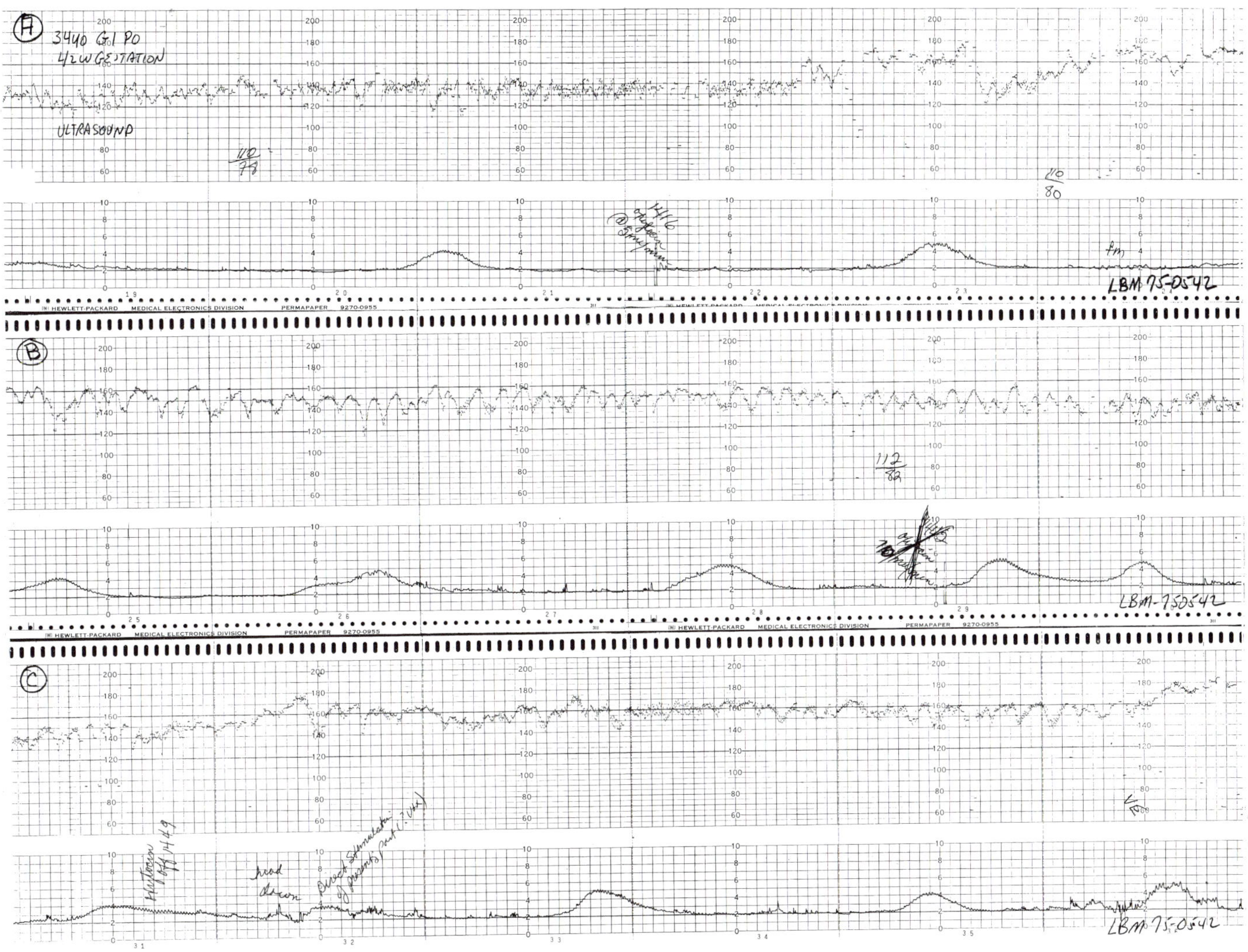

Figure 6.36. As seen in **Panel B**, exaggerated long-term variability may resemble sinusoidal heart rate patterns. The presence of short-term variability within the pattern and the normal patterns before and after **Panel B** distinguish this pseudosinusoidal pattern from a true sinusoidal one.

The ability to correctly recognize and manage a sinusoidal pattern unrelated to previous analgesia use is of critical importance, as the presence of sinusoidal heart rate alone qualifies as a category III tracing. It is a visually distinct, smooth, sine wave-like undulating pattern in the FHR baseline with a cycle frequency of 3 to 5 per minute that persists for 20 minutes. The amplitude is typically 5 to 15 bpm.[24]

The exact pathophysiology of sinusoidal heart rate remains unknown. The association of fetal anemia with the sinusoidal heart rate is well documented for the human fetus. Young et al[25] clinically demonstrated an inverse correlation between sinusoidal heart rate amplitude and fetal pH. A derangement of nervous control of the heart secondary to central or peripheral ischemia is hypothesized to result in sinusoidal heart rate. Murata et al[26] have reported in an animal model an association between sinusoidal heart rate and plasma arginine vasopressin concentration. Chemical or surgical vagotomy with a subsequent infusion of arginine vasopressin produces a sinusoidal pattern. Arginine vasopressin is elevated following hemorrhage or acidosis, and perhaps secondary to direct or indirect effects of this hormone on calcium transfer in the sinus node, sinusoidal heart rate results.

Wandering Baseline

A very rare FHR abnormality is seen when it is impossible to establish the baseline. Although falling within the defined normal limits of 120 to 160 bpm, this

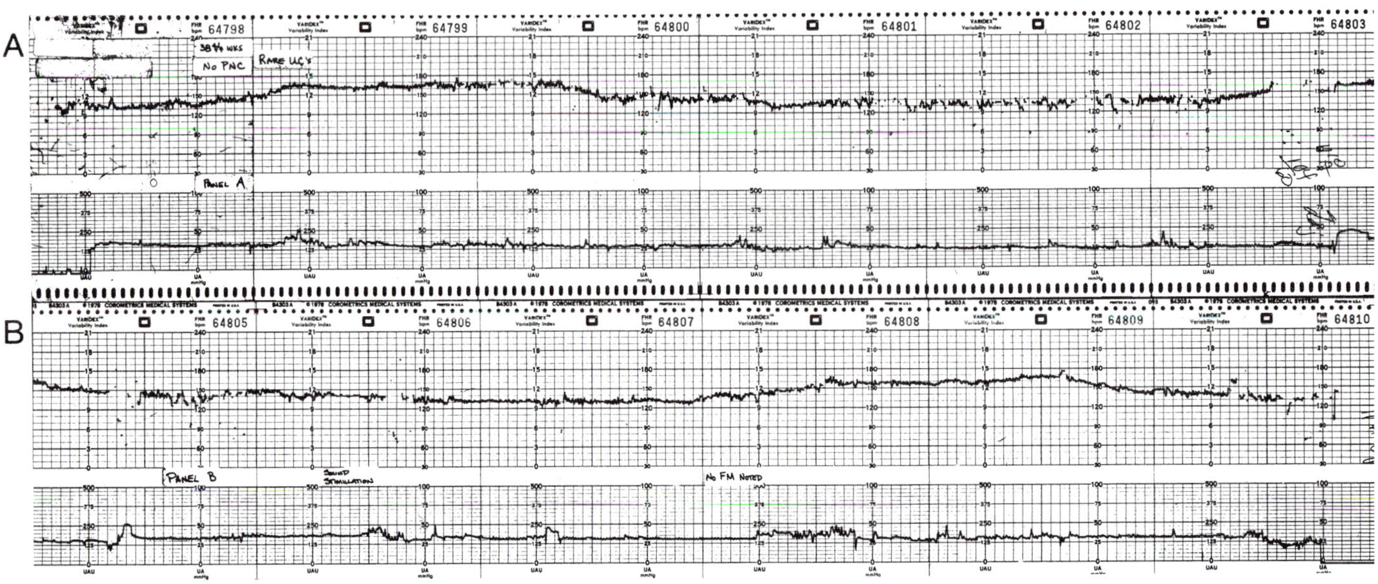

Figure 6.37. As seen in **Panel A**, when evaluated in early labor, this patient was thought to have a prolonged acceleration signifying the absence of fetal acidosis. However, as the monitoring continued, there was no evidence of true reactivity (**Panel B**). The patient stated that fetal movement had been decreased for 2 weeks. A biophysical profile found no evidence of fetal breathing, tone, or movement. Artificial rupture of membranes revealed thick yellow meconium. Subsequently, persistent late decelerations were noted and an emergency cesarean section was performed. The infant was depressed (Apgar scores 2 and 3 at 1 and 5 minutes) but not acidotic (umbilical pH 7.30). Seizure activity was noted in the delivery room. A head computed tomography scan and ultrasound revealed a large cystic area in the left brain consistent with a porencephalic cyst. This example of a wandering baseline resulted from significant preexisting central nervous system insult.

baseline wanders and does not remain steady. This rare abnormality is seen in the absence of STV and is highly suggestive of a neurologically abnormal fetus. This wandering baseline will occasionally be seen as a preterminal event (Fig. 6.37).

CONCLUSION

A knowledge of the physiology and pathophysiology of the FHR, coupled with experience in pattern recognition, is essential for the appropriate use of electronic FHR monitoring. Pattern recognition is a process of recognizing FHR changes, such as decelerations, that suggest the type of pathophysiologic process occurring, determining how the fetus is tolerating that process at any given moment by such parameters as variability and baseline heart rate, and prognosticating how long such a process might be allowed to continue without significant fetal depression or damage by the severity, repetitiveness, and duration of the pattern. Unfortunately, such a process is difficult to analyze quantitatively, making the task of pattern recognition and integration all the more important.

REFERENCES

1. National Institutes of Child Health and Human Development Research Planning Workshop. Electronic fetal heart rate monitoring: research guidelines for interpretation. *Am J Obstet Gynecol.* 1997;177(6):1385-1390.
2. Macones GA, Hankins GD, Spong CY, Hauth J, Moore T. The 2008 National Institute of Child Health and Human Development workshop report on electronic fetal monitoring: update on definitions, interpretation, and research guidelines. *Obstet Gynecol.* 2008;112(3):661-666.
3. Young B, Katz M, Klein S, Silverman F. Fetal blood and tissue pH with moderate bradycardia. *Am J Obstet Gynecol.* 1979;135(1):45-47.
4. Shenker L. Fetal cardiac arrhythmias. *Obstet Gynecol Surv.* 1979;34(8):561-572.
5. Dildy GA, Loucks CA, Clark SL. Intrapartum fetal pulse oximetry in the presence of fetal cardiac arrhythmia. *Am J Obstet Gynecol.* 1993;169(6):1609-1611.
6. Marsh TD, Lagrew DC, Cook LN, Lavery JP. Unexplained fetal baseline bradycardia in congenital panhypopituitarism. *Am J Obstet Gynecol.* 1987;156(4):977-979.
7. Druzin ML, Ikenoue T, Murata Y, Socol M, Martin CB. A possible mechanism for the increase in fetal heart rate variability following hypoxemia. Presented at the *Society for Gynecologic Investigation*, San Diego, California, 1979.

8. Paul RH, Suidan AK, Yeh SY, Schifrin BS, Hon EH. Clinical fetal monitoring. VII. The evaluation and significance of intrapartum baseline FHR variability. *Am J Obstet Gynecol.* 1975;123(2): 206-210.
9. Bowes W, Gabbe S, Bowes C. Fetal heart rate monitoring in premature infants weighing 1500 grams or less. *Am J Obstet Gynecol.* 1980;137(7):791-796.
10. Garite TJ, Linzey EM, Freeman RK, Dorchester W. Fetal heart rate patterns and fetal distress in fetuses with congenital anomalies. *Obstet Gynecol.* 1979;53(6):716-720.
11. Cahill AG, Tuuli MG, Stout MJ, López JD, Macones GA. A prospective cohort study of fetal heart rate monitoring: deceleration area is predictive of fetal acidemia. *Am J Obstet Gynecol.* 2018;218(5): 523.e1-523.e12.
12. Hurtado-Sanchez MF, Perez-Melero D, Pinto-Ibanez A, González-Mesa E, Mozas-Moreno J, Puertas-Prieto A. Characteristics of heart rate tracings in preterm fetuses. *Medicina.* 2021;57(6):528.
13. Vintizileos AM, Campbell WA, Nochimson DJ, Weinbaum PJ. Degree of oligohydramnios and pregnancy outcome in patients with premature rupture of membranes. *Obstet Gynecol.* 1985;66(2):165-167.
14. Gamboa SM, Moros ML, Mancho JP, Moros CL, Mateo SC. Deceleration area and fetal acidemia. *J Matern Fetal Neonatal Med.* 2017;30(21): 2578-2584.
15. Kubli FW, Hon EH, Khazin AE, Takemura H. Observations on heart rate and pH in the human fetus during labor. *Am J Obstet Gynecol.* 1969;104(8):1190-1206.
16. Hamilton E, Warrick P, O'Keeffe D. Variable decelerations: do size and shape matter? *J Matern Fetal Neonatal Med.* 2012;25(6): 648-653.
17. Henigsman S, Garite T, Patillo C, Brewster W. Fetal pulse oximetry defines which variable decelerations with slow return to baseline are associated with hypoxia. *Am J Obstet Gynecol.* 2001;185:S131.
18. Goodlin RC, Lowe EW. A functional umbilical cord occlusion heart rate pattern: the significance of overshoot. *Obstet Gynecol.* 1974;43(1):22-30.
19. Shenker L. Clinical experience with fetal heart rate monitoring of 1000 patients in labor. *Am J Obstet Gynecol.* 1973;115(8): 1111-1116.
20. Kubli F, Ruttgers H, Haller U, Bogdan C, Ramzin M. Die antepartale fetale Herzfrequenz. II. Verhalten von Grundfrequenz, Fluktuation and Dezerationo bei antepartalem Fruchttod. *Z. Gerburtshilfe Perinatol.* 1972;176:309.
21. Angel J, Knuppel R, Lake M. Sinusoidal fetal heart rate patterns associated with intravenous butorphanol administration. *Am J Obstet Gynecol.* 1984;149(4):465-467.
22. Epstein H, Waxman A, Gleicher N, Lauersen NH. Meperidine induced sinusoidal fetal heart rate pattern and reversal with naloxone. *Obstet Gynecol.* 1982;59(6 Suppl):22S-25S.
23. Gleicher N, Runowicz C, Brown B. Sinusoidal fetal heart rate patterns in association with amnionitis. *Obstet Gynecol.* 1980;56(1):109-112.
24. Modanlou H, Freeman RK. Sinusoidal fetal heart rate pattern: its definition and clinical significance. *Am J Obstet Gynecol.* 1982;142(8):1033-1038.
25. Young B, Katz M, Wilson S. Sinusoidal fetal heart rate. I. Clinical significance. *Am J Obstet Gynecol.* 1980;136(5):587-593.
26. Murata Y, Miyake Y, Yamamoto T, et al. Experimentally produced sinusoidal fetal heart rate pattern in the chronically instrumented fetal lamb. *Am J Obstet Gynecol.* 1985;153(6):693.

CHAPTER 7

Umbilical Cord Blood Gases to Assess Fetal Condition at Birth

Rachel Wiley and Suneet Chauhan

The assessment of the fetal condition at birth was traditionally restricted to the Apgar score. It is interesting to note that this score, proposed originally by its namesake, Virginia Apgar, an anesthesiologist, was developed primarily to assess the need for newborn resuscitation.[1] However, as investigators became interested in the influence of the process of labor and delivery on the long-term development of affected newborns, investigators began to assess the utility of the Apgar score in predicting adverse neurologic development. It became apparent that low Apgar scores, except in the extreme, had little predictive ability for such adverse outcomes. For example, an Apgar score of 0 to 3 at 5 minutes only increases the risk of cerebral palsy (CP) by 1%, whereas with an Apgar score of 0 to 3 even at 10 minutes, 90% of children did not develop CP.[2,3] This should not be surprising as the primary complications in term babies, which are likely to adversely affect the long-term development of the brain, are hypoxia and acidosis (perinatal asphyxia). However, a low Apgar score is only a reflection of neurologic depression, of which acidosis may certainly be one cause, but is far from the only cause.

Other causes of newborn depression include drugs or anesthetic agents; anomalies affecting the fetal brain, lungs, airway, or heart; airway obstruction; sepsis; pulmonary hypoplasia; and even the resuscitation process itself, as with intubation and suctioning for meconium. Thus, there is an alternative for assessing the fetus at birth and that is the evaluation of umbilical cord blood gases. The assessment of the fetus for the presence, absence, and degree of acidosis at birth is not only potentially useful for the prediction of short- and long-term sequelae but also has other important implications. For the depressed baby who is not acidotic, it guides the pediatrician to look for other causes of depression. If the baby is acidotic, it will assist the pediatrician in tailoring resuscitative efforts. For the obstetrician, the assessment of umbilical blood gases will help, at least in retrospect, with the interpretation of the fetal heart rate (FHR) tracing, as will be discussed later in this chapter. In the case of a baby who later develops any neurologic dysfunction, the cord blood gases can be used to refute or confirm the possibility of perinatal asphyxia as a contributing cause, and this has implications for the treating neurologist as well as medical legal significance. Thus, the evaluation of umbilical cord blood gases has become an important and common method for evaluating a depressed baby at birth.

PHYSIOLOGY OF FETAL ACID-BASE BALANCE

pH is a logarithmic representation of the quantity of hydrogen ions in a fluid. In humans, it is critical that hydrogen ions are kept in a close balance both by the rate of production and by a process of either conversion or buffering with substances in blood and tissue, which prevents excess hydrogen ions from doing harm. The major buffers in blood are hemoglobin and bicarbonate. Hemoglobin essentially absorbs hydrogen ions and has a finite capacity to simply absorb acid and carry it to the kidneys where it can be excreted. In the fetus, the kidney's ability to excrete acid is relatively immature, and therefore, its role in acid buffering is minimal once the hemoglobin capacity has been saturated. The other major method of buffering excess H^+ is by the conversion of bicarbonate to carbonic acid (H_2CO_3) by the following formula:

$$H^+ + CO_2 \leftrightarrow H_2CO_3 \leftrightarrow CO_2 + H_2O$$

Under normal circumstances, the metabolism of sugars produces carbon dioxide (CO_2) and water, and CO_2 produced by the fetus is eliminated across the placenta. Under conditions of hypoxia, as with the adult, the fetus converts energy with a process known as anaerobic metabolism, which involves the conversion of sugars and fatty acids into pyruvic and lactic acids resulting in excess H^+ ion production and a lowering of the pH. To prevent harm from these hydrogen ions to cells, tissues, and organs, these excess H^+ ions must be buffered by the mechanisms described above. As the pH drops during such anaerobic metabolism, the shift in the equation results in reduced bicarbonate and loss of this buffering capacity. Thus, the H^+ content increases (a drop in pH), and when this falls out of the normally very tight range of safe pH, an *acidosis* results. This type of acidosis resulting from an increased production of hydrogen ions by anaerobic metabolism (or by the direct production of other organic acids as in diabetic ketoacidosis) is called *metabolic acidosis*. Both hydrogen ions and the bicarbonate that buffers them are highly charged ions and move very slowly across the placenta. Thus, with metabolic acidosis, the placenta's ability to clear hydrogen ions from the fetus or replenish bicarbonate from the mother is a relatively slow process, and a significant metabolic acidosis, when it is finally resolved, will take many hours for the placenta alone to reverse it.

The other type of acidosis seen in the fetus is known as *respiratory acidosis*. This results from an inability to clear from the bloodstream the normally produced CO_2. In the fetus, the putative etiology for this is compression or other reduction in flow in the umbilical cord vessels; although if the mother develops a respiratory acidosis, the fetus will accumulate more CO_2, and the gradient is changed as well. The fetus, as with the adult, produces CO_2 as a result of oxidative metabolism of sugars and fatty acids under normal well-oxygenated circumstances. The CO_2 produced by the fetus cannot be eliminated, as in the adult, through the lungs, so it is eliminated through the placenta into the maternal circulation and out of the maternal respiratory tract. As long as there is normal umbilical blood flow, placental exchange, and maternal respiration, the CO_2 diffuses very rapidly across the placenta. Normal umbilical arterial pCO_2 (reflecting that blood exiting the fetus to the placenta) has a value of about 50 mm Hg, whereas the venous pCO_2 exiting the placenta has a value of about 40 mm Hg. This relatively large difference demonstrates how rapidly CO_2 is cleared through the placenta. A respiratory acidosis reflecting retained CO_2 in the fetus, purportedly caused by umbilical cord compression or other obstruction to umbilical blood flow, will clear very rapidly when the compression is released as the CO_2 in the umbilical artery is rapidly diffused across the placenta, the equilibrium of the equation is shifted away from the production of hydrogen ions, and the pH moves toward normal.

When the pH is low, it is important to distinguish between respiratory acidosis and metabolic acidosis; the bicarbonate value that can be measured is not an accurate reflection in and of itself. The concept of base excess or base deficit is used for this purpose. The pH value and the measured pCO_2 are plotted on a curve known as the Siggaard-Andersen nomogram (Fig. 7.1). Now that measurement of the pH and pCO_2 is automated, this calculation is most commonly done on the same instrument that has a computer built in for this purpose. As seen in Figure 7.1, a line is drawn through the pCO_2 (Point E) and the pH (Point A), and the base excess is read from the plot at Point C. The plot is variable based on the fetal hemoglobin concentration, and the base excess is read from the plot. An elevated base excess for an umbilical cord is >–9, and thus a low pH with an elevated base excess would be indicative of a metabolic acidosis and a low pH with a normal base excess would be a respiratory acidosis. In the latter case, the pCO_2 would be elevated, and in the former, the pCO_2 would be normal. A mixed respiratory and metabolic acidosis will have both an elevated base excess and an elevated pCO_2. The clinical picture of the baby at birth with respiratory acidosis, depending on the severity, will be a low 1-minute Apgar score and, following resuscitation, a relatively normal 5-minute Apgar score, as the efforts of resuscitation will clear the elevated CO_2 rapidly and allow the pH to return to normal. A metabolic acidosis, when relatively severe, will be reflected in both low 1- and 5-minute Apgar scores. This is because with resuscitation, only after oxygen (O_2) reaches the cells and tissues is the anaerobic metabolism reversed and buffers are restored that the pH becomes normal, and this process takes considerably longer.

An additional marker that can be used to discern metabolic status at the time of delivery is umbilical cord arterial lactate, however not all laboratories include this as part of a standard umbilical cord gas analysis. As fetal compromise develops, fetal lactate increases early in the hypoxic pathway and persists longer than low fetal pH after normal oxygenation status is restored. Fetal lactate has been shown to be more predictive of neonatal morbidity, however utility is limited by the lack of universality in reporting.[4]

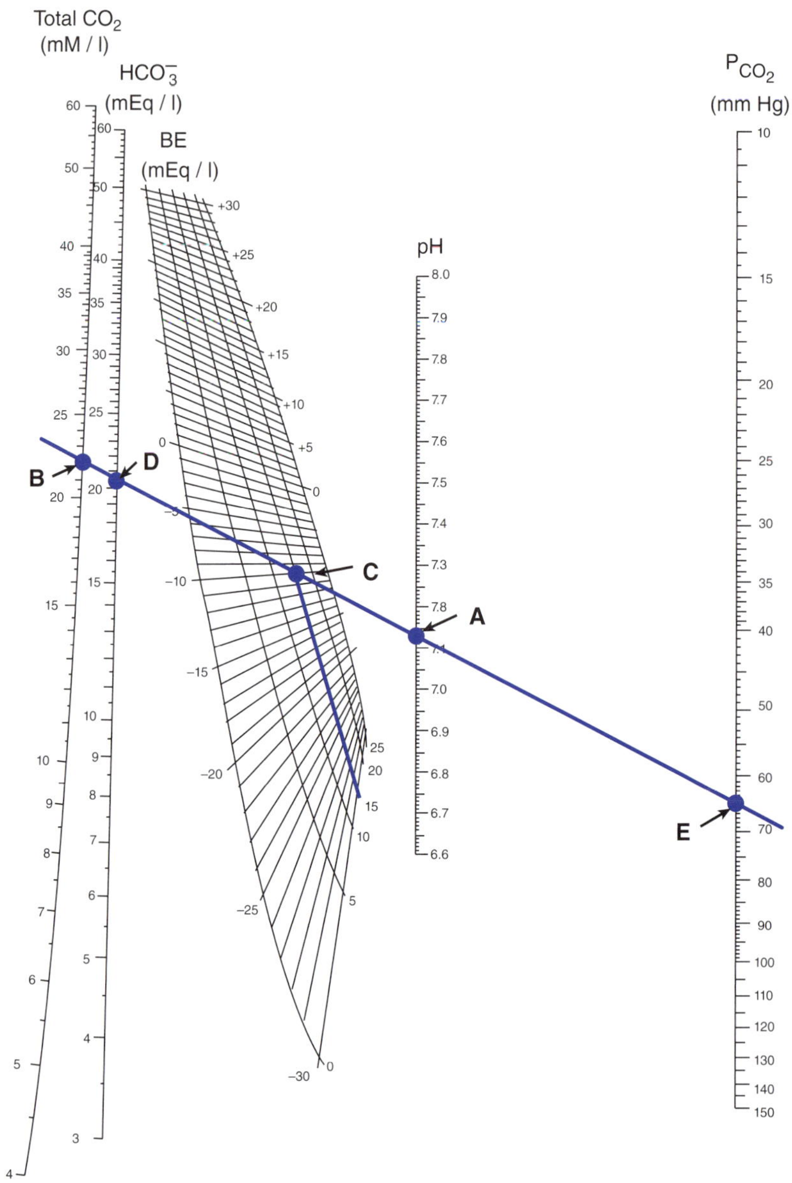

Figure 7.1. This is the Siggaard-Andersen nomogram used to calculate base excess (or base deficit, the negative of base excess). A line is drawn through the pCO_2 (Point E) and the pH (Point A), and the base excess is read from the plot at Point C. The plot is variable based on the fetal hemoglobin concentration, and the base excess is read from the plot.

TABLE 7.1 Terminology used to describe blood gases in the fetus
■ Acidemia—increased H^+ in blood
■ Acidosis—increased H^+ in tissue
■ Asphyxia—hypoxia with metabolic acidosis
■ Base deficit—[HCO_3] below normal
■ Base excess—[HCO_3] above normal (the negative of base deficit)
■ Hypoxemia—decreased O_2 in blood
■ Hypoxia—decreased O_2 in tissue
■ pH—negative log of [H^+]

It is important to review the terminology as this is often confusing, and care must be used to express the status of fetal blood gases and their results as accurately as possible (Table 7.1).

Technique for Obtaining Umbilical Cord Blood Gases

To collect umbilical cord blood for analysis, a doubly clamped segment of the cord is cut away from the placenta immediately after delivery of the baby. A delay in clamping the cord segment to obtain cord blood gases can significantly alter the pH and pCO_2. However, delayed cord clamping of 30 to 60 seconds has been recommended by multiple international organizations, and it appears that the magnitude of changes in this frame of time is not clinically significant in vaginally delivered, term, healthy singletons.[5] The blood samples can be obtained with disposable plastic syringes that have been flushed with heparin (1000 U per cm^3). It is important to carefully expel all the heparin from the syringes, as heparin can alter the pH. Samples are obtained from both the umbilical artery and vein whenever possible. Umbilical arterial blood is often more difficult to obtain. If this proves to be the case, blood can be obtained from an artery on the surface of the placenta. The arteries are identified as they override the vein on the placental surface. Samples should be carefully labeled as an umbilical artery or vein and with the time they are obtained. The samples are stable either in the clamped segment of the cord or in the syringe for up to 60 minutes and do not have to be transported to the laboratory on ice.

Normal Cord Blood Gas Values

The blood from the umbilical artery reflects information on the blood returning to the placenta from the fetus, so it is most informative about the state of the fetus at the time of delivery. Blood from the venous side will be useful in confirming the accuracy of the values obtained from the artery and, as will be discussed, if an acidosis does exist confirming whether the acidosis is metabolic or respiratory. The values that are most important are the pH and the pCO_2. The pO_2 is only useful in confirming that the specimen obtained was actually from the umbilical cord and not from an umbilical venous catheter obtained from the newborn sometime later, as fetal pO_2 is substantially lower than newborn values. The pO_2 in and of itself is not informative because the level fluctuates so much from minute to minute, especially in the final minutes before birth, and even very vigorous and subsequently normal fetuses can have very low pO_2 values.

Normal values for the umbilical cord artery and vein are shown in Table 7.2.[5-8] Values for term and preterm babies are similar.[9]

It should be pointed out that these normal values have been derived for the most part from babies who have experienced labor and delivery. The labor process itself is associated with a decrease in pH and elevation of base excess (Fig. 7.2).[10] Blood gas values obtained from cordocentesis or from babies delivered electively by cesarean section without labor confirm this general trend toward a lower pH and higher base excess

TABLE 7.2 Normal values for umbilical cord blood gases

	Mean value	Normal range
Artery		
pH	7.26	7.15-7.38
pCO_2	50	35-70
Base excess	–3.0	–2 to –9
Venous		
pH	7.34	7.20-7.41
pCO_2	40	33-50
Base excess	–2.6	–1 to –8

Values are a composite of four studies evaluating cord blood gases in babies with normal Apgar scores and normal newborn courses.[5-8]

as labor progresses, as values obtained from nonlaboring patients and via cordocentesis show higher pH and lower base excess values (Table 7.3).[11-14] Thus, if a baby is delivered by cesarean section without labor, or in early labor, the normal values will be somewhat different, with the pH somewhat higher and the base excess somewhat lower.

Correlating Umbilical Cord Blood Gases with FHR Patterns

Continuous fetal monitoring was introduced in an attempt to provide a screening test to predict the acid-base status of the fetus, in order to allow early intervention. However, intrapartum fetal monitoring has low sensitivity to predict asphyxia.[15] There are well-established proposed mechanisms for the pathophysiology of FHR patterns that have been formulated in animals, and to some degree, have agreement in human studies. For example, it is well established that the trigger for late decelerations is a fall in fetal pO_2, usually caused by inadequate exchange or delivery of O_2 within the placenta. As with the adult lung, the placenta's capacity for exchanging CO_2 far exceeds its ability to exchange O_2. Thus, with late decelerations, if the O_2 delivered to the baby is insufficient to support aerobic metabolism, anaerobic metabolism results in a buildup of organic acids, and metabolic acidosis results. In such a case, the cord gases will exhibit a low pH, a normal pCO_2, and an elevated base deficit that exceeds 9. As metabolic acidosis is only slowly corrected by the placenta, the blood gases in the umbilical vein will be similar to those in the umbilical artery.[15]

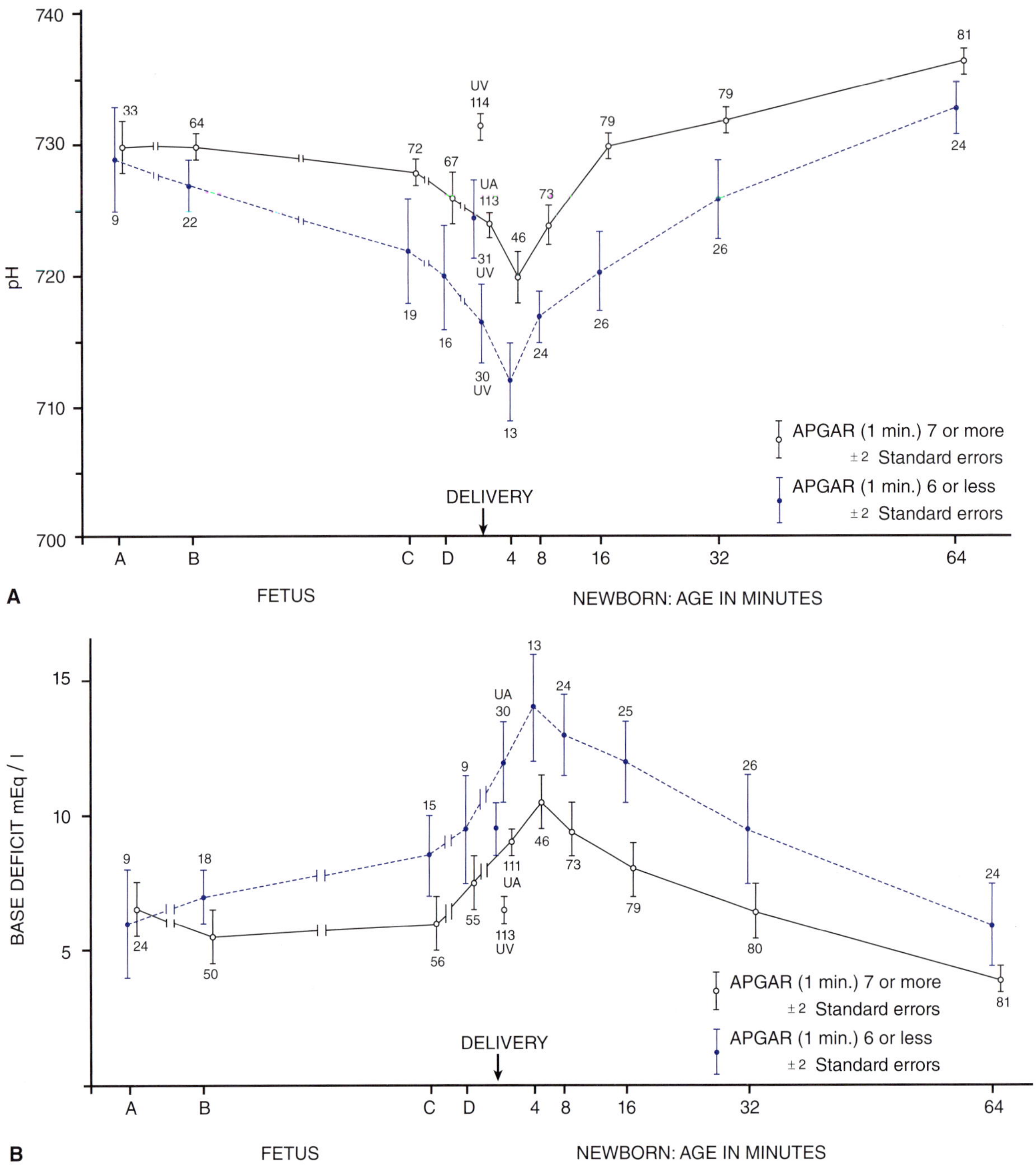

Figure 7.2. **A.** Normal pH (*solid line*) during labor, at delivery, and in the early newborn period is shown. In addition, the *dotted line* represents pH from fetuses and newborns delivered with 1-minute Apgar scores of 6 or less. Point A is early labor, B is at 5-cm dilation, C is at complete dilation, and D is just prior to delivery. **B.** The *dark line* is the normal of base deficit in labor, and the *dotted line* represents the base deficit from depressed babies in labor. **B** is the normal course of base deficit (base excess is the negative of base deficit) in labor and in the early newborn period. As in A, the *dotted line* is from depressed newborns. (From Modanlou H, Yeh SY, Hon EH, Forsythe A. Fetal and neonatal biochemistry and Apgar scores. *Am J Obstet Gynecol*. 1973; 117(7):942.)

TABLE 7.3 Normal fetal blood gases and pH obtained by cordocentesis

Parameter (mean value)	22 week	28 week	34 week	40 week
UV (Ph)	7.416	7.407	3.398	7.388
UV (Po_2)	47.6	42.0	36.3	30.6
UV (PCO_2)	33.6	34.9	36.2	37.5
UV (HCO_3)	22.3	23.0	23.7	24.3
UA (pH)	7.390	7.379	7.368	7.357
UA (PO_2)	28.3	26.3	24.3	22.3
UA pressure (mm Hg)	3.8	5.2	6.5	—

From Creasy RK, Resnik R. *Maternal-Fetal Medicine: Principles and Practice.* 5th ed. Elsevier, Inc.; 2004.

In the case of variable decelerations, most often caused by umbilical cord compression, if the frequency and duration of the cord compression is severe enough, as in airway obstruction in the adult, accumulation of CO_2 will be the first event. When looking at neonates with fetal acidosis at birth, variable declarations were considered to be significant if the depth was at least 60 beats per minute, the lowest value was 60 or less or the duration was 60 or longer.[16] If severe enough, this will result in respiratory acidosis.[17] If even more severe and the fetus can progress to an O_2 deficit as well, a combined respiratory and metabolic acidosis will result. In the former case of the respiratory acidosis, there will be a low pH, an elevation of pCO_2, and a normal base excess. A combined respiratory and metabolic acidosis would result in the umbilical artery in a low pH, an elevated pCO_2, and a base deficit of >9. Interestingly with a respiratory acidosis caused by umbilical cord compression, most often there will be a disparity in pCO_2, and thus the pH, between the umbilical artery and vein. This occurs because, as previously explained, CO_2 can be rapidly cleared in the placenta and the pCO_2 in the umbilical vein will be considerably lower than in the artery as the blood flows through the placenta and the CO_2 diffuses into the maternal circulation. Thus, the artery will have a lower pH and a more elevated pCO_2, and the vein will have a lower or more normal pCO_2 and the pH will have risen back toward normal. However, with most variable decelerations, there will be no significant changes in fetal blood gas analysis unless recurrent.[18]

One of the major disadvantages of FHR monitoring is that interpretations of FHR tracings are subjective, with significant intraoperative variability. Although the National Institute for Child Health and Human Development has developed standardized definitions of tracings for research purposes, there is still poor predictability between FHR tracings and birth outcomes or cord gas analysis. Despite imperfect prediction of asphyxia, mean values of pH and base excess have been shown to decrease with worsening tracing, and the duration of >30 minutes of category III tracings is predictive of pH <7.0.[19] Category II tracings produce a highly heterogenous grouping of cord gas values, however one of the most significant parameters to predict acidemia may be the presence or absence of minimal variability rather than a particular deceleration pattern.[20] Continuous FHR monitoring is not a precise tool in the identification of acidemia, or necessarily predictive of neonatal outcomes, and continuous monitoring does not reliably produce statistically significant decreases in fetal acidemia or neurologic outcomes.[21] However, knowledge of the FHR pattern in conjunction with the umbilical artery and vein blood gases may provide insights into the possible reasons for acidosis, guide the clinician to evaluate their interpretation of the pattern, and can assist the with determining the etiology of newborn depression and help guide resuscitation.

Recently Zullo et al[21] reported the results of a systematic review meta-analysis of FHR tracing within the last 30 to 120 min of the delivery among ~47,000 non-anomalous singletons at 37 weeks or more. Overall, the tracings before delivery were characterized as being category I for 12,866 (27.0%) participants, category II for 34,730 (72.9%), and category III for 52 (0.1%) of the individuals. The rates of neonatal acidosis with category I, II, or III before delivery are described in Table 7.4. It's notable that category III occurs infrequently and even then, the majority of the newborns do not have neonatal acidosis.

TABLE 7.4 Three-tiered categorization of fetal heart rate tracing and umbilical arterial acid-base

	Category I	Category II	Category III	OR (95% CI); P; I^2		
				I vs. II	I vs. III	II vs. III
UA pH <7.00	1/1189 (0.08%; 0.00%-0.54%)	16/7275 (0.22%; 0.13%-0.27%)	19/52 (36.53%; 23.97%-51.09%)	2.85 (0.41,19.55); 0.29; 21%	**161.56 (25.18, 1036.42); 0.00001;** 0%	**42.29 (14.29-125.10); <0.00001;** 29%
UA pH <7.00 and BE <−12 mmol/L	1/1189 (0.08%; 0.00%-0.54%)	12/7275 (0.16%; 0.09%-0.29%)	16/52 (30.8%; 19.12%-45.26%)	2.04 (0.37,11.13); 0.43; 0%	**65.64 (20.05, 214.85); <0.00001;** 0%	12.21 (0.70-211.97); 0.09; NA

OR, odds ratio; CI, confidence intervals; UA, umbilical artery.
Data presented as *N* (%; 95% confidence intervals).
Bolded, if 95% confidence intervals did not cross integer 1 or if P < .05.

Correlation of Umbilical Blood Gases with Long-Term Outcome

As covered in Chapter 3, neurologic damage resulting from intrapartum asphyxia is only one of the many causes of CP and other encephalopathies. Prior to using umbilical cord blood gas assessment, it was common to base the prognosis of the fetus on the Apgar score and thus the need for resuscitation. Subsequent to the realization of the poor predictive value of the Apgar score as well as its nonspecific nature for understanding the cause of any depression, it became a practice to utilize umbilical cord pH in assessing fetal status at birth. As should be apparent now, the problem with using pH alone, especially when using pH alone from the umbilical artery, is that an elevated pCO_2 causing a respiratory acidosis cannot be distinguished from a metabolic acidosis. Because respiratory acidosis has virtually no correlation with, and thus is not a cause of, neurologic damage,[15] a pH alone is often not sufficient information upon which to base prognostication. Despite the incomplete information, pH <7.0 is significantly associated with neonatal morbidity and mortality and CP in childhood, and neonates with low cord pH should have increased surveillance.[22]

It was previously thought that the addition of the base deficit added additional predictive value to the prediction of adverse outcomes, however more recent data suggests that base deficit provides no additional predictive power.[23] It is likely that neonates with higher base deficits are more likely to be acidemic, however there may be some additional information added by arterial lactate values.[4] Overall, the ability of umbilical cord gas analysis to predict adverse outcomes is weak, with most neonates with neurologic morbidity having normal cord gas values.[24,25]

WHICH PATIENTS SHOULD HAVE UMBILICAL CORD BLOOD GAS ASSESSMENT?

There is some controversy in the United States over whether all babies should have an assessment of umbilical cord blood gases or just selected babies either depressed or at risk for hypoxia and acidosis. The argument in favor of testing all babies is that it may be of utility in defending against an allegation of failure to deliver a baby earlier and preventing an acidosis in a situation that results in a lawsuit. Universal gases may identify neonates who require higher levels of care, however it is important to note that a baby with a normal Apgar score, even when a low pH is found (probably mostly caused by laboratory error), shows no difference in the immediate neonatal outcome, including complications and duration of stay, than a baby with a normal Apgar score and a normal pH…. Despite the burdensome nature of the practice, the potential advantage of "universal" umbilical acid-base is that it is available in cases when needed and it is useful for clinical investigations.[26-28]

The American Congress of Obstetricians and Gynecologists (ACOG) recommends cord blood sampling and analysis on babies with cesarean section for suspected fetal compromise, those with low 5-minute Apgar scores, with severe intrauterine growth restriction, and with abnormal FHR tracings and on babies

TABLE 7.5 Indications for umbilical cord pH: a proposed checklist

■ Premature delivery <34 week
■ Moderate or thick meconium
■ Any of the following nonreassuring patterns with 1 h of delivery: Persistent late decelerations Fetal tachycardia Absent variability (≤5 beats per minute) Severe variable decelerations Recurrent prolonged decelerations Bradycardia
■ Intrapartum vaginal bleeding more than "bloody show"
■ Maternal fever (≥100.4°F)
■ Apgar score <7 at 1 and/or 5 min
■ Unexpected fetal anomaly
■ Instrumented vaginal delivery
■ Shoulder dystocia
■ Breech or other malpresentation delivered vaginally
■ Any nonelective cesarean section
■ Fetal growth restriction
■ Maternal thyroid disease

from mothers with maternal thyroid disease, intrapartum fever, and multifetal gestations. Because "abnormal FHR tracings" can be ambiguous, and because this means category II FHR tracings can be ambiguous, an alternative list of indications for umbilical cord sampling and testing is provided in Table 7.5. The potential pitfall of selective blood sampling is that the labor and delivery staff may not obtain the blood sample for the indications that ACOG recommends.

SUMMARY

Umbilical cord blood gas analysis is one of the most specific and accurate methods of determining the condition of the baby at birth. An understanding of the physiologic basis of umbilical cord blood gases and their correlation with FHR patterns will enhance one's ability to predict and understand the baby's status at birth and in retrospect improve and validate the interpretation of the FHR pattern that preceded birth. Selected babies who are depressed at birth or otherwise at risk for acidosis should be sampled immediately following delivery. Both umbilical arterial and venous blood should be obtained whenever possible and should be analyzed for pH and pCO_2 and a base deficit/excess calculated.

REFERENCES

1. Apgar V. A proposal for a new method of evaluation of the newborn infant. *Curr Res Anesth Analg.* 1953;32(4):260-267.
2. Nelson KB, Ellenberg JH. Apgar score as a predictor of chronic neurologic disability. *Pediatrics.* 1981;68(1):36–44.
3. Stanley FJ. Cerebral palsy trends: implications for prenatal care. *Acta Obstet Gynecol Scan.* 1994;73(1):5-9.
4. Tuuli MG, Stout MG, Shanks A, Odibo AO, Macones GA, Cahill AG. Umbilical cord arterial lactate compared with pH for predicting neonatal morbidity at term. *Obstet Gynecol.* 2014;124(4):756061.
5. Thorp JA, Boylan PC, Parisis VM, Creasy RK. Routine umbilical cord blood gas determinations? *Am J Obstet Gynecol.* 1989;161(3):600-605.
6. Yeomans ER, Hauth JC, Gilstrap LC, Strickland DM. Umbilical cord pH, pCO_2, and bicarbonate following uncomplicated vaginal deliveries. *Am J Obstet Gynecol.* 1985;151(6):798-800.
7. Riley RJ, Johnson JWC. Collecting and analyzing cord blood gases. *Clin Obstet Gynecol.* 1993;36(1):13-23.
8. Nudelman MJ, Belogolovsky E, Jegatheesan P, Govindaswami B, Song D. Effect of delayed cord clamping on umbilical blood gas values in term newborns. *Obstet Gynecol.* 2020;135(3):576-582.
9. Ramin SM, Gilstrap LC, Leveno KJ, Burris J, Little BB. Umbilical artery acid-base status in the preterm infant. *Obstet Gynecol.* 1989;74(2):256-258.
10. Modanlou H, Yeh SY, Hon EH, Forsythe A. Fetal and neonatal biochemistry and Apgar scores. *Am J Obstet Gynecol.* 1973;117(7):942-951.
11. Soothill PW, Nicolaides KH, Rodeck CH, Campbell S. Effect of gestational age on fetal and intervillous blood gas and acid-base values in human pregnancy. *Fetal Ther.* 1986;1(4):168-175.
12. Nicolaides KH, Economides DL, Soothill PW. Blood gases, pH and lactate in appropriate and small for gestational age fetuses. *Am J Obstet Gynecol.* 1989;161(4):996-1001.
13. Weiner CP, Sipes SL, Wenstrom K. The effect of fetal age upon normal fetal laboratory values and venous pressure. *Obstet Gynecol.* 1992;79(5 (Pt 1)):713-718.
14. Tuuli MG, Stout MJ, Macones GA, Cahill AG. Umbilical cord venous lactate for predicting arterial lactic acidemia and neonatal morbidity at term. *Obstet Gynecol.* 2016;127(4):674-680. doi:10.1097/AOG.0000000000001339.
15. Jensen OHR, Narverud G. Fetal heart rate decelerations and umbilical cord blood gas values. *Eur J Obstet Gynecol Reprod Biol.* 1994;53(2):103-106.
16. Hamilton E, Warrick P, O'Keeffe D. Variable decelerations: do size and shape matter? *J Matern.-Fetal Neonatal Med.* 2011;25(6):648-653. Hankins GDV, Snyder RR, Hauth JC, Gilstrap LC 3rd, Hammond T. Nuchal cords and neonatal outcome. *Obstet Gynecol.* 1987;70(5):687-691.

17. Soncini E, Paganelli S, Vezzani C, Gargano G, La Sala GB. Intrapartum fetal heart rate monitoring: evaluation of a standardized system of interpretation for prediction of metabolic acidosis at delivery and neonatal neurological morbidity. *J Matern.-Fetal Neonatal Med.* 2014;27(14):1465-1469.
18. Cahill AG, Roehl KA, Odibo AO, Macones GA. Association and prediction of neonatal acidemia. *Am J Obstet Gynecol.* 2012;207(3):206.e1-206.e8. doi: 10.1016/j.ajog.2012.06.046.
19. Williams KP, Galerneau F. Intrapartum fetal heart rate patterns in the prediction of neonatal acidemia. *Am J Obstet Gynecol.* 2003;188(3):820-823.
20. Alfirevic Z, Devane D, Gyte GM, Cuthbert A. Continuous cardiotocography (CTG) as a form of electronic fetal monitoring (EFM) for fetal assessment during labor. *Cochrane Database Syst Rev.* 2017;2(2):CD006066.
21. Zullo F, Di Mascio D, Raghuraman N, et al. Three-tiered fetal heart rate interpretation system and adverse neonatal and maternal outcomes: a systematic review and meta-analysis. *Am J Obstet Gynecol.* 2023;229(4):377-387.
22. Malin GL, Morris RK, Khan KS. Strength of association between umbilical cord pH and perinatal and long term outcomes: systematic review and meta-analysis. *BMJ.* 2010;340:c1471.
23. Knutzen L, Sirko E, Impey L. The significance of base deficit in academic term neonates. *Am J Obstet Gynecol.* 2015;213(3):373.e1-373.e7.
24. Myrhaug HT, Kaasen A, Pay ASD, et al. Umbilical cord blood acid-base analysis at birth and long term neurodevelopmental outcomes in children: a systemic review and meta-analysis. *BJOG.* 2023;130(10):1156-1166.
25. Yeh P, Emary K, Impey L. The relationship between umbilical cord arterial pH and serious adverse neonatal outcome: analysis of 51,519 consecutive validated samples. *BJOG.* 2012;119(7):824-831.
26. Watkins VY, Frolova AI, Stout MJ, et al. The relationship between maternal anemia and umbilical cord oxygen content at delivery. *Am J Obstst Gynecol MFM.* 2021;3(1):100270.
27. Beermann SE, Watkins VY, Frolova AI, Raghuraman N, Cahill AG. The relationship between maternal anemia and electronic fetal monitoring patterns. *Am J Obstet Gynecol.* 2023;229(4):449.e1-449.e6.
28. Bligard KH, Cameo T, McCallum KN, et al. The association of fetal acidemia with adverse neonatal outcomes at the time of scheduled cesarean delivery. *Am J Obstet Gynecol.* 2022;227(2):265.e1-265.e8.

CHAPTER 8

Clinical Management of Category II and Category III Fetal Heart Rate Patterns

Christy Gandhi and Uma M. Reddy

The process of labor and delivery can often be the most stressful period for the fetus in pregnancies. During a uterine contraction, there is a transient hypoperfusion of uteroplacental blood flow, which is accompanied by a temporary impairment of transplacental gas exchange. Analgesics, oligohydramnios, chorioamnionitis, and placental insufficiency are some other common intrapartum stressors that can contribute to fetal hypoxia and acidemia.[1] The aim of intrapartum fetal heart rate (FHR) monitoring is to detect fetal hypoxia and acidemia early enough to allow clinicians an opportunity for resuscitation interventions, corrective efforts, and ultimately operative delivery if abnormal FHR patterns persist. Given the stressors in labor, abnormalities in intrapartum FHR patterns are commonly encountered.

ACID-BASE STATUS

The interpretation of intrapartum FHR surveillance relies on the fundamental understanding of fetal acid-base physiology. Fetal acid-base balance is achieved through aerobic metabolism in which the oxidation of glucose requires oxygen and produces carbon dioxide. This gas exchange occurs across the placenta and relies on normal maternal acid-base status, maternal circulation, uteroplacental blood flow, and umbilical blood flow. There are three types of neonatal acidemia: metabolic, respiratory, and mixed. Metabolic acidosis usually refers to a prolonged state of acidemia, typically from prolonged hypoxia necessitating reliance on anaerobic metabolism, which results in the loss of bicarbonate for the buffering of the fixed organic acids and high base deficit. Respiratory acidosis is typically over a shorter time interval such that not much buffering with bicarbonate occurs. Mixed acidosis is a combination of the two.

Maternal acid-base status can also adversely affect fetal acid-base status, as seen in maternal diabetic ketoacidosis or eclampsia. In these settings, the FHR tracing can show prolonged decelerations and even demonstrate a terminal bradycardia appearance. With the correction of the maternal acid-base status and treatment of the underlying maternal etiology, the fetal acid-base status normalizes and the FHR abnormalities improve.

FHR MONITORING LIMITATIONS

Discussion of limitations of FHR monitoring prior to the review of intrapartum management of abnormal FHR tracings will help provide context when understanding the development of various approaches. A reactive and reassuring FHR pattern often correlates with a low likelihood of fetal acidemia and is a reliable sign of fetal well-being. The opposite, however, is not always the case. When the FHR pattern shows diminished variability or with decelerations, the fetus can very well be vigorous and not acidotic at birth.[2] Therefore, rather than using the imprecise term "fetal distress" to describe abnormalities in the FHR pattern, the more appropriate term "nonreassuring fetal status" should be used; as in, a "reassuring" clinical impression cannot be made from the abnormal FHR pattern.

Given the limitations of electronic FHR monitoring, particularly intra- and interobserver variability, the *Eunice Kennedy Shriver* National Institute for Child Health and Human Development, the American College of Obstetrics & Gynecologists, and the Society for Maternal Fetal Medicine convened a workshop to

TABLE 8.1 **Intrapartum electronic fetal monitoring categories**

Category I Normal	Fetal heart rate tracing that includes all of the following: ■ Baseline 110-160 bpm ■ Moderate variability ■ Absence of variable or late decelerations. Early decelerations can be present ■ Accelerations can be present or absent
Category II Indeterminate	FHR tracing that cannot be classified as category I or III

Category III
Abnormal
	Either
	■ Absent variability with
	  ■ recurrent late or variable decelerations
	  ■ bradycardia
	■ Sinusoidal pattern

revise the guidelines and created a universal three-tiered interpretation system (Table 8.1).[3] These definitions of categories are only reserved for intrapartum FHR tracings and should not be used for those not in labor.

CATEGORY I FHR MANAGEMENT

Category I FHR tracings are defined as the normal baseline of 110 to 160 beats per minute (bpm), have moderate baseline variability, and no variable or late decelerations. Early decelerations, which represent a physiologic response from head compression, and accelerations could be absent or present in this category. Category I FHR tracings are strongly predictive of normal fetal acid-base status, and therefore no interventions are indicated.

CATEGORY III FHR MANAGEMENT

Category III FHR tracings include absent baseline variability with recurrent late decelerations, recurrent variable decelerations, or bradycardia. Recurrent decelerations are defined as those occurring with ≥50% of uterine contractions in a 20-minute segment. A sinusoidal FHR pattern also qualifies as a category III FHR tracing and is defined as having a visually apparent smooth wave-like undulating pattern in the FHR baseline with a cycle frequency of 3 to 5 per minute that persists for 20 minutes. Sinusoidal patterns are very rare and are seen in the context of fetal anemia, medications (such as meperidine, alphaprodine, butorphanol, and nalbuphine hydrochloride), and severe fetal hypoxia.[4]

Category III FHR tracings are highly concerning for fetal acidemia and are associated with an increased risk of neonatal neurologic sequelae.[5,6] Category III FHR tracings require urgent evaluation and simultaneous preparation for operative delivery. If there is no prompt improvement in the tracing with resuscitative measures, expedited delivery is recommended.

CATEGORY II FHR MANAGEMENT

Category II refers to patterns that cannot be classified into category I or III.[3] Identification, surveillance, and management of category I and category III tracings can be relatively straightforward with either expectant management and observation in category I settings or urgent intervention in category III settings. The majority of fetuses in labor, however, will demonstrate a category II pattern at one point or another.[7] Category II tracings encompass a wide range of patterns; the management of such tracings can also be broad and would depend on the stage in labor, the presence of other risk factors that elevate concern for fetal well-being, and the absence of other reassuring features. Along with interobserver variability in FHR interpretation, there is substantial variation in management of intrapartum category II tracings. Additionally, a given fetus may have more than one pathologic process and therefore more than one type of FHR abnormality. Therefore, several algorithms on the management of category II tracings, including the implementation of resuscitation measures, have been proposed and adopted by hospital labor and delivery units. Even statewide initiatives in maternal mortality and morbidity review committees have adopted such algorithms to standardize the approach to category II FHR tracings to support intended vaginal births.[8] Figure 8.1 is an algorithm published by Clark et al[9] in 2013 that has been commonly adapted across many hospitals and state perinatal quality collaboratives.

Generally, the first step of most algorithms is to assess moderate variability and fetal heart accelerations. Fetal heart rate accelerations are defined as 15 beats above baseline lasting at least 15 seconds in pregnancies greater than 32 weeks' gestation and 10 beats above baseline over 10 seconds in pregnancies less

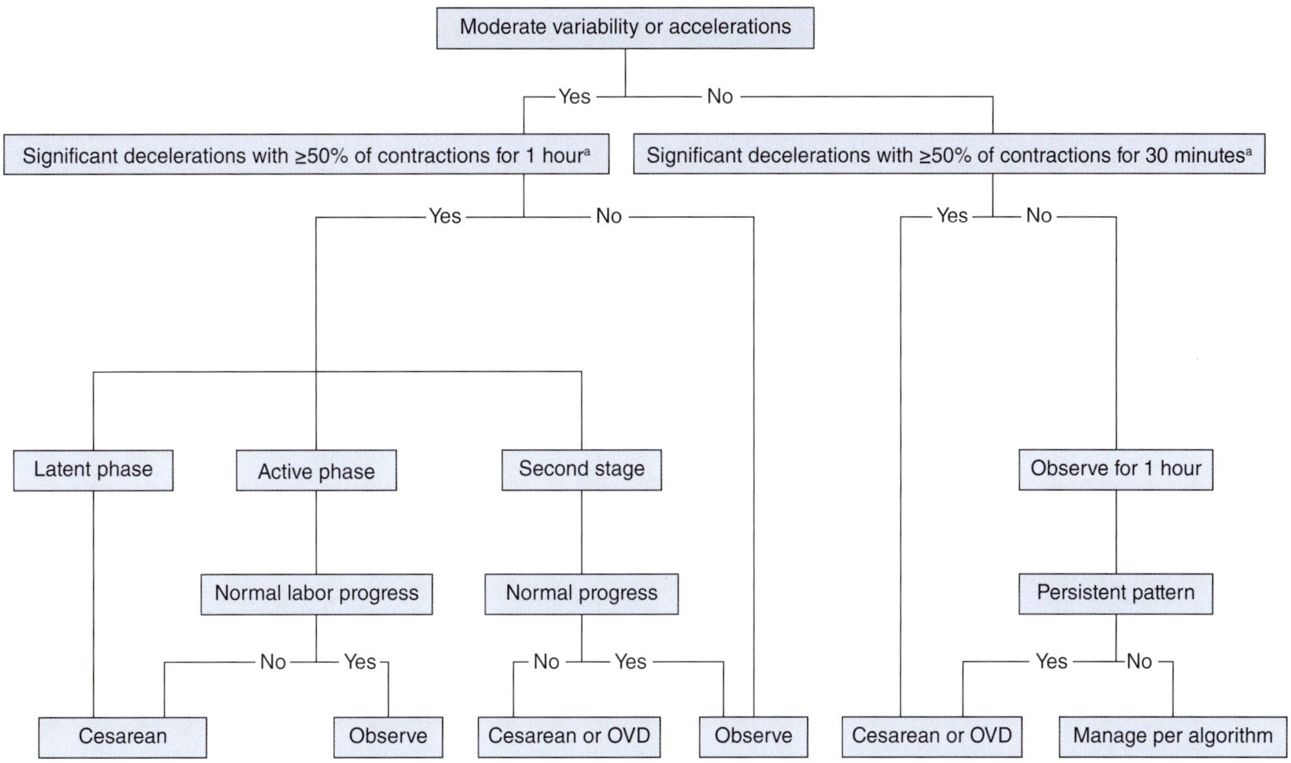

Figure 8.1. A proposed algorithm on management of category I fetal heart rate tracings. OVD: Operative vaginal delivery. Note: [a]Decelerations that have not resolved with appropriate conservative corrective measures, which may include maternal position changes, intravenous fluid administration, correction of hypotension, reduction or discontinuation of the uterine stimulation, administration of uterine relaxant, amnioinfusion, and/or changes in second stage breathing and pushing techniques. (Reproduced with permission from Clark SL, Nageotte MP, Garite TJ, et al. Intrapartum management of category II fetal heart rate tracings: towards standardization of care. *Am J Obstet Gynecol.* 2013;209(2):89-97.)

than 32 weeks' gestation. The presence of accelerations excludes fetal acidemia. Accelerations in response to fetal scalp stimulation are supportive evidence suggesting the absence of fetal acidosis and can be elicited to provide intrapartum reassurance. Typically, baseline variability and accelerations are reliably depressed before a level of fetal acidemia associated with neurologic injury is reached. Of note, variability within decelerations alone cannot be used to exclude fetal acidemia.[10]

Once moderate variability and/or fetal heart accelerations are confirmed, which thereby rules out the presence of clinically significant fetal metabolic acidemia, the focus is shifted on identifying the likelihood of developing fetal acidemia intrapartum by assessing the nature and frequency of significant decelerations. Examples of significant decelerations include variable decelerations lasting longer than 60 seconds and reaching a nadir of less than 60 bpm below baseline or reaching an absolute nadir of less than 60 bpm regardless of baseline. Other examples of significant decelerations include any form of late or prolonged decelerations.[9,11] When significant decelerations occur for greater than 50% of contractions for 1 hour despite conservative corrective measures, in the setting of moderate variability and/or accelerations, intervention via operative delivery may be warranted if active labor is not normally progressing. If this occurs during the second stage of labor, an operative vaginal delivery either via forceps or vacuum assistance can be considered per provider experience and patient eligibility. Otherwise, delivery may be most expedited via a cesarean section. If active labor or second stage labor is progressing normally, then clinicians may closely observe the tracing as long as reassuring signs of moderate variability and accelerations persist.

Significant fetal metabolic acidemia cannot be excluded in cases where there is no moderate variability or accelerations and where there are significant late decelerations. Absent variability with recurrent

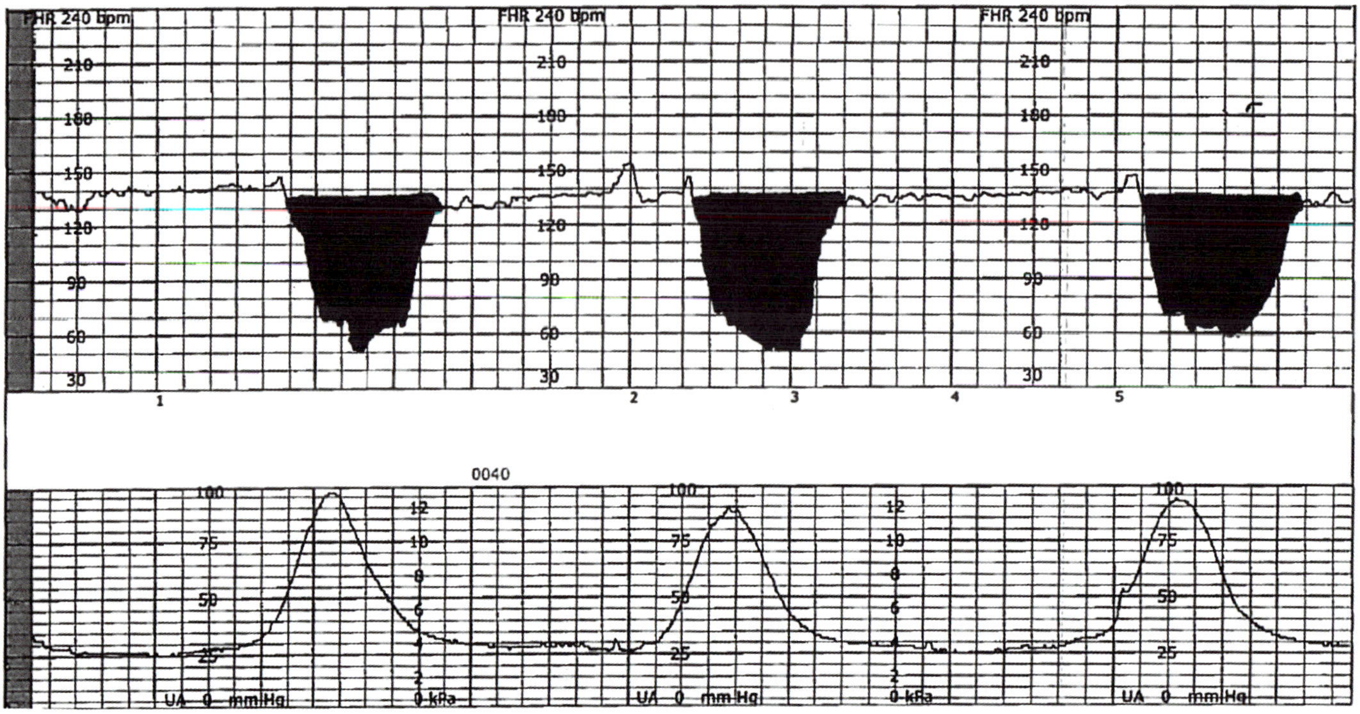

Figure 8.2. Shaded region represents the deceleration area that is estimated by width of the widest aspect of deceleration (below the baseline) measured in seconds, multiplied by the maximum depth below the baseline, divided by 2. (Reproduced from Cahill AG, Tuuli MG, Stout MJ, López JD, Macones GA. A prospective cohort study of fetal heart rate monitoring: deceleration area is predictive of fetal acidemia. *Am J Obstet Gynecol.* 2018;218(5):523.e521-523.e512.)

decelerations qualifies as category III FHR and urgent delivery is necessitated. Absent variability reliably correlates with a high degree of severe fetal acidemia and is typically preceded by minimal variability in scenarios of progressive fetal acidemia. Nevertheless, delivery should not be significantly delayed in the setting of minimal variability because criteria for absent variability has not been met. There is considerable interobserver variation in interpreting absent versus minimal variability.[12] Therefore, some algorithms chose to treat persistent minimal variability and absent variability similarly. When significant decelerations occur for greater than 50% of contractions for 30 minutes despite conservative corrective measures, in the setting of minimal variability or no accelerations, expedited intervention via operative delivery may be warranted even if labor is progressing normally.

A recent study has suggested that the total declaration area, which was defined as a function of the length of time of the deceleration multiplied by the maximum depth below the baseline, in the final 120 minutes of electronic fetal monitoring prior to a full-term delivery, may be the most predictive FHR pattern for acidemia (see Figure 8.2).[5]

CONSERVATIVE CORRECTIVE MEASURES

Ensure the Accuracy of FHR Tracing

Confirm that the monitor is accurately displaying the FHR tracing by verifying that it differs from maternal pulse. With maternal tachycardia, the maternal heart rate pattern can deceptively resemble a normal FHR pattern, with normal-appearing baseline rate and variability. In this setting, an increase in maternal heart rate during uterine contractions can be mistaken for FHR accelerations.

Generally, the external FHR monitors are reliable. Yet, if there is poor FHR signal quality or interference from a tachycardic maternal heart rate, the placement of a fetal scalp electrode should be considered.

Maternal Repositioning and Intravenous Fluid Hydration

Repositioning the patient on a lateral side could help alleviate any compression of the umbilical cord that is causing variable decelerations and/or improve uteroplacental hypoperfusion that could be responsible for late decelerations.

No randomized trials have evaluated the effect of intravenous (IV) fluid boluses alone on FHR abnormalities. An IV fluid bolus of a crystalloid solution (either lactated ringers or normal saline) can improve uteroplacental blood flow if the patient is slightly dehydrated, especially in the setting of restricted oral intake while admitted in labor. A prospective study concluded that an IV fluid bolus of one liter crystalloid is effective in improving fetal oxygen saturation.[13] Fluid administration should be done with caution in patients at risk of volume overload.

Maternal hypotension secondary to recent neuraxial anesthesia placement is corrected with IV fluid replacement and administration of an alpha-adrenergic agonists, such as ephedrine or phenylephrine. In the setting of maternal hypotension, the uteroplacental hypoperfusion leads to FHR decelerations that resolve once blood flow is improved. In anticipation of maternal hypotension from neuraxial anesthesia, many institutions administer a prophylactic IV fluid bolus prior to epidural placement.[14]

Amnioinfusion

Amnioinfusion is the process of instilling fluid (either lactated ringers or normal saline) back into the amniotic cavity to help alleviate umbilical cord compression or tightening, which results in variable decelerations. Typically, umbilical cord compression occurs in cases of oligohydramnios or after rupture of membranes. Nuchal cords cause cord tightening, especially as the fetus descends into the pelvis. The rapid phase of descent usually begins between 8 and 10 cm of dilation so variable decelerations from the nuchal cord can be seen at this stage.[2] Several studies have demonstrated the benefit of amnioinfusion in resolving recurrent variable decelerations and reducing cesarean sections for nonreassuring FHR tracing.[15]

A recent systematic review and meta-analysis of 24 randomized studies with 5994 participants demonstrated that in the setting of meconium-stained amniotic fluid, prophylactic transcervical amnioinfusion was associated with the reduction of meconium aspiration syndrome by 67% and improved secondary outcomes that included neonatal acidosis, cesarean delivery for FHR abnormalities, and neonatal intensive care unit (NICU) admission.[16]

During an amnioinfusion, crystalloid fluid is instilled back into the amniotic cavity through an intrauterine pressure catheter (IUPC). IUPC allows for improved tocometry monitoring in patients who are difficult to monitor transabdominally along with the assessment of contraction adequacy. In a retrospective cohort study of over 6000 subjects, patients with an IUPC had a twofold increased risk of intrapartum or postpartum fever than patients without IUPC (adjusted odds ratio [AOR] 2.4, 95% CI 1.8-3.2).[17]

Maternal Oxygen Administration

Maternal oxygen supplementation is only beneficial when treating respiratory conditions leading to maternal hypoxia with an oxygen saturation of <95%. In the setting of normal maternal oxygen levels, oxygen supplementation has no proven benefit in fetal resuscitation. One study published as a secondary analysis of a randomized trial in which 114 patients with term pregnancies in active labor with category II electronic FHR were assigned to 10 L/min of oxygen by face mask or room air until delivery. Trained obstetrical research nurses who were blinded to this allocation examined the FHR tracing, and there was no difference in the resolution of decelerations within 60 minutes between the two groups. The time to resolution of recurrent decelerations was also similar between the room air and oxygen groups. This study concluded that intrapartum maternal oxygen administration for category II FHR patterns did not yield resolution within 60 minutes or hasten the resolution of recurrent decelerations.[18] Consequently, ACOG has stated that the routine use of oxygen supplementation in individuals with normal oxygen saturation is not recommended for fetal intrauterine resuscitation.[19]

Decrease Uterine Contractions/Tocolytics

Uterine contractions transiently decrease placental perfusion and temporarily impair transplacental gas exchange. Frequent contractions can lead to fetal hypoxia that is sensed by the chemoreceptors and triggers a vagal response as a transient deceleration. A decrease in the frequency of uterine contractions by adjusting oxytocin infusions or administering tocolytics, especially in the setting of tachysystole, can provide a temporary break from the impaired transplacental gas exchange. A systematic review and meta-analysis of 4 randomized controlled trials and included 605 singleton pregnancies with nonreassuring FHR tracing concluded that acute tocolysis with beta agonists, compared with emergency delivery, was associated with improved neonatal acid-base status (reduced prevalence of base deficit >12 mmol/L: odds ratio [OR] 0.61,

95% CI 0.37-0.99) and reduced NICU admission (OR 0.42, 95% CI 0.22-0.78). Despite tocolytics being associated with an increase in the time-to-delivery interval (beta-2 agonists mean difference, 17.62 minutes; 95% CI 15.66-19.58), there was no reduction in the cesarean delivery rate. The systematic review and meta-analysis also concluded that beta-2-agonists were most effective tocolytic agents compared with atosiban and nitric oxide donors.[20]

During the second stage, the patient can be instructed to pause pushing for a brief period of time or push with every other contraction.

Algorithm limitations:

- Algorithms cannot predict a sudden deterioration of fetal status because of a sentinel event, such as placental abruption, umbilical cord prolapse, or uterine rupture. These algorithms are designed to address the progressive intrapartum acidemia from contractions and the process of labor, and therefore algorithms should not be used in the setting of vaginal bleeding or scarred uterus in which clinical suspicion for placental abruption or uterine rupture is high, respectively.
- The algorithm attempts to find a balance between identifying and delivering fetuses that are at risk of significant damaging acidemia who may need expedited delivery versus identifying fetuses with FHR patterns that suggest minimal risk of significant acidemia prior to delivery, and thereby avoiding unnecessary intervention. Algorithms should find a balance in allowing patients with minimal risk of significant acidemia the opportunity of a vaginal delivery while also recommending operative deliveries in pregnancies with intrapartum FHR tracing at risk of significantly damaging acidemia.
- Fetal tachycardia is not typically included in these algorithms.
- Marked variability is also not factored into these algorithms.
- The presence of prolonged decelerations is not typically included in these algorithms given the broad definition.

INTRAPARTUM CONSIDERATIONS

FHR tracings should not be interpreted in isolation. Incorporating factors such as labor progress, stage of labor, diagnosis of chorioamnionitis, and placental abruption is crucial when interpreting FHR tracings to make a clinical impression on fetal status. For example, although observation may be acceptable for a category II tracing in the late second stage of labor, a cesarean delivery may be indicated for that same tracing if in the latent phase. Another example includes management of an 8-minute prolonged deceleration after an epidural placement versus a trial of labor after a cesarean (TOLAC). The context is extremely important.

Neuraxial Anesthesia

Maternal hypotension after the placement of epidural or combined spinal-epidural analgesia often responds with IV fluid bolus and alpha-adrenergic agonists, such as ephedrine or phenylephrine. Along with maternal hypotension that can lead to uteroplacental hypoperfusion and subsequent FHR tracing abnormalities, the rapid onset of pain relief from neuraxial analgesia may trigger a sudden imbalance of maternal catecholamines, which results in dysfunctional uterine hypertonia.[21] According to one systematic review and meta-analysis of 17 trials, including almost 4000 parturients, combined spinal-epidural analgesia was associated with a higher risk of nonreassuring FHR tracings than epidural analgesia alone.[22] A more recent study demonstrated no difference in FHR abnormalities between those with a combined spinal epidural versus epidural alone in laboring patients at risk for uteroplacental insufficiency.[23] Nevertheless, continuous intrapartum FHR monitoring immediately before and after the placement of neuraxial analgesia is commonly performed.

Placental Dysfunction

Common obstetric conditions because of placental dysfunction include oligohydramnios and fetal growth restriction (FGR), especially if complicated by abnormal umbilical artery dopplers. Pregnancies with preexisting chronic placental insufficiency, as evidenced by oligohydramnios or abnormal umbilical artery dopplers, may be less likely to tolerate uterine contractions. This concern is further heightened in the setting of prostaglandin use caused by the known adverse effect of uterine tachysystole from these cervical ripening agents.[24,25] In pregnancies complicated by FGR with abnormal umbilical artery dopplers, late decelerations may be noted in the FHR tracing.[26] A secondary analysis of a randomized trial compared FHR patterns during the last hour of labor between small for gestational age (SGA) and appropriate for gestational age neonates,[27] and cesarean delivery for fetal indications was found to be significantly more common for SGA neonates (7% vs. 4%; $P < .001$). With oligohydramnios, variable decelerations may also be present on the intrapartum FHR tracing. Variable decelerations from oligohydramnios may improve after an amnioinfusion.

Intraamniotic Infection

Intraamniotic infection (IAI), also known as chorioamnionitis, is an infection with resultant inflammation of the amniotic fluid, placenta, fetus, fetal membranes, or decidua.[28] If there is maternal fever, fetal temperature will increase, which may result in fetal tachycardia and/or loss of variability. Increased oxygen and metabolic demands caused by IAI may result in late decelerations. Therefore, septic fetuses may demonstrate tachycardia, loss of variability, and absence of accelerations. Resuscitative intrapartum efforts involve maternal IV fluid repletion, antipyretics to reduce maternal temperature, and prompt antibiotic administration.

Magnesium

Continuous magnesium sulfate infusion is commonly administered during labor for eclampsia risk reduction or fetal neuroprotection. Magnesium sulfate crosses the placenta with levels detectable in the newborn. Magnesium exposure is associated with a lower FHR baseline within the normal range and decreased variability[29] without an increased incidence of significant adverse neonatal effect.[29,30]

Prematurity

Many of the pathologic causes of premature delivery (preeclampsia, FGR, preterm rupture of membranes, etc) are often also associated with an increased likelihood of fetal hypoxia and resultant FHR abnormalities. Premature infants are not only more likely exposed to scenarios that are associated with fetal hypoxia but are also more likely to endure severe morbidity from prematurity, and even mortality, if born acidotic.

FHR patterns in a preterm gestation differ slightly from those at term gestations. The preterm FHR baseline will still be within the normal range of 110 to 160 bpm; yet it tends to be at a higher end of the range, whereas the FHR baseline of a term fetus is rarely above 155 bpm. Before 32 weeks of gestation, accelerations are defined as 10 beats above baseline for 10 seconds. Furthermore, the variability is somewhat diminished in extreme prematurity.[31] The FHR pattern in prematurity is likely a reflection of fetal immaturity and the resulting interplay between the parasympathetic and sympathetic systems.

CASE STUDIES

Case 1

Figure 8.3 is an FHR tracing of a nulliparous patient undergoing an elective induction of labor at 39 weeks of gestation. She is currently at 5 cm dilated and 80% effaced. Her tracing is category I with normal baseline, moderate

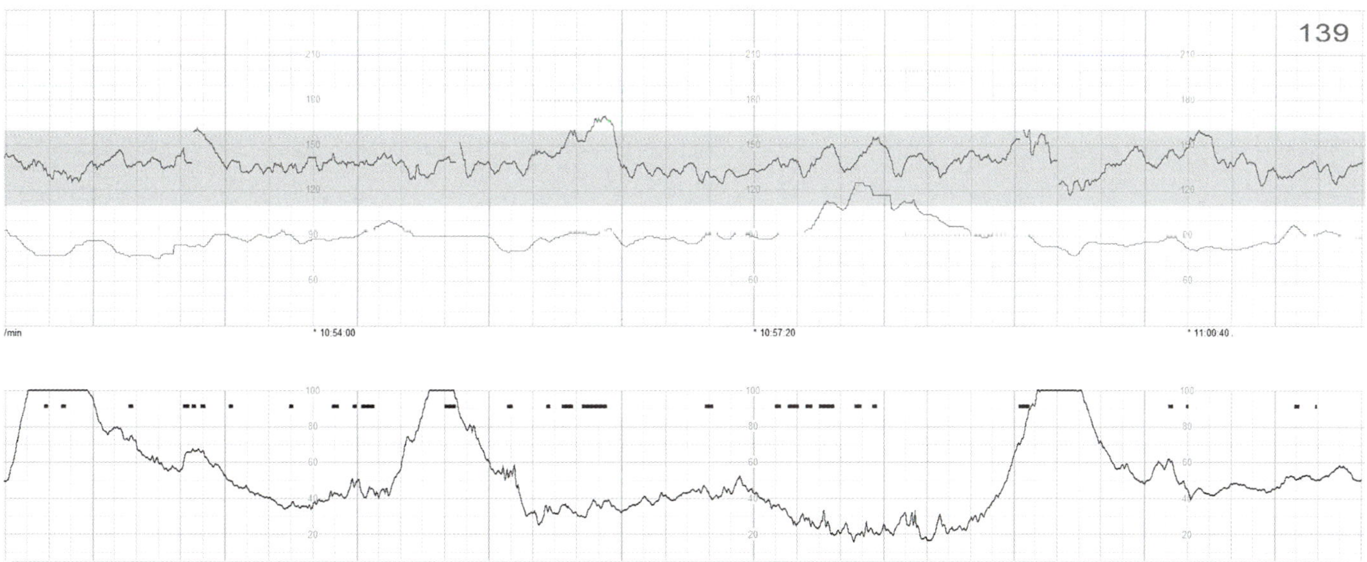

Figure 8.3. Case 1.

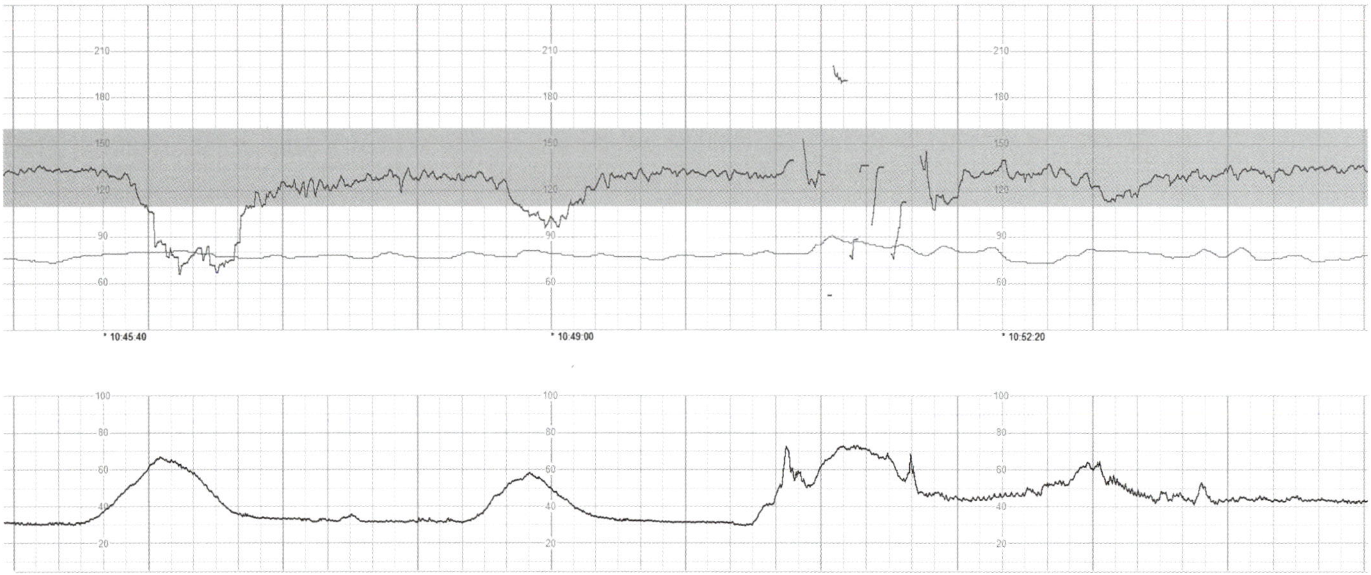

Figure 8.4. Case 2. Maternal repositioning helped improve the variable decelerations.

variability, numerous accelerations, and no decelerations, all of which exclude the presence of fetal acidemia. Based on the reassuring FHR tracing, labor augmentation and efforts toward a vaginal delivery can continue.

Case 2

This is an FHR tracing of a multiparous patient with two prior full-term vaginal deliveries who is 37 weeks' gestation being induced for gestational hypertension diagnosed a week prior. Her cervix was checked after the cervical ripening balloon had expelled, and she was noted to be 3 cm dilated and 50% effaced. Artificial rupture of membranes was performed, and the oxytocin infusion rate continued to be appropriately increased per the local hospital protocol. The FHR tracing continued to be category I until approximately 2 hours later when the tracing transitioned to below. The baseline heart rate is normal with moderate variability, and recurrent variable decelerations are noted as shown in Figure 8.4.

Maternal repositioning temporarily relieved the depth of the variable deceleration as noted in the last few contractions; yet, the variable decelerations resumed shortly after as shown in Figure 8.5.

These variable decelerations occur with greater than half the contractions; yet they are not considered

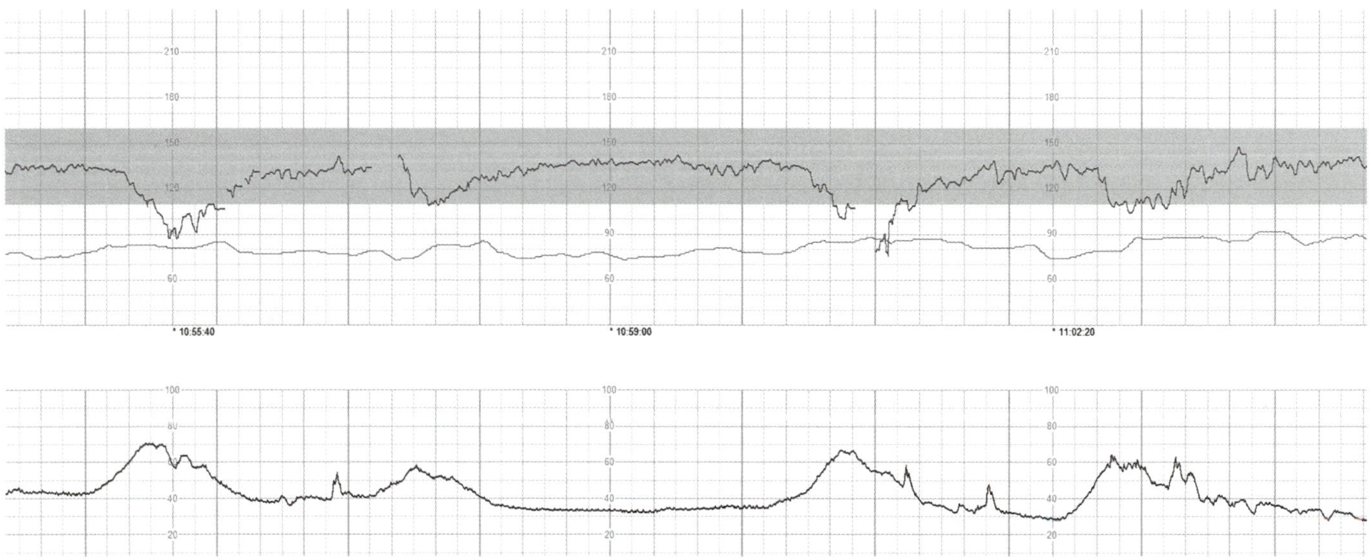

Figure 8.5. Case 2. Variable decelerations resumed.

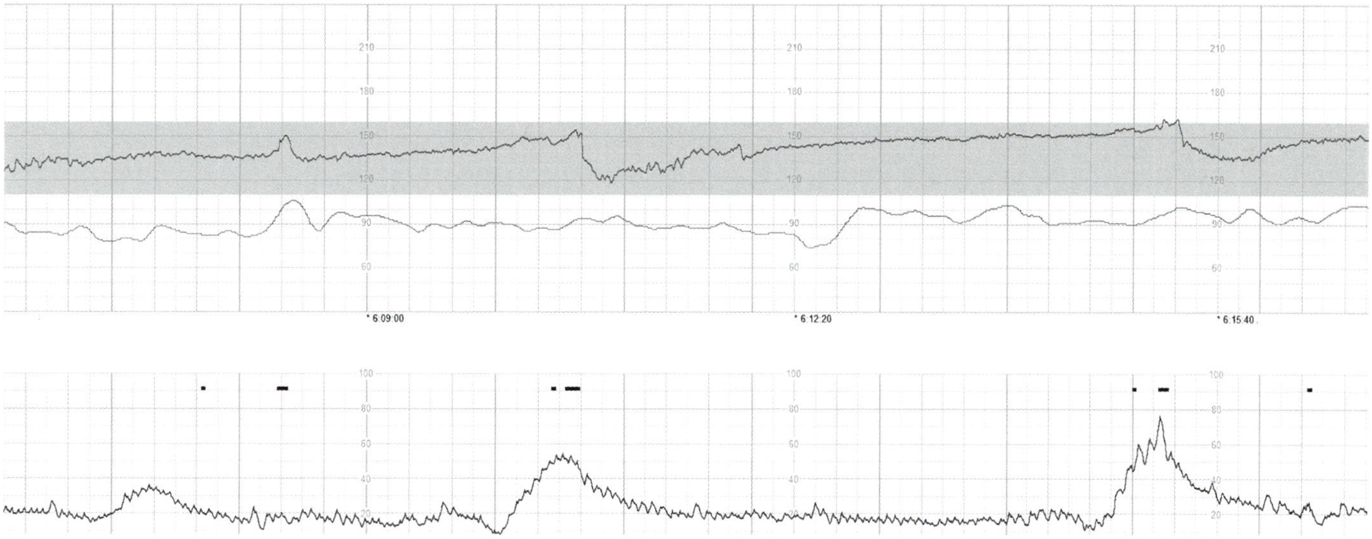

Figure 8.6. Case 3. Category II tracing at the time of intraamniotic infection diagnosis.

to be significant. Significant variable decelerations are typically defined as variable decelerations lasting longer than 60 seconds and reaching a nadir more than 60 beats below baseline or less than 60 bpm, regardless of baseline.[14] Cervical examination at this time was noted to be 5 cm and 80% effaced. An amnioinfusion was started, which relieved the variable decelerations as the patient transitioned to active labor. She had a successful vaginal delivery with newborn's Apgar scores of 8 and 9.

Case 3

This case is of nulliparous patient at 38 weeks of gestation who presented with spontaneous prelabor rupture of membranes and is undergoing labor augmentation. The amniotic fluid had been ruptured for approximately 6 hours prior to the patient's arrival, and the cervical dilation was about 4 cm and 80% effaced. Labor augmentation with oxytocin infusion had been started. Maternal fever to 39.1°C was noted approximately 10 hours after the reported spontaneous rupture of membranes, and the FHR tracing demonstrated recurrent late decelerations with periods of minimal variability in between the decelerations as noted in Figure 8.6. Antibiotics, antipyretics, and IV fluid resuscitation were started for suspected IAI in the setting of maternal fever and leukocytosis.

The FHR tracing improved to category I after resuscitative measures were taken as demonstrated in Figure 8.7.

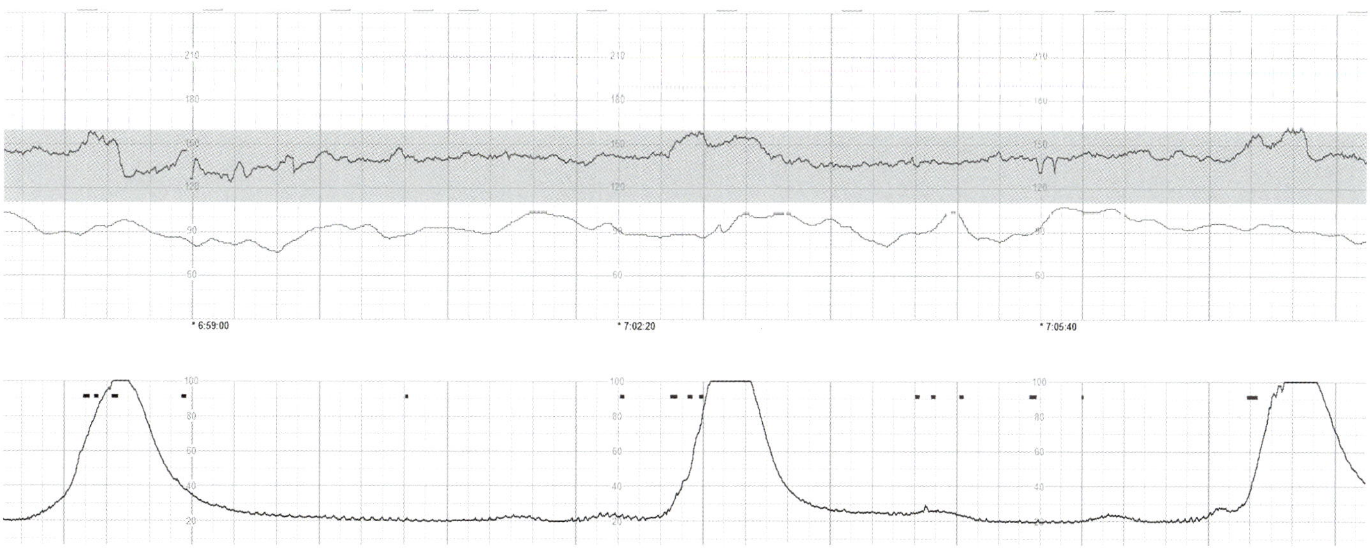

Figure 8.7. Case 3. Category I tracing after resuscitative measures and initiation of antibiotics.

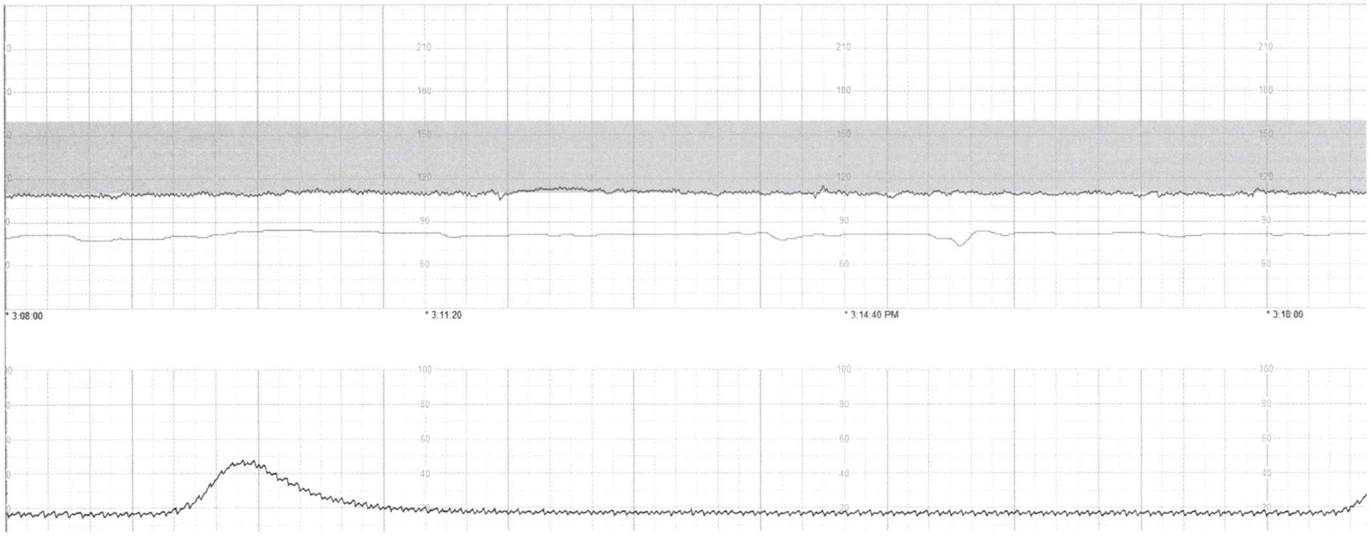

Figure 8.8. Case 4. The effect of magnesium infusion on fetal heart tracing.

Case 4

This is a case of a multiparous patient undergoing an induction of labor at 34 weeks' gestation for severe preeclampsia. Magnesium infusion for the reduction of eclampsia was running. Notice the low baseline at 110 bpm with diminished variability, as shown in Figure 8.8.

Acceleration is elicited with scalp stimulation, noted in Figure 8.9.

Case 5

This is a case of a nulliparous patient undergoing an induction of labor. After the expulsion of the cervical ripening balloon, the cervical exam was 2 cm dilated and 50% effaced. The amniotic membranes were artificially ruptured at that time and the tracing quickly deteriorated as shown in Figure 8.10. A cord prolapse was palpated on reexamination, and the patient was expeditiously moved to the operating room for an emergent cesarean section.

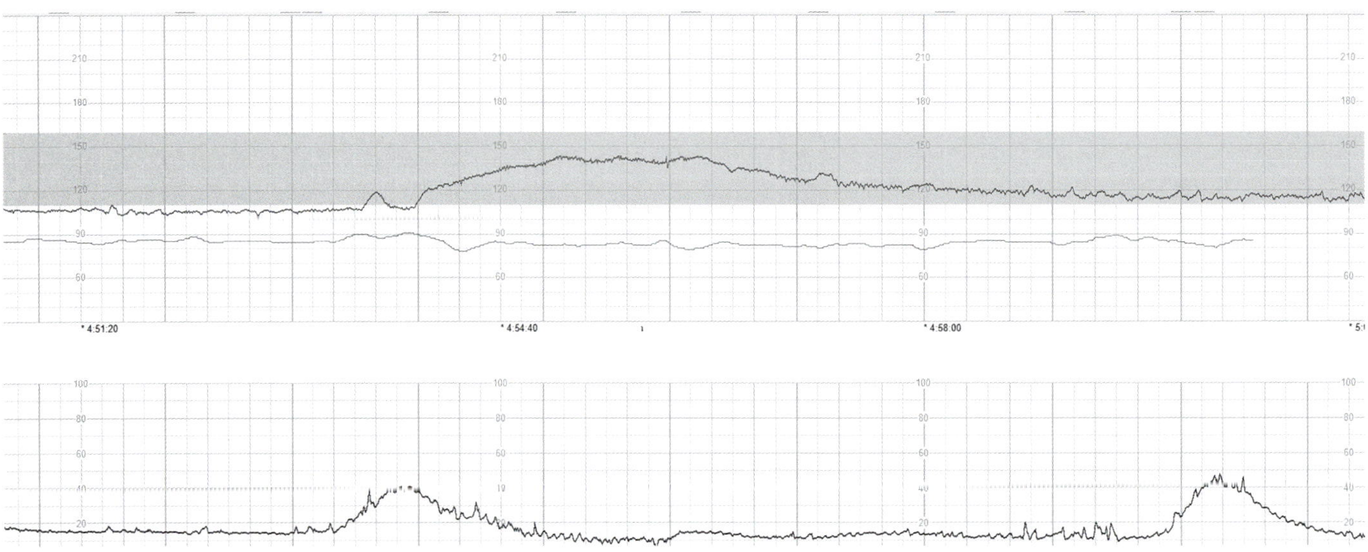

Figure 8.9. Case 4. Scalp stimulation elicits an acceleration.

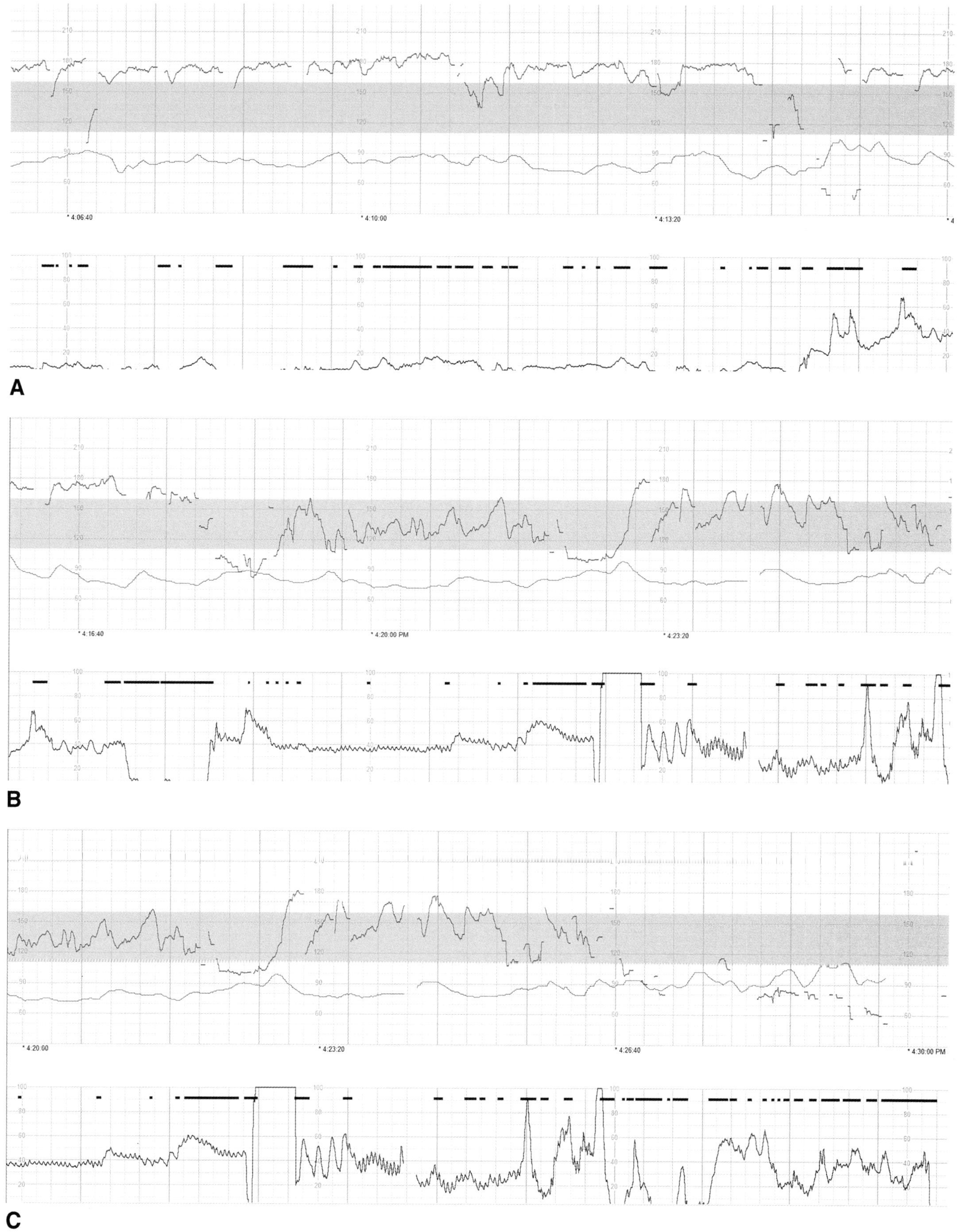

Figure 8.10. Case 5. Fetal heart rate tracing in the setting of cord prolapse.

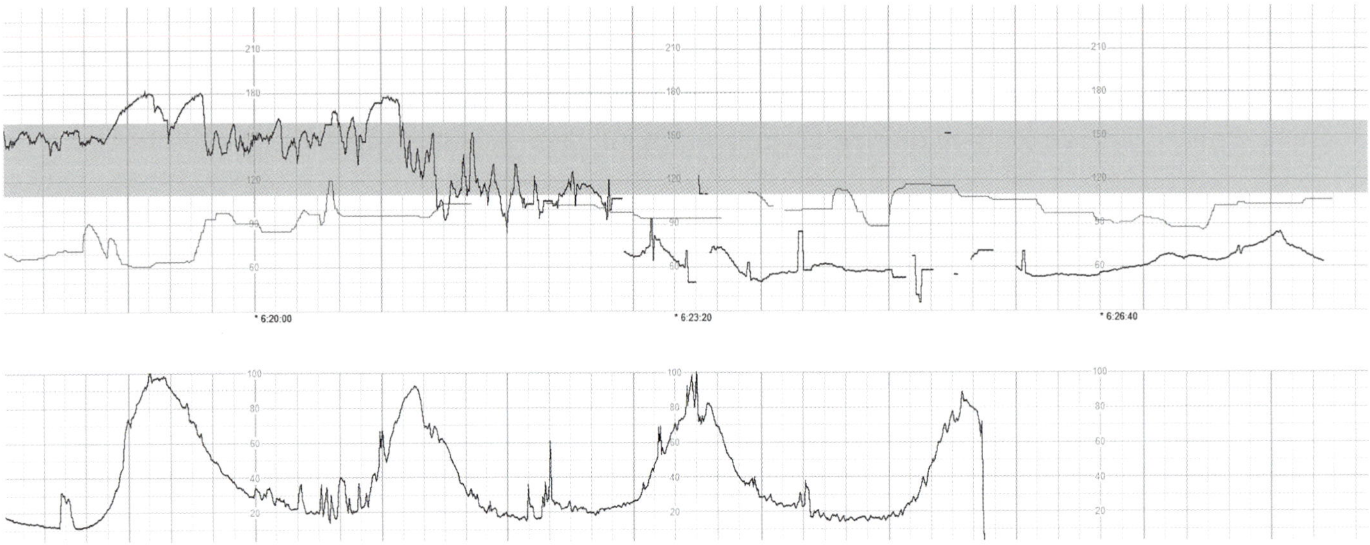

Figure 8.11. Case 6. Fetal heart tracing in a uterine rupture.

Case 6

Figure 8.11 is a case of a multiparous patient who is undergoing spontaneous labor of a term singleton pregnancy. Her first pregnancy was a vaginal delivery of dichorionic twins at 36 weeks' gestation and her second pregnancy was a cesarean section of triplets one year ago. This is a short interval pregnancy, and patient desires TOLAC. The FHR tracing was category I, and the patient progressed to 8 cm dilated until she felt a sudden onset of abdominal pain despite having good neuraxial analgesia prior. The FHR tracing during the onset of the abdominal pain was noted to be below and loss of fetal station was appreciated on vaginal exam. There was high clinical suspicion for uterine rupture, and therefore the patient was emergently moved to the operating room for a cesarean delivery.

SUMMARY

Management of intrapartum category II and category III FHR patterns is a complex process with a goal of erring on the side of avoiding fetal death and morbidity. Limitations of electronic fetal monitoring include variability in interpretation amongst providers and lack of consistent scientific evidence that the intervention of any type of intrapartum FHR abnormalities reduces the risk of cerebral palsy or neurologic impairment. Protocols have been proposed and implemented in various labor and delivery units across the country to standardize the interpretation and management of intrapartum FHR tracings. Ongoing research is needed to assess the effectiveness of these standardized protocols in improving the practice variability and neonatal neurologic outcomes.

REFERENCES

1. ACOG Practice Bulletin No. 116: Management of intrapartum fetal heart tracings. *Obstet Gynecol.* 2010;116(5):1232-1240.
2. Freeman RK, Garite TJ, Nageotte MP, Miller LA, eds. Clinical management of abnormal fetal heart rate patterns. In: *Fetal Heart Rate Monitoring.* 4th ed. Williams & Wilkins; 2012:chap. 8;119-155.
3. Macones GA, Hankins GD, Spong CY, Hauth J, Moore T. The 2008 National Institute of Child Health and Human Development workshop report on electronic fetal monitoring: update on definitions, interpretation, and research guidelines. *Obstet Gynecol.* 2008;112(3):661-666.
4. Modanlou HD, Murata Y. Sinusoidal heart rate pattern: reappraisal of its definition and clinical significance. *J Obstet Gynaecol Res.* 2004;30(3):169-180.
5. Cahill AG, Tuuli MG, Stout MJ, López JD, Macones GA. A prospective cohort study of fetal heart rate monitoring: deceleration area is predictive of fetal acidemia. *Am J Obstet Gynecol.* 2018;218(5):523.e521-523.e512.
6. Frey HA, Liu X, Lynch CD, et al. An evaluation of fetal heart rate characteristics associated with neonatal encephalopathy: a case-control study. *BJOG.* 2018;125(11):1480-1487.
7. Jackson M, Holmgren CM, Esplin MS, Henry E, Varner MW. Frequency of fetal heart rate categories and short-term neonatal outcome. *Obstet Gynecol.* 2011;118(4):803-808.
8. Smith H, Peterson N, Lagrew D, Main E. *Toolkit to Support Vaginal Birth and Reduce Primary Cesareans: A Quality Improvement Toolkit.* California Maternal Quality Care Collaborative; 2016.

9. Clark SL, Nageotte MP, Garite TJ, et al. Intrapartum management of category II fetal heart rate tracings: towards standardization of care. *Am J Obstet Gynecol.* 2013;209(2):89-97.
10. Cahill AG, Roehl KA, Odibo AO, Macones GA. Association of atypical decelerations with acidemia. *Obstet Gynecol.* 2012;120(6):1387-1393.
11. Hamilton E, Warrick P, O'Keeffe D. Variable decelerations: do size and shape matter? *J Matern Fetal Neonatal Med.* 2012; 25(6):648-653.
12. Blackwell SC, Grobman WA, Antoniewicz L, Hutchinson M, Bannerman CG. Interobserver and intraobserver reliability of the NICHD 3-Tier Fetal Heart Rate Interpretation System. *Am J Obstet Gynecol.* 2011;205(4):378.e371-e375.
13. Simpson KR, James DC. Efficacy of intrauterine resuscitation techniques in improving fetal oxygen status during labor. *Obstet Gynecol.* 2005;105(6):1362-1368.
14. Mahfouz A, Monaghan S, Zacharzewski A. Intrauterine fetal resuscitation. *Anaesth Intensive Care Med.* 2022;23(6):336-340.
15. Hofmeyr GJ, Lawrie TA. Amnioinfusion for potential or suspected umbilical cord compression in labour. *Cochrane Database Syst Rev.* 2012;1:CD000013.
16. Davis JD, Sanchez-Ramos L, McKinney JA, Lin L, Kaunitz AM. Intrapartum amnioinfusion reduces meconium aspiration syndrome and improves neonatal outcomes in patients with meconium-stained fluid: a systematic review and meta-analysis. *Am J Obstet Gynecol.* 2023;228(5S):S1179-S1191.e19.
17. Harper LM, Shanks AL, Tuuli MG, Roehl KA, Cahill AG. The risks and benefits of internal monitors in laboring patients. *Am J Obstet Gynecol.* 2013;209(1):38.e1-6.
18. Raghuraman N, Lopez JD, Carter EB, et al. The effect of intrapartum oxygen supplementation on category II fetal monitoring. *Am J Obstet Gynecol.* 2020;223(6):905.e1-905.e7.
19. ACOG Practice Advisory. Oxygen supplementation in the setting of category II or III fetal heart tracings. *Obstet & Gynecol.* 2022;139(3):476.
20. Xodo S, de Heus R, Berghella V, Londero AP. Acute tocolysis for intrapartum nonreassuring fetal status: how often does it prevent cesarean delivery? A systematic review and meta-analysis of randomized controlled trials. *Am J Obstet Gynecol MFM.* 2022;4(5):100639.
21. Abrão KC, Francisco RPV, Miyadahira S, Cicarelli DD, Zugaib M. Elevation of uterine basal tone and fetal heart rate abnormalities after labor analgesia: a randomized controlled trial. *Obstet Gynecol.* 2009;113(1):41-47.
22. Hattler J, Klimek M, Rossaint R, Heesen M. The effect of combined spinal-epidural versus epidural analgesia in laboring women on nonreassuring fetal heart rate tracings: systematic review and meta-analysis. *Anesth Analg.* 2016;123(4):955-964.
23. Maetzold E, Lambers DS, Devaiah CG, Habli M. The effect of combined spinal epidural versus epidural analgesia on fetal heart rate in laboring patients at risk for uteroplacental insufficiency. *J Matern Fetal Neonatal Med.* 2022;35(1):46-51.
24. Al-Hafez L, Bicocca MJ, Chauhan SP, Berghella V. Prostaglandins for induction in pregnancies with fetal growth restriction. *Am J Obstet Gynecol MFM.* 2022;4(2):100538.
25. Horowitz KM, Feldman D. Fetal growth restriction: risk factors for unplanned primary cesarean delivery. *J Matern Fetal Neonatal Med.* 2015;28(18):2131-2134.
26. Epplin KA, Tuuli MG, Odibo AO, Roehl KA, Macones GA, Cahill AG. Effect of growth restriction on fetal heart rate patterns in the second stage of labor. *Am J Perinatol.* 2015;32(4):873-878.
27. Chauhan SP, Weiner SJ, Saade GR, et al. Intrapartum fetal heart rate tracing among small-for-gestational age compared with appropriate-for-gestational-age neonates. *Obstet Gynecol.* 2018; 132(4):1019-1025.
28. ACOG Committee Opinion No. 712: Intrapartum management of intraamniotic infection. *Obstet Gynecol.* 2017;130(2):e95-e101.
29. Duffy CR, Odibo AO, Roehl KA, Macones GA, Cahill AG. Effect of magnesium sulfate on fetal heart rate patterns in the second stage of labor. *Obstet Gynecol.* 2012;119(6):1129-1136.
30. Stewart AM, Macones GA, Odibo AO, Colvin R, Cahill AG. Changes in fetal heart tracing characteristics after magnesium exposure. *Am J Perinatol.* 2014;31(10):869-874.
31. Westgren M, Holmquist P, Svenningsen NW, Ingemarsson I. Intrapartum fetal monitoring in preterm deliveries: prospective study. *Obstet Gynecol.* 1982;60(1):99-106.

CHAPTER 9 Adjunctive Tools for Intrapartum Fetal Heart Rate Monitoring

Lorene Atkins Temming and Ngina K. Connors

INTRODUCTION

The majority of fetal heart rate (FHR) patterns seen in labor will evolve into category II tracings that are neither clearly indicative of fetal hypoxia (category III) nor clearly not associated with fetal hypoxia (category I).[1,2] Although electronic fetal monitoring (EFM) has a high sensitivity for intrapartum fetal hypoxia and acidosis, there is also a high false positive rate that approaches 60%, leading to many unnecessary cesarean deliveries or operative vaginal births.[3,4] Indeed, some patterns seen in category II tracings, such as milder degrees of variable decelerations with average variability, are unlikely to be indicative of a deteriorating or concerning status.[5] In those cases, although interventions such as fluid and position change may be warranted, these patterns can be watched to be sure they do not deteriorate into one that is more concerning. Other patterns seen in category II tracings, such as recurrent late decelerations with moderate or reduced variability, may be more likely to be associated with some degree of hypoxia. In these cases, the obstetrical team must evaluate if the hypoxia is severe enough that the fetus is becoming acidotic and decide if intervention by cesarean section or operative vaginal delivery is warranted.

Unfortunately, EFM is limited because there are many other variables that affect the FHR and may mimic the changes that occur when hypoxia and resulting acidosis are present. Thus, in the case of indeterminate tracings, adjunctive methods for more specifically assessing fetal well-being and the degree of hypoxia and/or fetal acidosis would be useful. This chapter will describe both past, current, and future potential adjunctive methods to FHR monitoring for intrapartum fetal assessment.

FETAL SCALP SAMPLING

Historically, fetal scalp blood sampling was the most commonly used intrapartum adjunctive test for fetal well-being. Traditionally, candidates for fetal scalp blood sampling are patients who are in labor with ruptured membranes and cervical dilation sufficient to allow the introduction of the endoscope (usually 2- to 3-cm dilated) and with the fetal head at a station that is within 2 cm of the ischial spines. Generally, fetal scalp blood sampling was limited to patients who have EFM suggestive of hypoxia or to clarify a confusing pattern such as absent variability without decelerations of accelerations.

Briefly, fetal scalp sampling involves the use of an endoscope and a small blade on a long handle to make a small incision on the fetal scalp. Then, heparinized capillary tubes are used to collect fetal blood for blood gas analysis.

A pH of 7.25 or greater indicates the absence of acidosis; the pattern can be safely watched unless it worsens. A value between 7.20 and 7.25 is equivocal and needs to be repeated immediately, whereas a value of <7.20 is consistent with acidosis and warrants operative intervention unless delivery is imminent. Because respiratory acidosis alone would not be an indication for delivery, whenever possible, the fetal pCO_2 should be simultaneously measured. Only if an acidosis appears to be metabolic should a low pH be considered potentially harmful to the fetus.

There are several challenges with fetal scalp blood sampling. Many factors, including contamination with amniotic fluid, error caused by contamination of the sample with air, and sampling from the scalp affected by fetal vasoconstriction and caput may impact the reliability and predictive value of scalp sampling.[6] Additionally, concerns have been raised regarding the risk of continued bleeding from the fetal scalp causing significant fetal hemorrhage.[7] A recent review of 12 articles reported 37 cases of severe complications following fetal blood sampling, including 2 cases of fetal death. However, the same review cited a registry of 25,000 patients without severe complications.[7]

Early studies on the correlation between EFM patterns and fetal scalp blood pH revealed a general correlation.[8] However, many subsequent observational and randomized studies have called into question the utility of fetal scalp blood sampling. One systematic review and meta-analysis which evaluated heterogeneous studies of modest quality with somewhat inconsistent results concluded that fetal scalp blood sampling in conjunction with EFM could reduce the risk of operative delivery.[7] However, a recent, large multicenter observational study in the UK concluded that as an adjunct tool to cardiotocography, fetal scalp blood sampling offered limited value to predict neonatal acidemia, low Apgar Scores, and admission to NICU.[9] A recent Cochrane review demonstrated that when EFM is combined with fetal blood sampling, although there is no difference in rates of cerebral palsy or perinatal mortality, there is a decrease in neonatal acidemia and seizures with an accompanying increase in rates of cesarean delivery and operative vaginal delivery.[3]

There are some recent data demonstrating that fetal scalp lactate may be more feasible to obtain than pH as it requires a smaller sample. Some studies have shown that lactate levels have higher sensitivity and specificity than scalp pH; although others suggest that when compared to pH, scalp lactate assessment does not show a difference in neonatal outcomes and may increase cesarean deliveries.[10,11]

Experts disagree on the utility of scalp sampling, with some arguing that risks outweigh potential benefits and that fetal scalp sampling may cause harm, whereas others contend it may reduce the risk of operative vaginal delivery.[12,13] Even formal guidelines on the use of fetal scalp blood sampling conflict. The American College of Obstetricians and Gynecologists (ACOG) practice bulletin for management principles of EFM concludes that when a category III FHR tracing is persistent, a scalp blood sample for pH or lactate may be considered and may provide additional information.[14] The Society of Obstetricians and Gynaecologists of Canada (SOGC) recommends that if available, fetal scalp blood sampling for assessment of fetal acidemia is recommended in women with concerning EFM at gestations >34 weeks when delivery is not imminent, or if digital fetal scalp stimulation does not result in an acceleratory FHR response.[15] A recent update of the National Institute for Health and Care Excellence (NICE) United Kingdom guideline for fetal monitoring in labor removed recommendations about fetal blood sampling after finding no evidence that fetal blood sampling with EFM improves outcomes and that it may be associated with reduced 5-minute APGAR score caused by sampling procedure delaying birth.[16] The International Federation of Gyneacology and Obstetrics (FIGO) states that fetal blood sampling may be used in the case of suspicious EFM.[17] Overall, the practical challenges involved with fetal scalp sampling mean that it is virtually unavailable in the United States. Fetal blood sampling does continue to be used in Canada, Europe, and internationally.

FETAL STIMULATION TESTS

Given the concerns with fetal scalp blood sampling, fetal stimulation has been proposed as a less invasive alternative approach. First described by Clark et al in 1982, evidence suggests that manipulation of the fetal scalp for 15 seconds during a vaginal examination can be used to evaluate acidemia.[18] If the FHR reacts with an acceleration of 15 beats per minute amplitude lasting 15 seconds in duration, the likelihood of acidemia is greatly decreased and we can be reassured regarding fetal well-being.[14,19] Fetal stimulation has been described using Allis clamp scalp stimulation, vibroacoustic stimulation, and fetal scalp puncture. When vibroacoustic stimulation is performed, it is applied continuously for 3 to 5 seconds to the maternal abdomen over the fetal head.[19] Of note, it is inappropriate to use fetal stimulation during a deceleration. During an ongoing prolonged deceleration or bradycardia, data is lacking in the literature to help understand whether the presence or absence of an acceleration has the same meaning. More importantly, even if the acceleration does mean the absence of acidosis at that point, there is no assurance that, in the face of potentially rapidly deteriorating oxygenation, a few minutes later the fetus would not become acidotic.

Several studies have looked at fetal stimulation and its association with fetal hypoxia. A meta-analysis by Skupski et al examined positive and negative likelihood ratios of the various methods of fetal stimulation. Likelihood ratios and 95% CIs for the prediction of fetal acidemia given a positive test were: scalp puncture

TABLE 9.1 **Post-test probability of acidemia after fetal stimulation**

Type of stimulation	Negative LR (95% CI)	Positive LR	Post-test probability if negative (%)	Post-test probability if positive (%)
Vibroacoustic	0.20 (0.11,0.37)	5.06 (2.69, 9.50)	2.4	38.5
Scalp Puncture	0.12 (0.02,0.78)	8.54 (1.28, 56.96)	1.5	51.4
Allis clamp	0.10 (0.01,0.68)	10.4 (1.47, 73.6)	1.2	56.2
Digital	0.03 (0.01,0.31)	15.68 (3.22,76.24)	0.7	66.0

Assumes baseline prevalence of fetal acidemia of 11.0% in laboring patients.
Data from Skupski et al[19,20]

8.54 (CI 1.28, 56.96), Allis clamp 10.4 (CI 1.47, 73.61), vibroacoustic stimulation 5.06 (CI 2.69, 9.50), and digital 15.68 (CI 3.22, 76.24). For a negative test, these were: scalp puncture 0.12 (CI 0.02, 0.78), Allis clamp 0.10 (CI 0.01, 0.68), vibroacoustic stimulation 0.20 (CI 0.11, 0.37), and digital 0.06 (CI 0.01, 0.31).[19] The prevalence of fetal acidemia in the meta-analysis was 11%, and these likelihood ratios can be used to calculate the post-test probabilities, as shown in Table 9.1. With a positive test, which would result in no acceleration after stimulation, the probability of acidemia ranges from 38.5% with vibroacoustic stimulation to 66.0% with digital scalp simulation.[19,20] With a negative test, or when there is acceleration after stimulation, the probability of acidemia decreases to 2.4% with vibroacoustic stimulation to 0.7% with digital scalp stimulation[19,20] (see Table 9.1).

Several studies have compared fetal manipulation, typically with digital scalp stimulation, to EFM alone. A recent Cochrane review included four trials with a total of 1280 women.[21] Although there was a trend toward fetal manual manipulation decreasing the incidence of nonreactive EFM compared to mock or no stimulation, this difference was not statistically significant.[21] When digital scalp stimulation was compared to vibroacoustic stimulation, there was no difference in the incidence of nonreactive EFM or the need for contraction-stress test.[21] A more recent randomized controlled trial compared manual fetal stimulation to no stimulation in a group of laboring women with EFM abnormalities and found similar results, with no change in the rate of cesarean delivery, cord pH, or Apgar scores between the two groups.[22]

Fetal scalp simulation has also been compared with fetal blood sampling. An early study by Elimian et al evaluated if digital scalp stimulation could decrease the need for fetal blood sampling. In the study, all patients with accelerations of 15 beats per minute or more lasting 15 seconds or more had a scalp pH >7.20.[23] When accelerations were defined less strictly as 10 beats per minute for 10 seconds, more reactive responses were obtained and all had a pH >7.20.[23] Of the nonreactive responses, those with variability were less likely to have a pH of <7.20.[23] They concluded that the scalp stimulation test could decrease the need for fetal scalp blood sampling by 47% and assessment of FHR variability before scalp stimulation could decrease further the need for scalp blood sampling by 73%.[23] A more recent Cochrane review was equivocal in its findings, concluding that there is very low-certainty evidence available which makes it unclear whether stimulating the fetal scalp is a safe and effective way to confirm fetal well-being in labor.[24] A pilot study assessed the feasibility of conducting an RCT comparing the impact on cesarean delivery of digital fetal scalp stimulation compared to fetal blood sampling, and the trial developed from this pilot, the Fetal Intrapartum Randomized Scalp Stimulation Trial (FIRSST NCT05306756), is ongoing.[25,26]

In summary, fetal manipulation may augment the interpretation of EFM and be useful in decreasing suspicion to fetal acidemia. However, the overall benefit, particularly in comparison to fetal blood sampling, is unclear. Digital scalp stimulation is the least invasive method which requires no additional equipment and has the best predictive value of the fetal stimulation tests. ACOG recommends that in the setting of concerning category II tracing if the improvement is not noted with interventions including maternal repositioning and fluid bolus, additional assessment with digital scalp or vibroacoustic stimulation should be done.[5] Similarly, SOGC and NICE guidelines recommend that digital fetal scalp stimulation be performed in response to atypical EFM and that absence of accelerations in response should lead to fetal scalp blood sampling if available or prompt delivery if scalp sampling is not available or if sampling shows concern for acidemia.[15,16] FIGO encourages the use of fetal scalp stimulation in the setting of reduced variability on EFM and discourages its use in other patterns.[17]

FETAL PULSE OXIMETRY

Monitoring of oxygen saturation using pulse oximetry is pervasive in children and adults in the operating room and other settings. Pulse oximetry relies on the principle that deoxyhemoglobin absorbs red light (735 nm), whereas oxyhemoglobin absorbs infrared light (890 nm).[27] The pulse oximeter contains two low-voltage, light-emitting diodes as light sources and one photodetector. Red and near-infrared light are alternately shined on tissue and the absorption of transmitted or reflected light is measured; using standard curves, the oximeter calculates the relative amounts of saturated and unsaturated hemoglobin to determine percent oxygenation. The oxygen saturation is determined at the peak of the pulse wave (equal to light absorbed by arterial and venous blood and surrounding tissue) and the nadir of the pulse wave (light absorbed only by venous blood and tissue). The amount of light absorbed at the nadir is subtracted from the amount absorbed at the peak, yielding the amount of light absorbed by arterial blood. This ratio is used to calculate percent oxygenation (Fig. 9.1).[27]

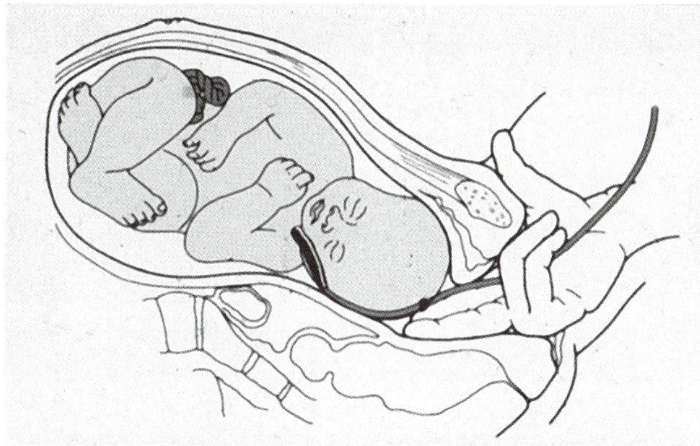

Figure 9.2. Picture of a pulse oximeter probe inserted transcervically to ultimately lodge against the fetal cheek. The catheter is inserted much like an intrauterine pressure catheter. The sensor is held against the fetal cheek by the pressure provided by the uterine wall and pelvic sidewall.

A fetal pulse oximeter was designed that seemed to be a safe and minimally invasive way to directly measure fetal oxygenation in labor. A specialized sensor is inserted through the dilated cervix after ruptured membranes and positioned against the fetal face (Fig. 9.2). Once in contact with the fetal skin, the device measures fetal oxygen saturation during labor. The level of fetal oxygen saturation ($FSpO_2$) in labor is normally only approximately 40% to 55%, and human studies validated 30% as a critical value below which, when combined with abnormal EFM, there is a high risk of hypoxia and fetal acidosis.[28,29]

Several trials evaluated the use of fetal pulse oximetry. The first randomized controlled trial, published

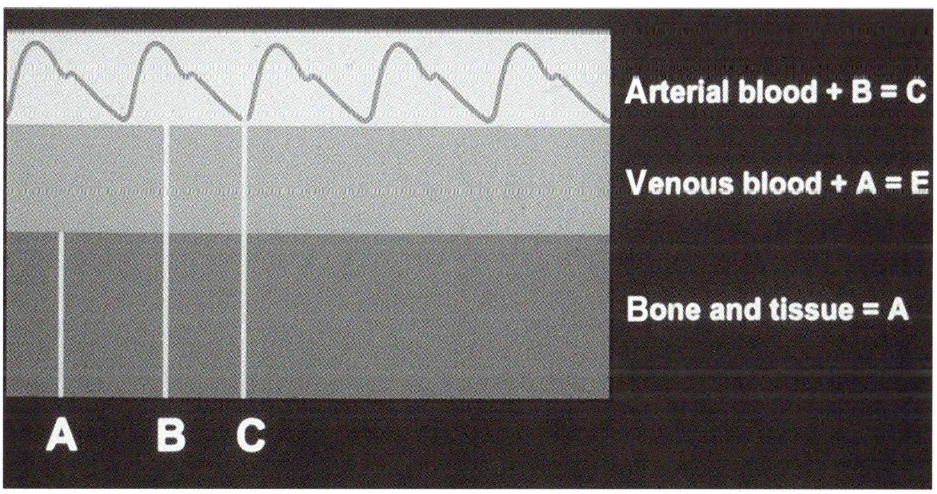

Figure 9.1. This figure illustrates how the pulse wave is used to separate the light absorption of arterial blood from the venous blood and surrounding tissue.

by Garite et al in 2000, randomized 1010 patients in active labor with abnormal EFM patterns to EFM alone or EFM with pulse oximetry.[30] Although this study demonstrated a reduction in cesarean delivery because of nonreassuring fetal status in those with fetal pulse oximetry, there was no overall difference in cesarean delivery rate between the two groups because the rate of cesareans caused by labor dystocia was increased in the group with fetal pulse oximetry.[30] This raised questions as to whether nonreassuring fetal status precedes dystocia or if the pulse oximeter itself interfered with labor progression.

Subsequent studies comparing EFM alone to EFM plus pulse oximetry in women in labor with nonreassuring fetal heart patterns yielded similar results. The FOREMOST trial, which was done at four large hospitals in Australia, randomized 600 women and found that fetal pulse oximetry was associated with a lower rate of cesarean delivery for nonreassuring fetal status. However, the overall cesarean rate was comparable between the two groups, and there were no differences in neonatal outcomes.[31] Klauser et al randomized 360 women at the University of Mississippi Medical Center and found that the overall rate of cesarean delivery, as well as the rates of cesarean for nonreassuring fetal heart-rate tracing and for dystocia, was similar between the two groups.[32] Although decision-to-incision time was approximately 10 minutes shorter in the fetal pulse oximetry arm, there were no statistically significant differences in neonatal outcomes.[32]

A large Maternal Fetal Medicine Units Network (MFMU) trial aimed to evaluate the efficacy and safety of fetal pulse oximetry. Women were randomized to masked versus unmasked fetal pulse oximetry in addition to EFM.[33] Although the trial originally planned to enroll 10,000 women, ultimately 5553 women were randomized before the trial was stopped for already having adequate power to detect a difference in the primary outcome, cesarean delivery.[33] The results of the MFMU network trial demonstrated no difference in overall cesarean rate or in cesarean for nonreassuring fetal status in the two groups. These results held true for the subgroup of women with nonreassuring EFM prior to randomization.[33] There was also no difference in neonatal outcomes.[33]

A recent Cochrane review that included seven trials found that there was no difference in overall cesarean delivery rate when fetal pulse oximetry was used in addition to EFM.[34] This review did demonstrate a reduction in cesarean delivery for nonreassuring fetal status when only the four trials that enrolled patients with nonreassuring EFM were included.[34] Nonetheless, with no clear evidence for benefit, the Food and Drug Administration did not approve the use of a fetal pulse oximeter in the United States, and it was removed from the market by its manufacturer.[27] Thus, fetal pulse oximetry is no longer used in clinical practice in the US or internationally, with ACOG, NICE, and FIGO guidelines not mentioning its use and SOGC guidelines specifically recommending against the use of fetal pulse oximetry.[5,15-17]

FETAL ELECTROCARDIOGRAPHIC ST SEGMENT ANALYSIS

A more recent development in technology to assist in managing and more accurately detecting fetal hypoxia and acidosis in labor has been the introduction of fetal electrocardiographic (ECG) analysis. This technology, known as fetal ST segment waveform analysis (STAN) and marketed by Neoventa of Sweden, is a combination of FHR interpretation and ST analysis (Fig. 9.3). The ST analysis is based on changes in the fetal ECG waveform caused by myocardial adaptation to oxygen deficiency. The analysis is conducted using the

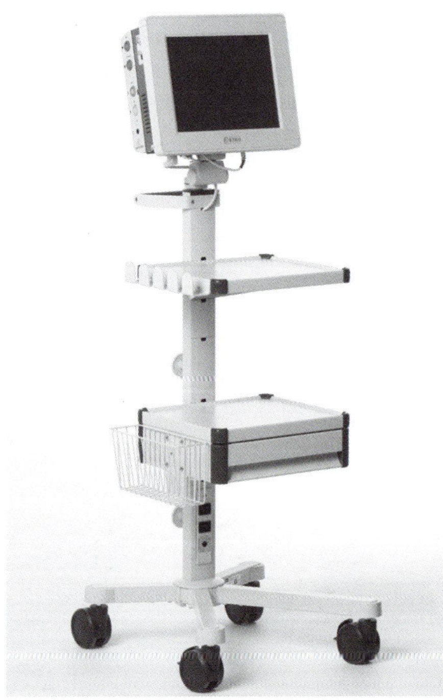

Figure 9.3. This is the device marketed by Neoventa of Sweden that contains an FHR monitor and a computer that analyzes the fetal ECG and alerts the clinician to various changes in the ECG waveform that suggest fetal hypoxia.

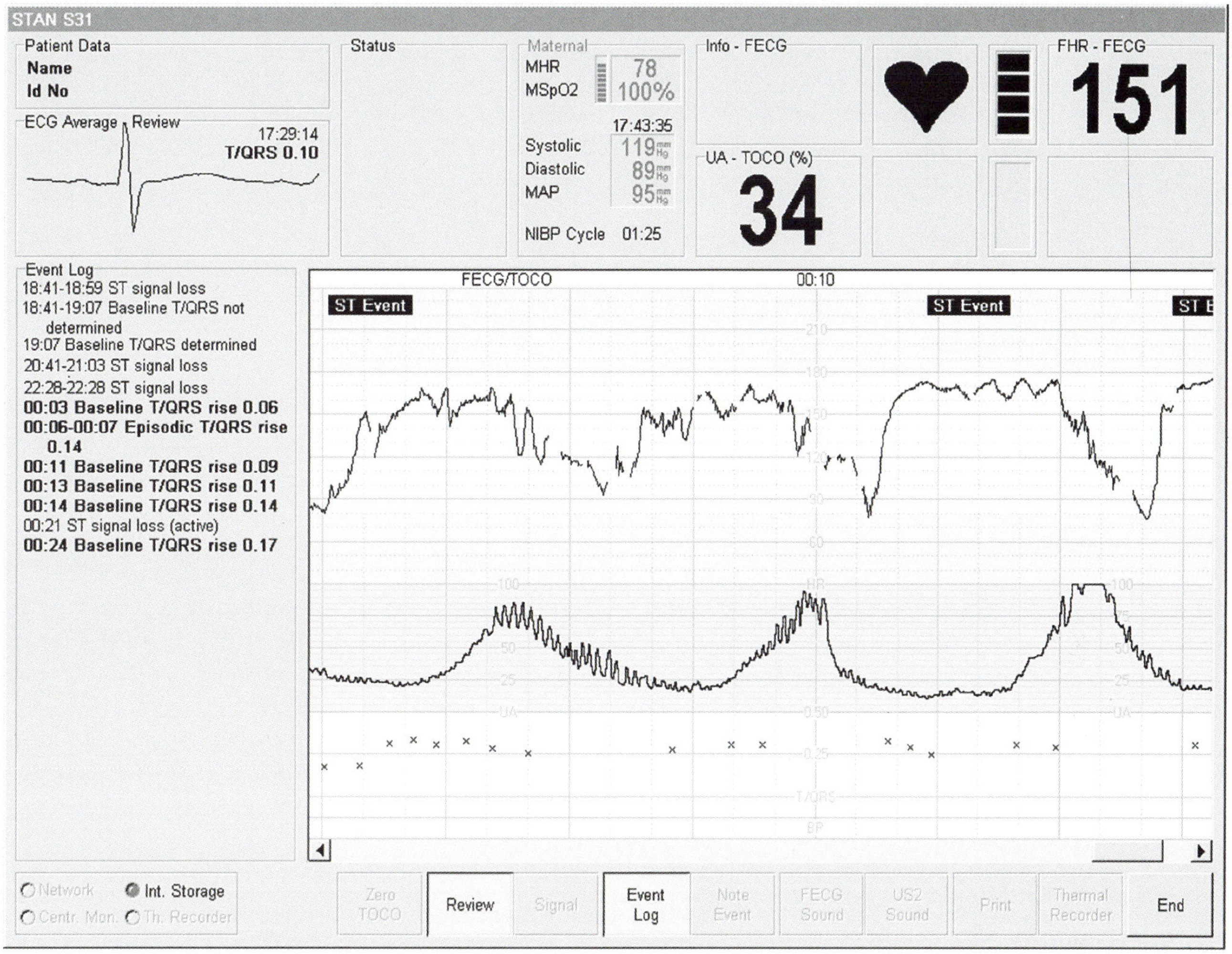

Figure 9.4. This is the tracing produced by the STAN monitor. Deep decelerations late in timing possibly suggestive of hypoxia are confirmed by several "ST events," which the ECG waveform analysis has concluded as also suggestive of fetal hypoxia.

computerized real-time analysis of the ST segment and T-wave patterns and intervals of the fetal ECG. STAN incorporates this analysis with EFM and categorizes tracings accordingly (Fig. 9.4). A complete description of the STAN categories and their management is beyond the scope of this chapter. However, in the US, EFM is categorized into green, yellow, and red categories, whereas in Europe they are categorized into green, yellow, orange, and red, where green is reassuring and red indicates the need for imminent delivery. Yellow zone tracings in the US and yellow and orange zone tracings in Europe have a complex management scheme that incorporates the presence or absence of ST changes and the degree of baseline T/QRS increase.[27] This technology aims to provide useful information for indeterminate EFM tracings and potentially decrease neonatal acidemia and operative deliveries.

The Plymouth trial, which was the first large randomized trial to compare EFM alone to EFM with ST waveform analysis, was conducted in England and demonstrated the promise of ST waveform analysis as an adjunct.[35] It showed a 43% reduction in operative interventions for fetal distress and a trend toward a decrease in metabolic acidosis and low Apgar score.[35] Similarly promising results were found in a subsequent Swedish randomized trial that showed decreased operative interventions and decreased metabolic acidosis when ST segment analysis was used.[36] However, a number of concerns were raised about both the conduct and analysis of this trial that has called its results into question.[27]

Subsequent studies of fetal ECG as an adjunct to EFM failed to demonstrate benefit. Finnish, Dutch, and French randomized trials did not show a change in neonatal acidosis with the use of ST segment analysis nor did they demonstrate a decrease in operative deliveries or a change in neonatal outcomes.[37-39] Of note, the Dutch trial did show a reduction in cases of metabolic acidosis defined as a base deficit in the blood greater than 12, but not by pH.[38] All three of those trials showed a reduced need for fetal blood sampling when fetal ECG was added.[37-39]

A comprehensive US randomized controlled trial was undertaken by the MFMU Network after a pilot stage and extensive training on the STAN technology.[40] Ultimately, 11,108 patients were randomized at 26 hospitals to either open or masked fetal ST analysis monitoring.[40] There was no difference in the primary outcome that was a composite including intrapartum fetal death, neonatal death, an Apgar score of <3 at 5 minutes, neonatal seizure, umbilical artery pH less than 7.05 with a base deficit greater than 12 mmol/L, neonatal intubation, or neonatal encephalopathy.[40] When examining individual components of the composite, Apgar score <3 at 5 minutes was reduced in the open group. There were no significant differences in the rate of cesarean delivery or operative deliveries between groups.[40]

A subsequent Cochrane systematic review and another meta-analysis both conclude that fetal ECG does not decrease cesarean deliveries, operative deliveries, metabolic acidosis, or adverse neonatal outcomes.[4,41] The Cochrane review did demonstrate decreased rates of fetal blood sampling when fetal ECG was added.[4] An individual participant data meta-analysis of four trials including 12,987 women also did not show any decrease in acidosis or cesarean delivery, although it did show a decrease in operative vaginal delivery as well as fetal blood sampling.[42] However, a meta-analysis by Blix et al reported that STAN monitoring decreased metabolic acidosis and had a minor reduction in operative vaginal deliveries as well as a reduction in fetal blood sampling. The authors concluded that 401 women would need to be monitored with STAN to prevent one case of metabolic acidosis.[43] The conflicting findings of these meta-analyses may be that Blix et al used revised data from the Swedish and Dutch trials and used trial sequential analysis rather than traditional meta-analysis.[43-45]

In summary, most data currently available regarding fetal ECG as an adjunct to EFM do not support its regular use at this time. Proponents of STAN technology cite the combination of low- and high-risk populations used in various trials and the relative rarity of adverse outcomes and lack of power in trials to advocate that more evaluation is required before fetal ECG technology is entirely rejected.[46] ACOG and NICE guidelines do not currently mention the use of fetal ECG as an adjunct, whereas SOGC guidelines recommend against the use of ST waveform analysis at this time, and FIGO guidelines indicate that further research is needed to evaluate if changing management guidelines based on fetal ECG output could improve the performance of the technique before it is widely used.[5,15-17]

FUTURE DIRECTIONS

There are several other potential adjunctive tools to FHR monitoring that have emerged recently and are promising areas for future study.

Artificial Intelligence

Medical artificial intelligence (AI) is rapidly developing in various specialties. Machine learning is a basic method that uses data, learns from the data, and makes decisions or predictions by itself.[47] Fetal monitoring, which is traditionally interpreted by practitioners, has been found to have low inter- and intra-rater reliability and is an area where AI and machine learning could be useful. AI could potentially help humans decide when an intervention is needed to prevent fetal hypoxia.

Several studies have demonstrated the benefit of AI in principle. Warrick et al found that a combination of an identification system and EFM baseline heart rate could be a good detector of fetal distress.[48] The system recognized half of the pathologic cases (missed by clinical observation) with a low percentage of false positives.[48] Similarly, Fergus et al used machine learning as a decision support tool and found that a deep learning classifier reached 94% sensitivity and 91% specificity, for an area under the curve of 0.99.[49] Zhao et al designed a computer-aided diagnosis system integrated with an advanced deep learning algorithm to detect fetal hypoxia.[50] They used an open-access database to test the performance using umbilical artery pH as the gold standard to distinguish normal and pathologic fetuses.[50] They demonstrated that their computer-aided diagnosis system had 99% sensitivity, 98% specificity, and an area under the curve of 0.987 for predicting acidosis.[50]

However, the results of clinical trials have been less promising. A Cochrane systematic review of AI for fetal assessment in labor found only one study to include and was underpowered to evaluate the association between the use of AI and its impact on outcomes including cesarean delivery and adverse neonatal outcomes.[51] Balaya et al conducted a more recent systematic review and meta-analysis which evaluated inter-rater reliability between human and AI interpretations of EFM and the impact of AI-assisted EFM interpretation on outcomes.[52] Inter-rater reliability between AI and human interpretation was moderate in the six studies that evaluated it, with a weighted means Cohen's Kappa of 0.49 (0.32-0.66).[52] In the three randomized trials that evaluated the impact of machine learning on outcomes of 55,064 patients, AI interpretation of EFM during labor did not improve neonatal outcomes in terms of neonatal acidosis, cord blood pH <7.15 to 7.20, 5-minute Apgar score <7, mode of delivery, neonatal intensive care unit admission, neonatal seizures, or perinatal death.[52]

Total Deceleration Area

Additionally, there are several ways to evaluate EFM outside of standard NICHD descriptions that could be combined with AI and serve as an adjunct to EFM. Cahill et al found that the total deceleration area, described as the depth multiplied by the duration of the deceleration in the 30 minutes preceding delivery had the best predictive ability for fetal acidemia when compared to patterns of repetitive late decelerations, repetitive prolonged decelerations, and repetitive variable decelerations.[53] Several subsequent studies have evaluated and confirmed the inverse association of increasing total deceleration area to decreasing cord pH.[54-57] Moreover, another recent case-controlled study confirmed the association of increased total deceleration area with neonatal encephalopathy.[58] Future efforts may be directed at the development of a computerized real-time analysis of deceleration areas on fetal monitoring as a more valid adjunctive clinical tool in predicting adverse neonatal outcomes.

Fetal Reserve Index

Another approach to evaluate EFM beyond standard classifications has been developed by Evans et al and is known as the "Fetal Reserve Index."[59] This was developed prospectively to incorporate both the context of EFM as well as quantifiable components of the tracing. The index includes eight defined factors which include FHR, baseline variability, accelerations, decelerations, increased uterine activity, maternal risk factors, obstetrical risk factors, and fetal risk factors. Each factor is scored as 1 if normal/present or 0 if not. These metrics are combined into a Fetal Reserve Index that may change over time and can progress from a green to yellow to red zone.[59] Multiple studies have shown that when compared with NICHD/ACOG categories, the Fetal Reserve Index more accurately identifies babies born with cerebral palsy and could also reduce the rates of emergency cesarean delivery and vaginal operative deliveries.[59] Similar to the total deceleration area, the Fetal Reserve Index could be validated in future studies and combined with computerized real-time analysis or machine learning to create a clinical tool that would function as an adjunct to fetal monitoring.

CONCLUSION

In conclusion, although EFM continues to be the gold standard for assessing fetal well-being, its use is fraught with limitations. Nearly all clinicians have had the experience of performing an operative delivery for a nonreassuring fetal tracing, only to deliver an infant with Apgars of 9 and 9 who is not acidotic. Conversely, many have experienced the delivery of a compromised infant with a tracing that did not appear to be too alarming. The patient and clinician would certainly benefit from a reliable adjunct method to EFM that can definitively answer the question of whether the fetus is experiencing hypoxia or acidosis during labor. Currently, for any additional information, practitioners in the US are relegated to fetal response to stimulation, whether manually or by vibroacoustic means. Unfortunately, attempts with fetal pulse oximetry as well as STAN technology have not proven to be effective. As the medical field evolves with the use of AI, hopefully, a clinically meaningful algorithm will be developed to assist clinicians in one of the most difficult areas of decision-making.

REFERENCES

1. Macones, GA, Hankins GDV, Spong CY, Hauth J, Moore T. The 2008 National Institute of Child Health and Human Development workshop report on electronic fetal monitoring: update on definitions, interpretation, and research guidelines. *Obstet Gynecol.* 2008;112(3):661-666.
2. Cahill AG, Spain J. Intrapartum fetal monitoring. *Clin Obstet Gynecol.* 2015;58(2):263-268.
3. Alfirevic Z, Devane D, Gyte GM, Cuthbert A. Continuous cardiotocography (CTG) as a form of electronic fetal monitoring (EFM) for fetal assessment during labour. *Cochrane Database Syst Rev.* 2017;2019(5).

4. Neilson JP. Fetal electrocardiogram (ECG) for fetal monitoring during labour. *Cochrane Database Syst Rev*. 2015;2015(12): CD000116.
5. American College of Obstetricians and Gynecologists. Practice bulletin no. 116: management of intrapartum FHR tracings. *Obstet Gynecol*. 2010;116(5):1232-1240.
6. Sherman DJ, Arieli S, Raziel A, Bukovsky I. The effect of sampling technique on measurement of fetal blood pH and gases: an in vitro system. *Am J Obstet Gynecol*. 1994;171(4):1125-1128.
7. Jørgensen JS, Weber T. Fetal scalp blood sampling in labor: a review. *Acta Obstet Gynecol Scand*. 2014;93(6):548-555.
8. Clark SL, Paul RH. Intrapartum fetal surveillance: the role of fetal scalp blood sampling. *Am J Obstet Gynecol*. 1985;153(7):717-720.
9. Al Wattar BH, Lakhiani A, Sacco A, et al. Evaluating the value of intrapartum fetal scalp blood sampling to predict adverse neonatal outcomes: a UK multicentre observational study. *Eur J Obstet Gynecol Biol*. 2019;240:62-67.
10. Kruger K, Hallberg B, Blennow M, Kublickas M, Westgren M. Predictive value of fetal scalp blood lactate concentration and pH as markers of neurologic disability. *Am J Obstet Gynecol*. 1999; 181(5 Pt 1):1072-1078.
11. Stål I, Wennerholm UB, Nordstrom L, Ladfors L, Wiberg-Itzel E. Fetal scalp blood sampling during second stage of labor: analyzing lactate or pH? A secondary analysis of a randomized controlled trial. *J Matern Fetal Neonatal Med*. 2022;35(6):1100-1107.
12. Chandraharan E. Fetal scalp blood sampling should be abandoned: FOR: FBS does not fulfil the principle of first do no harm. *BJOG*. 2016;123(11):1770-1770.
13. Stener Jørgensen J. Fetal scalp blood sampling should be abandoned: AGAINST: fetal scalp blood sampling in conjunction with electronic fetal monitoring reduces the risk of unnecessary operative delivery. *BJOG*. 2016;123(11):1771-1771.
14. ACOG Practice Bulletin No. 106: Intrapartum fetal heart rate monitoring: nomenclature, interpretation, and general management principles. *Obstet Gynecol*. 2009;114(1):192-202.
15. Liston R, Sawchuck D, Young D. Fetal health surveillance: antepartum and intrapartum consensus guideline. *J Obstet Gynaecol Can*. 2007;29(9 Suppl 4):S3-56.
16. O'Heney J, McAllister S, Maresh M, Blott M. Fetal monitoring in labour: summary and update of NICE guidance. *BMJ*. 2022; 379:o2854.
17. Visser GH, Ayres-De-Campos D; FIGO Intrapartum Fetal Monitoring Expert Consensus Panel. FIGO consensus guidelines on intrapartum fetal monitoring: adjunctive technologies. *Int J Gynaecol Obstet*. 2015;131(1):25-29.
18. Clark SL, Gimovsky ML, Miller FC. Fetal heart rate response to scalp blood sampling. *Am J Obstet Gynecol*. 1982;144(6):706-708.
19. Skupski DW, Rosenberg CR, Eglinton GS. Intrapartum fetal stimulation tests: a meta-analysis. *Obstet Gynecol*. 2002;99(1): 129-134.
20. Grimes DA, Schulz KF. Refining clinical diagnosis with likelihood ratios. *Lancet*. 2005;365(9469):1500-1505.
21. Tan KH, Sabapathy A, Wei X. Fetal manipulation for facilitating tests of fetal wellbeing. *Cochrane Database Syst Rev*. 2013;(12): CD003396.
22. Tahmina S, Daniel M, Krishnan L. Manual fetal stimulation during intrapartum fetal surveillance: a randomized controlled trial. *Am J Obstet Gynecol MFM*. 2022;4(2):100574.
23. Elimian A, Figueroa R, Tejani N. Intrapartum assessment of fetal well-being: a comparison of scalp stimulation with scalp blood pH sampling. *Obstet Gynecol*. 1997;89(3):373-376.
24. Murphy DJ, Devane D, Molloy E, Shahabuddin Y. Fetal scalp stimulation for assessing fetal well-being during labour. *Cochrane Database Syst Rev*. 2023;1(1):Cd013808.
25. Hughes O, Murphy DJ. Comparing second-line tests to assess fetal wellbeing in labor: a feasibility study and pilot randomized controlled trial. *J Matern Fetal Neonatal Med*. 2022;35(1):91-99.
26. Murphy DJ, Shahabuddin Y, Yambasu S, et al. Digital fetal scalp stimulation (dFSS) versus fetal blood sampling (FBS) to assess fetal wellbeing in labour—a multi-centre randomised controlled trial: Fetal Intrapartum Randomised Scalp Stimulation Trial (FIRSST NCT05306756). *Trials*. 2022;23(1):848.
27. Bloom SL, Belfort M, Saade G. What we have learned about intrapartum fetal monitoring trials in the MFMU Network. *Seminars in Perinatology*. 2016;40(5):307-317.
28. Dildy GA, Thorp JA, Yeast JD, Clark SL. The relationship between oxygen saturation and pH in umbilical blood: implications for intrapartum fetal oxygen saturation monitoring. *Am J Obstet Gynecol*. 1996;175(3 Pt 1):682-687.
29. Goffinet F, Langer B, Carbonne B, et al. Multicenter study on the clinical value of fetal pulse oximetry. I. Methodologic evaluation. The French Study Group on Fetal Pulse Oximetry. *Am J Obstet Gynecol*. 1997;177(5):1238-1246.
30. Garite TJ, Dildy GA, McNamara H, et al. A multicenter controlled trial of fetal pulse oximetry in the intrapartum management of nonreassuring fetal heart rate patterns. *Am J Obstet Gynecol*. 2000;183(5):1049-1058.
31. East CE, Brennecke SP, King JF, Chan FY, Colditz PB; FOREMOST Study Group. The effect of intrapartum fetal pulse oximetry, in the presence of a nonreassuring fetal heart rate pattern, on operative delivery rates: a multicenter, randomized, controlled trial (the FOREMOST trial). *Am J Obstet Gynecol*. 2006;194(3):606.e1-606.e16.
32. Klauser CK, Christensen EE, Chauhan SP, et al. Use of fetal pulse oximetry among high-risk women in labor: a randomized clinical trial. *Am J Obstet Gynecol*. 2005;192(6):1810-1817; discussion 1817-9.
33. Bloom SL, Spong CY, Thom E, et al; National Institute of Child Health and Human Development Maternal-Fetal Medicine Units Network. Fetal pulse oximetry and cesarean delivery. *N Engl J Med*. 2006;355(21):2195-2202.
34. East CE, Begg L, Colditz PB, Lau R. Fetal pulse oximetry for fetal assessment in labour. *Cochrane Database Syst Rev*. 2014;2014(10): CD004075.
35. Westgate J, Harris M, Curnow JS, Greene KR. Plymouth randomized trial of cardiotocogram only versus ST waveform plus cardiotocogram for intrapartum monitoring in 2400 cases. *Am J Obstet Gynecol*. 1993;169(5):1151-1160.
36. Amer-Wåhlin I, Hellsten C, Norén H, et al. Cardiotocography only versus cardiotocography plus ST analysis of fetal

electrocardiogram for intrapartum fetal monitoring: a Swedish randomised controlled trial. *Lancet.* 2001;358(9281):534-538.

37. Ojala K, Vääräsmäki M, Mäkikallio K, Valkama M, Tekay A. A comparison of intrapartum automated fetal electrocardiography and conventional cardiotocography: a randomised controlled study. *BJOG.* 2006;113(4):419-423.
38. Westerhuis M, Visser GHA, Moons KGM, et al. Cardiotocography plus ST analysis of fetal electrocardiogram compared with cardiotocography only for intrapartum monitoring: a randomized controlled trial. *Obstet Gynecol.* 2010;115(6):1173-1180.
39. Vayssière C, David E, Meyer N, et al. A French randomized controlled trial of ST-segment analysis in a population with abnormal cardiotocograms during labor. *Am J Obstet Gynecol.* 2007;197(3):299.e1-299.e6.
40. Belfort MA, Saade GR, Thom E, et al; Eunice Kennedy Shriver National Institute of Child Health and Human Development Maternal-Fetal Medicine Units Network. A randomized trial of intrapartum fetal ECG ST-segment analysis. *N Engl J Med.* 2015;373(7):632-641.
41. Saccone G, Schuit E, Amer-Wåhlin I, Xodo S, Berghella V. Electrocardiogram ST analysis during labor: a systematic review and meta-analysis of randomized controlled trials. *Obstet Gynecol.* 2016;127(1):127-135.
42. Schuit E, Amer-Wahlin I, Ojala K, et al. Effectiveness of electronic fetal monitoring with additional ST analysis in vertex singleton pregnancies at >36 weeks of gestation: an individual participant data metaanalysis. *Am J Obstet Gynecol.* 2013;208(3):187.e1-187.e13.
43. Blix E, Brurberg KG, Reierth E, Reinar LM, Øian P. ST waveform analysis versus cardiotocography alone for intrapartum fetal monitoring: a systematic review and meta-analysis of randomized trials. *Acta Obstet Gynecol Scand.* 2016;95(1):16-27.
44. Westerhuis M, Visser GHA, Moons KGM, et al. Cardiotocography plus ST analysis of fetal electrocardiogram compared with cardiotocography only for intrapartum monitoring: a randomized controlled trial. *Obstet Gynecol.* 2011;117(2 Pt 1):406-407.
45. Amer-Wåhlin I, Kjellmer I, Maršál K, Olofsson P, Rosén KG. Swedish randomized controlled trial of cardiotocography only versus cardiotocography plus ST analysis of fetal electrocardiogram revisited: analysis of data according to standard versus modified intention-to-treat principle. *Acta Obstet Gynecol Scand.* 2011;90(9):990-996.
46. Xodo S, Saccone G, Schuit E, Amer-Wåhlin I, Berghella V. Why STAN might not be dead. *J Matern Fetal Neonatal Med.* 2017;30(19):2306-2308.
47. Kim HY, Cho GJ, Kwon HS. Applications of artificial intelligence in obstetrics. *Ultrasonography,* 2023;42(1):2-9.
48. Warrick PA, Hamilton EF, Precup D, Kearney RE. Classification of normal and hypoxic fetuses from systems modeling of intrapartum cardiotocography. *IEEE Trans Biomed Eng.* 2010;57(4):771-779.
49. Fergus P, Hussain A, Al-Jumeily D, Huang DS, Bouguila N. Classification of caesarean section and normal vaginal deliveries using foetal heart rate signals and advanced machine learning algorithms. *Biomed Eng Online.* 2017;16(1):89.
50. Zhao Z, Zhang Y, Comert Z, Deng Y. Computer-aided diagnosis system of fetal hypoxia incorporating recurrence plot with convolutional neural network. *Front Physiol.* 2019;10:255.
51. Lutomski JE, Meaney S, Greene RA, Ryan AC, Devane D; Cochrane Pregnancy and Childbirth Group. Expert systems for fetal assessment in labour. *Cochrane Database Syst Rev.* 2015;2015(4):CD010708.
52. Balayla J, Shrem G. Use of artificial intelligence (AI) in the interpretation of intrapartum fetal heart rate (FHR) tracings: a systematic review and meta-analysis. *Arch Gynecol Obstet.* 2019;300(1):7-14.
53. Cahill AG, Roehl KA, Odibo AO, Macones GA. Association and prediction of neonatal acidemia. *Am J Obstet Gynecol.* 2012;207(3):206.e1-206.e8.
54. Cohen G, Ravid D, Gnaiem N, et al. The impact of total deceleration area and fetal growth on neonatal acidemia in vacuum extraction deliveries. *Children.* 2023;10(5):776.
55. Talmor M, Rotem R, Wientraub AY, Salem SY. The correlation between total deceleration and acceleration surface areas on electronic fetal monitoring and neonatal cord blood pH in postdate pregnancies. *Int J Gynecol Obstet.* 2023;161(3):870-876.
56. Matmor Loeub S, Weintraub AY, Rotem R, Geva Y, Salem SY. Correlation between total deceleration area and fetal cord blood pH in neonates complicated with meconium-stained amniotic fluid at term. *Int J Gynecol Obstet.* 2022;159(3):974-978.
57. Gyllencreutz E, Varli IH, Lindqvist PG, Holzmann M. Variable deceleration features and intrapartum fetal academia: the role of deceleration area. *Eur J Obstet Gynecol Reprod Biol.* 2021;267:192-197.
58. Geva Y, Salem SY, Geva N, et al. Intrapartum deceleration and acceleration areas are associated with neonatal encephalopathy. *Int J Gynecol Obstet.* 2023;161(3):1061-1068.
59. Evans MI, Britt DW, Evans SM, Devoe LD. Improving the interpretation of electronic fetal monitoring: the fetal reserve index. *Am J Obstet Gynecol.* 2023;228(5s):S1129-S1143.

CHAPTER 10 Antepartum Fetal Monitoring

Xiao-Yu Wang and Heather Frey

Antepartum fetal death affects 5.7 in 1000 pregnancies in the US as of 2020.[1,2] The causes of fetal death can include obstetric complications, placental disease, fetal growth restriction, congenital and genetic abnormalities, infection, and cord accidents.[1,3] An ideal test for assessing the antepartum fetus would allow intervention before fetal morbidity or mortality. It makes sense to extend intrapartum fetal heart rate monitoring to antepartum monitoring for the goal of reducing the risk of intrauterine fetal demise or adverse neurologic outcomes. The difficulty of antenatal monitoring is balancing the risks of prematurity with the risks of fetal morbidity and mortality.

Throughout the history of antenatal fetal assessment, several tests and procedures have been used. In practice, current methods include:

1. Fetal movement counting
2. Assessment of fetal growth
3. Antepartum fetal heart rate testing
4. Biophysical profile (BPP) testing
5. Doppler velocimetry

PHYSIOLOGY AND PATHOPHYSIOLOGY

Fetal assessment relies on evidence of fetal compromise prior to intrauterine fetal demise. The risk for fetal compromise depends on a variety of maternal, placental, and fetal factors that can impact the delivery of nutritive and/or respiratory substances to the developing fetus as well as the clearance of toxic substances. Deteriorations in this pathway caused by poor placental function are broadly termed uteroplacental insufficiency (UPI). Figure 10.1 demonstrates a theoretical scheme for which declining placental function might cause fetal compromise leading to asphyxiation and death. The increased risk of intrauterine fetal demise from many different maternal and fetal conditions may be mediated by UPI. Maternal diseases such as diabetes, chronic hypertension, and thrombophilias as well as diseases of pregnancy such as preeclampsia have been associated with changes in placental blood flow and release of proinflammatory agents.[4-6] Fetal conditions including a variety of both genetic and acquired may influence placental function. Additionally, fetal anemia from causes such as alloimmunization can lead to respiratory compromise by affecting the fetal uptake of oxygen.[7] Regardless of the underlying etiology, the central goal of fetal monitoring is to identify pregnancies at risk for fetal compromise from UPI and intervene before asphyxiation and fetal death occur.

INDICATIONS AND TIMING OF TESTING INITIATION

Several maternal, fetal, and obstetrical factors that have increased risk for intrauterine fetal demise have been identified. The decision on when to initiate testing and frequency of testing relies on a balance on when delivery may be beneficial to perinatal outcomes. This is a balance between the risk of intrauterine fetal demise and the risks of prematurity. Antenatal testing should not be initiated if delivery does not convey a benefit. Shared decision-making between the patient and clinician on the timing and interval of antenatal testing should be employed. Suggested indications and gestational ages of initiation of antenatal testing are listed in Table 10.1.[8] Recommendations for the timing and frequency of testing are based largely on expert opinion but reflect the

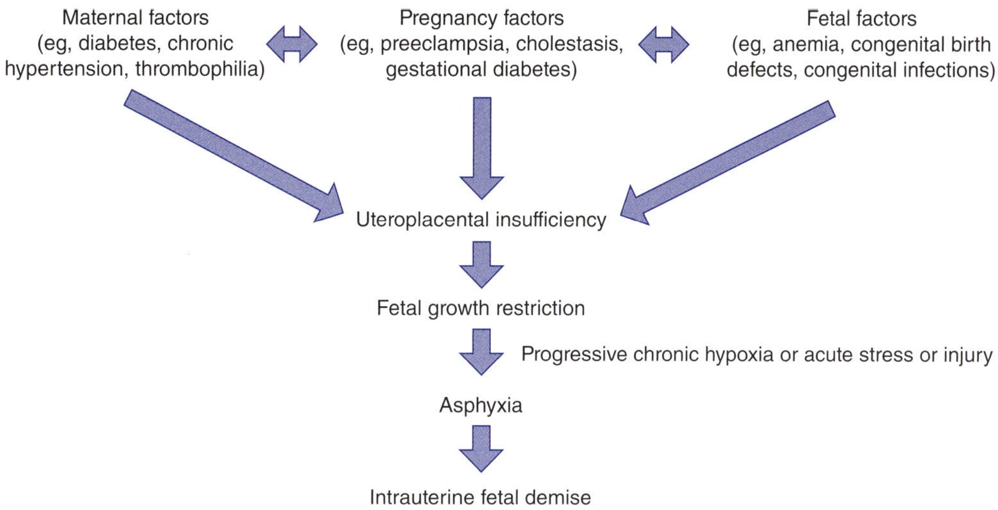

Figure 10.1. Theoretical scheme of fetal deterioration with progressive uteroplacental insufficiency.

TABLE 10.1 Indications and gestational age for antenatal testing[a]

Indication	Gestational age of initiation of testing
High risk	32 weeks or at diagnosis
Chronic hypertension on antihypertensives	32 weeks
Pregestational diabetes or gestational diabetes controlled on medications	32 weeks
Systemic lupus erythematosus	32 weeks
Antiphospholipid syndrome	32 weeks
Renal disease	32 weeks
Sickle cell anemia	32 weeks
Hypertensive disorders of pregnancy	At diagnosis
Intrahepatic cholestasis of pregnancy	At diagnosis
Chronic placental abruption	At diagnosis
Fetal growth restriction	At diagnosis or 32 weeks depending on Doppler assessment
Monochorionic-diamniotic gestation	32 weeks
Low risk	36 weeks or later
Gestational diabetes on no antidiabetic agents	40 weeks
Advanced maternal age	36 weeks
Obesity	34-36 weeks
In vitro fertilization	36 weeks
Postdate pregnancy	41 weeks
Dichorionic-diamniotic twin gestation	36 weeks

[a]Adapted from Indications for Outpatient Antenatal Fetal Surveillance: ACOG Committee Opinion, Number 828. *Obstet Gynecol.* 2021;137(6):e177-e197. doi: 10.1097/AOG.0000000000004407.

relative risk of stillbirth reported for a specific condition. Antenatal fetal monitoring for conditions such as poorly controlled diabetes, poorly controlled hypertension, or fetal growth restriction, which are associated with a higher risk for stillbirth at earlier gestational ages, is recommended earlier and more frequently than for lower risk conditions such as obesity or advanced maternal age. Frequency of testing can be individualized based on the testing modality used. Extremely high-risk conditions such as preeclampsia with severe features or fetal growth restriction with a reversed end-diastolic flow in the umbilical artery are such a high risk for fetal demise that inpatient management with at least daily antenatal testing is warranted.[8-10]

ANTENATAL FETAL MONITORING TESTS

Multiple methods for assessing fetal health have been developed and are commonly used in clinical practice. The overall test performance of the antenatal monitoring methods, including the nonstress test (NST), BPP, modified BPP, and contraction stress test (CST), is fairly similar with regard to their low-false positive rate. Thus, the choice of which test to use depends on a number of considerations including the indication for surveillance, available resources, and convenience.

FETAL MOVEMENT COUNTING

The most basic fetal assessment relies on maternal perception of fetal movement. Also known as "quickening," this can occur as early as the beginning of the second trimester.[11] Maternal perception of decreased fetal movement has been used as a sign of impending fetal death. It has been postulated that decreased fetal movement is an oxygen-sparing response to fetal hypoxia. In animal models, acute hypoxia has been shown to decrease forelimb movements and skeletal activity.[12,13]

Maternal assessment of fetal movement by itself requires no extra equipment and can be accomplished by individual patients at home. Therefore, protocols for fetal movement monitoring have been widely implemented to assess fetal well-being. Different thresholds for maternal assessment of fetal movement have been used. A commonly accepted recommendation is that 10 fetal movements or "kick counts" in 2 hours is considered normal and reassuring.[14,15] If decreased fetal motion is noted, the patient should present for urgent evaluation and another form of antenatal testing such as an NST should be performed to ensure fetal well-being.

Although there is an association between decreased fetal movements and adverse outcomes, there is unclear evidence that the implementation of such fetal movement awareness protocols prevents stillbirth. In 1980, Neldham et al showed a reduction in stillbirth using a daily fetal monitoring protocol. Moore and Piacquadio evaluated the implementation of a protocol based on 10 fetal movements within 2 hours at their center and showed an over a fourfold reduction of fetal mortality (44 per 1000 to 10 per 1000 pregnancies) with this method.[14] More recently, the AFFIRM trial was a large, multicenter step-wedged cluster randomized controlled trial involving 409,175 pregnancies. The intervention included formalized education modules for staff and the distribution of informational materials to patients. Rates of stillbirth and perinatal mortality were not reduced with the intervention.[16] A 2023 meta-analysis that included the AFFIRM trial demonstrated uncertain evidence for the use of fetal movement awareness techniques in reducing the risk of stillbirth. However, it did show some reduction in NICU admissions, Apgar score <7 at 5 minutes of life, and increased maternal-neonatal bonding and decreased maternal anxiety without increasing the risk of interventions in labor such as cesarean delivery.[15] Overall, fetal movement counting is a low-cost surveillance tool for low-risk pregnancies, and decreased fetal movement warrants further evaluation.

ASSESSMENT OF FETAL GROWTH

It is important to identify pregnancies at risk for fetal growth restriction given the risk for stillbirth and adverse neonatal outcomes.[17] Assessment of uterine growth with fundal height measurements can be a useful screening tool. The fundal height in centimeters, as measured from the pubic symphysis to the uterine fundus, should be equal to the weeks of gestation. The clinically relevant discrepancy of three or more centimeters in fundal height from the expected fundal height warrants further ultrasonographic evaluation. However, several things can affect this relationship including, but not limited to, maternal factors such as obesity, uterine fibroids, and fetal factors such as multiple gestations, abnormal fluid levels (polyhydramnios or oligohydramnios), low fetal station, or abnormal fetal lie. Therefore, ultrasound assessment of fetal growth is recommended in pregnancies complicated by maternal or fetal conditions at elevated risk for fetal growth abnormalities.

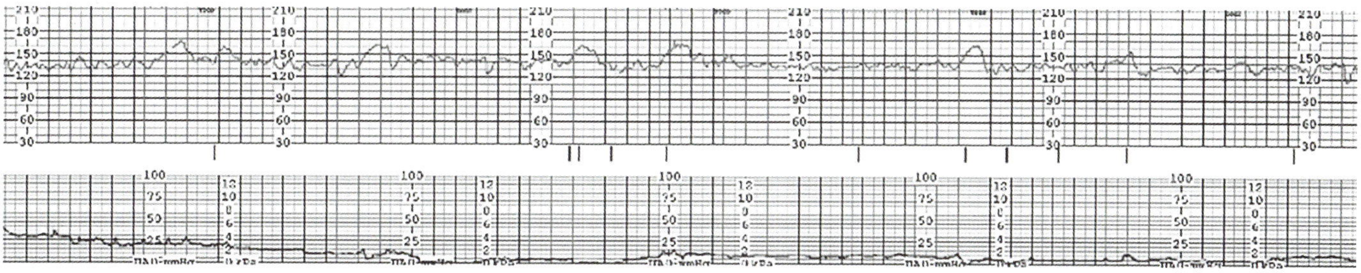

Figure 10.2. Reactive nonstress test of a 34-week fetus performed for diabetes.

Assessment of fetal growth is accomplished using four biometric parameters: biparietal diameter, head circumference, abdominal circumference, and femur length.[18] These biometric factors and others have been incorporated into fetal growth nomograms to establish an estimated fetal weight. In the US, the most commonly used method is the Hadlock formula, which was developed based on a study of 392 pregnancies in Texas.[19] Even when compared with newer customized growth standards such as the NICHD, WHO, and INTERGROWTH-21st standards, the Hadlock formula performed as well or better.[9,20]

NONSTRESS TESTING

The NST is currently the preferred form of antenatal fetal monitoring in many obstetric practices. The development of this antenatal testing method which relies on the interpretation of the fetal heart rate has its foundation in the work of Hammacher in 1966 and Kubli in 1969.[21,22] They observed that healthy fetuses have normal heart rate fluctuations and oscillations, and the absence of this variability indicated an increased risk of depressed neonates and perinatal mortality. Building upon these observations, Trierweiler et al later described the association between accelerations in fetal heart rate and fetal well-being.[23] The use of NST has been further refined to include parameters such as baseline heart rate, variability, accelerations, and decelerations. There are few contraindications to NSTs given the noninvasive nature of the test. However, in the setting of fetal arrhythmia, fetal well-being may be difficult to determine.

Test Performance and Interpretation

The test is performed with the patient placed in a semi-fowler or lateral recumbent position. External monitors for fetal heart rate and contractions are applied to the patient. Maternal vitals including heart rate should be noted. The use of ultrasound can be helpful to determine the optimal monitor placement.

NSTs are evaluated by the presence and absence of accelerations. An NST is considered reactive if there are two or more accelerations noted in a 20-minute period of continuous fetal heart tracing. An acceleration is defined as a rise in the fetal heart rate by at least 15 beats per minute (bpm) from the baseline with a duration of at least 15 seconds as measured from the start to rise in heart rate to return to the baseline (Figs. 10.2 and 10.3). In the setting of a reactive NST, the risk of stillbirth is 1.9 per 1000 (false negative rate) based on data from a multi-institutional prospective study.[24] However, the false positive rate has been estimated to exceed 55% (see Table 10.2).[25]

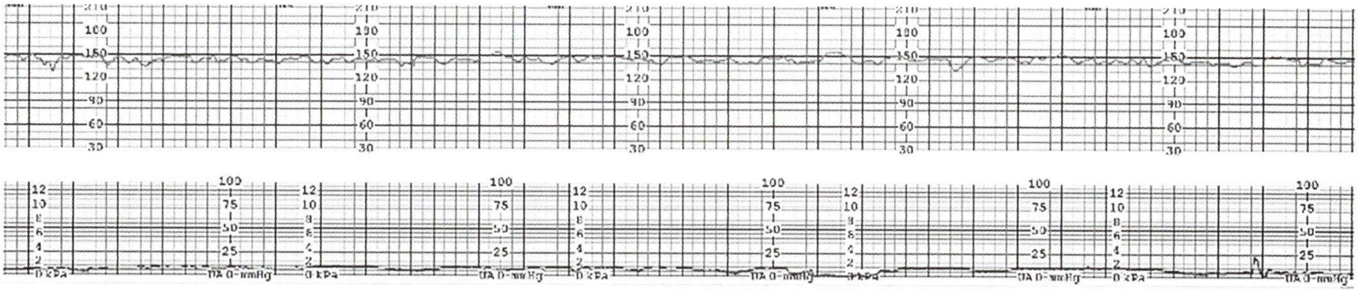

Figure 10.3. Reactive nonstress test of a 25-week fetus performed for preterm premature rupture of membranes.

TABLE 10.2 **False negative and false positive rates of antenatal testing[a]**

Test	False negative rate (%)	False positive rate (%)
NST	0.2-0.65	55-90
BPP	0.07-0.08	40-50
Modified BPP	0.08	60
CST	0.04	35-65

NST, nonstress test; BPP, biophysical profile; CST, contraction stress test.
[a]Adapted from Signore C, Freeman RK, Spong CY. Antenatal testing-a reevaluation: executive summary of a Eunice Kennedy Shriver National Institute of Child Health and Human Development workshop. *Obstet Gynecol.* 2009;113(3):687-701.

Nonreactive NSTs are common in preterm fetuses using the standard definition of accelerations (15 bpm)[26,27] because of the immaturity of the fetal autonomic system. A lower threshold for defining accelerations of a rise in the baseline by at least 10 bpm for at least 10 seconds for fetuses under 32 weeks has been adopted into clinical practice (refer to Fig. 10.4).[27,28] This is supported by studies comparing the standard acceleration criteria (15 bpm increase for 15 seconds) with the 10 bpm threshold in preterm infants, which demonstrated a decreased time to reactivity without increases in adverse perinatal outcomes.[29,30]

In addition to the determination of reactivity, information including the baseline heart rate and variability, as well as the presence or absence of decelerations and their relationship to contractions, should be recorded. Normal baseline fetal heart rate ranges between 120 and 160 bpm, but there is a trend toward lower baseline heart rates with increasing gestational age. Fetal heart rates outside of the normal range should prompt a thorough evaluation of the cause. Fetal tachycardia can be seen as a physiologic response to conditions such as fever, infection, hyperthyroidism, or in fetal tachyarrhythmias such as supraventricular tachycardia. Fetal bradycardia can be seen as a response to extreme fetal hypoxemia and impending fetal demise but also in fetal bradyarrhythmias such as atrioventricular block.

The presence of moderate baseline fetal heart rate variability between 6 and 25 bpm is reassuring for fetal well-being. Decelerations may be present either spontaneously or related to contractions (Fig. 10.4). Variable decelerations that are nonrepetitive and brief (less than 30 seconds) are not associated with fetal compromise.[31] Repetitive variable decelerations are concerning for a nonreassuring fetal status. Furthermore, spontaneous decelerations especially those longer than 1 minute are associated with increased risk for fetal distress.[32] Decelerations may occur even in the presence of a reactive NST.

Management

Reactive NSTs without decelerations are reassuring for fetal well-being. A nonreactive NST warrants further evaluation. Management options include extending the length of the NST until reactivity is established, or proceeding with a different form of antenatal testing such as BPP. Extending the duration of monitoring is one management option if the NST is nonreactive without other concerning features such as decelerations. Brown and Patrick assessed an extended duration of monitoring for 333 patients for nonreactive NSTs up to 120 minutes.[33] Reactivity was achieved by 20 minutes in 75% of NSTs, whereas <6% remained nonreactive if monitoring was extended to 40 minutes.

Use of vibroacoustic stimulation can also be employed to elicit accelerations. Devices such as electronic artificial larynx or other acoustic stimulators emit a short burst of sound for 1 to 3 seconds and vibrations to induce a neurologic response in the fetus. The use of vibroacoustic stimulation has been proven to be safe and effective. In a meta-analysis of 12 clinical trials, fetal vibroacoustic

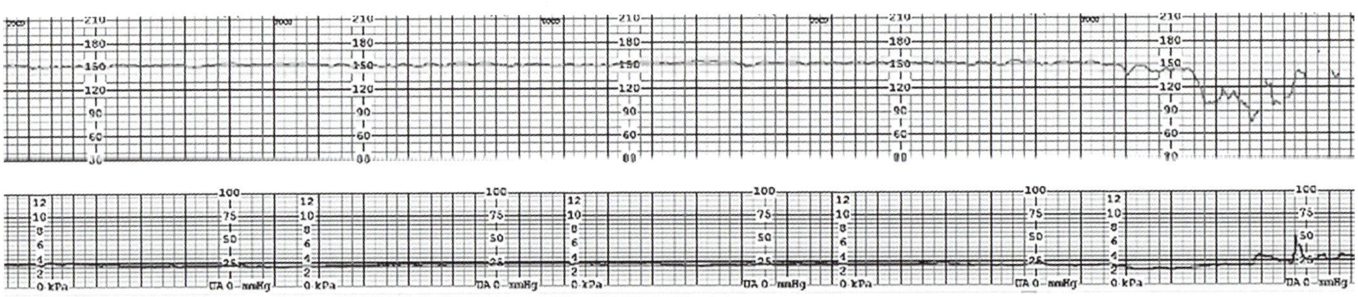

Figure 10.4. Nonreactive nonstress test of a 32-week fetus for chronic hypertension.

TABLE 10.3 Reversible causes of abnormal testing

Diabetic ketoacidosis
Maternal hypoxia
Maternal hypotension
Maternal acidosis
Sickle cell crisis
Asthma exacerbation

stimulation decreased the rate of nonreactive NST by 38% and reduced the length of NST testing time by about 7 minutes without decreasing the detection of fetal compromise.[34] Administration of a simple oral carbohydrate load, such as juice, to increase reactivity is a frequent practice, but the evidence to support the benefit of this approach is lacking.[35]

Because of the high false positive rate on nonreactive NSTs, the next best step is most often to proceed with another test, such as a BPP, to minimize the chance of unnecessary intervention (ie, delivery). However, factors including overall maternal and fetal health and gestational age may influence management. Reversible maternal conditions of fetal distress should be evaluated and corrected (Table 10.3). NSTs that are reactive (adequate accelerations) but with recurrent variable and/or late decelerations or long spontaneous decelerations should be considered nonreassuring and warrant additional evaluation that includes prolonged real-time fetal heart rate monitoring and assessment.

Other Patterns

Variable decelerations are suggestive of cord compression.[28,36] This can be seen in higher frequency in conditions such as oligohydramnios. An ultrasound evaluation for oligohydramnios should be performed to investigate the presence of oligohydramnios if repetitive variable decelerations are observed. Recurrent variable decelerations are concerning and should be evaluated similarly to late decelerations.

A sinusoidal pattern is a rare finding that is ominous for fetal distress and associated with a high incidence of perinatal morbidity and mortality. Sinusoidal patterns are characterized by a stable baseline heart rate of 120 to 160 with regular low amplitude oscillation of 5 to 15 bpm, with fixed or flat short-term variability, oscillation of the waveform above and below the baseline, and absence of periods of normal variability or reactivity.[37,38] Sinusoidal patterns can be associated with severe fetal anemia, such as with alloimmunization or fetal-maternal hemorrhage, or in cases of extreme fetal hypoxia and asphyxia.[37]

BIOPHYSICAL PROFILE

Developed by Manning and colleagues in 1980, the BPP is a common test for providing antepartum fetal assessment.[39] The BPP is comprised of five components: NST, fetal breathing, fetal movement, fetal tone, and amniotic fluid volume (Table 10.4). Each component is valued at two points. In large prospective studies, Manning et al demonstrated a clear association

TABLE 10.4 Biophysical profile scoring

Biophysical variable	Normal (score = 2)	Abnormal (score = 0)
1. NST	≥2 accelerations of ≥15 bpm for ≥15 s (or ≥10 bpm for ≥10 s for gestational age <32 weeks) in 20 min	>2 accelerations
2. Fetal breathing movements	≥1 episode of ≥30 s in 30 min	Absence or <30 s in 30 min
3. Gross body movements	≥3 discrete body/limb movements in 30 min	≤2 discrete body/limb movements in 30 min
4. Fetal tone	≥1 active extension/flexion of limb, trunk, or hand	Slow or absent fetal extension/flexion
5. Qualitative amniotic fluid volume	Deepest vertical pocket >2 cm	Deepest vertical pocket <2 cm

NST, nonstress test; bpm, beats per minute.
Modified from Manning FA, Platt LW, Sipos L. Antepartum fetal evaluation: development of a biophysical profile. *Am J Obstet Gynecol.* 1980;136(6):787-795, with permission.

between BPP score and perinatal mortality and morbidity, including a significant inverse relationship between BPP scores and fetal acidemia.[40,41] The risk of fetal demise within 1 week after a negative (normal) BPP is low (0.8/1000).[42]

Test Performance and Interpretation

The BPP requires sonographic evaluation by a healthcare provider with training in the performance of the test as well as an NST. The ultrasound assessment is conducted over 30 minutes. A quantitative measurement of fluid volume is performed. A deepest vertical pocket (DVP) greater than 2 cm is considered normal. Fetal breathing movements are defined by the presence of rhythmic breathing movements for 30 or more seconds. Fetal hiccups are a more forceful fetal diaphragmatic movement compared to breathing and are often considered equivalent to fetal breathing movement.[43,44] Fetal movement is defined by three or more discrete body or limb movements. The fetal tone is defined as observed active extension and flexion of the fetal spine or hand. The component of an NST can be performed separately from the ultrasound component either before or after the ultrasound. BPP scores are reported out of either 8 points or 10 points if an NST is performed as a part of the testing.

There are a number of factors that can influence BPP results. Variations in fetal activity are frequently related to the normal fetal wake-sleep cycle. Medications can also affect BPP parameters. Transient decreases in fetal movement and NST reactivity are observed after opioid administration and medications used to treat opioid-use disorder.[45] Reduced breathing movements and fetal heart rate reactivity may also be observed for 48 to 96 hours after antenatal corticosteroid administration.[46] Fetal maturity also affects BPP parameters. Fetal movement and tone are present very early in gestation, and fetal breathing may be observed as early as 20 to 22 weeks.[47] However, nonreactive NSTs are more frequently observed at earlier gestational ages. Similar to the NST, vibroacoustic stimulation can be used to elicit a fetal response during the sonographic portion of a BPP without compromising the validity of the test result.

The false negative rate of the BPP is 0.07% to 0.08% and it has false positive rate of 40% to 50%.[42,48] BPPs can be more time-consuming and require ultrasound capabilities, making them less efficient compared to NSTs. BPP can be useful as a follow-up test to a nonreactive NST as scores of 8 out of 10 are still reassuring for fetal well-being. Additionally, the BPP may be selected as the primary antenatal testing modality for practical reasons, such as when an ultrasound is also being performed for another purpose like fetal growth assessment and the tests can be done in conjunction.

Management

Normal BPP scores of 8 or 10 are reassuring for normal fetal status and low risk for fetal death. Scores of 0/10 or 2/10 are at high risk for fetal death and require prompt evaluation for delivery in the absence of reversible causes for fetal compromise such as maternal diabetic ketoacidosis or sepsis. BPP scores of 4/10 or less are abnormal and delivery may be indicated depending on the clinical situation. Equivocal scores of 6/10 warrant further evaluation with a repeat BPP within 24 hours. In one study, a follow-up BPP within 24 hours with a score of 6/10 was normal in 82% of cases.[49] For BPP scores of 6/10 with oligohydramnios, delivery may be considered even among preterm fetuses depending on other clinical conditions and gestational age (>32-34 weeks). Fetal heart rate reactivity and breathing movements are the most likely to be affected by fetal hypoxia, whereas loss of tone and absent fetal movements are later findings.[47] Thus, BPP results in which the NST is reactive or fetal breathing movement is present, but there is the abnormal tone or gross body movements should be viewed with some skepticism as causes other than hypoxia (eg, fetal wake-sleep cycle) are likely contributing to this result.

MODIFIED BPP

A modified BPP includes an NST and amniotic fluid volume assessment. A normal modified BPP is a reactive NST and normal amniotic fluid volume as measured by a DVP greater than or equal to 2 cm. An NST alone has a relatively higher false negative rate (fetal death risk following a normal test) relative to the BPP and CST.[50,51] However, the addition of a qualitative measure of amniotic fluid volume to the NST has been shown to have improved the predictive ability of the test with a false negative rate (0.8 per 1000 stillbirth rate) comparable to that of a CST and BPP.[52,53] It also maintains a similar false positive score of 60%. The benefit of the test is that the ultrasound component is simpler and quicker to perform when compared to a full BPP and CST and can improve the performance of the NST alone.

Amniotic Fluid Assessment

The evaluation of amniotic fluid quantity is an important component of the assessment of fetal status. It is incorporated into many antenatal testing strategies and is part of any ultrasound assessment of fetal growth. Although there are multiple potential causes of low amniotic fluid (eg, rupture of membranes and fetal genitourinary abnormality), chronic UPI leading to hypoxemia results in the distribution of blood flow away from organs such as the kidneys to the heart, brain, and adrenals. Reduced renal blood flow leads to oligohydramnios.

Normal amniotic fluid is defined as a DVP between 2 and 8 cm or an amniotic fluid index between 5 and 24 cm. The DVP is obtained by assessing the deepest pocket of fluid measuring at least 1-cm wide free of fetal parts or umbilical cord. AFI is a sum of the deepest pocket of fluid in each quadrant of the uterus. Oligohydramnios is defined as DVP less than 2 cm or AFI less than 5 cm. DVP as compared to AFI has the benefit of not overdiagnosing oligohydramnios leading to unnecessary testing or intervention and is not associated with worse fetal or neonatal outcomes.[54]

CONTRACTION STRESS TEST

The goal of the CST is to evaluate the fetal heart rate in response to uterine contractions. Uterine contractions may cause a transient decrease in blood flow and oxygen delivery to the fetus. A well-oxygenated fetus can tolerate this transient decreased perfusion, but a compromised and hypoxic fetus will manifest signs of fetal distress such as late decelerations.

In 1966, Hammacher studied 207 pregnancies in the antepartum period and found that late decelerations were associated with lower Apgar scores and a majority of stillbirths showed late decelerations with spontaneous contractions in the antepartum period.[22] Sanchez-Ramos et al found no deaths within a week of testing in the absence of late decelerations.[21,55-57] Ray et al performed the first US prospective trial of the oxytocin challenge test that would become adapted into the CST.[50]

The CST was once considered the gold standard test. However, there are significant barriers related to the time, cost, and inconvenience compared to other testing. By causing contractions, there is a theoretical risk of inducing labor. Additionally, there is a high frequency of equivocal testing for CSTs. There are also more contraindications for CST in situations that warrant avoidance of uterine stimulation (Table 10.5). As a result, the NST, BPP, and modified BPP have largely replaced the use of CST in clinical practice.

TABLE 10.5 Relative contraindications to the CST

Premature rupture of membranes
Prior non-lower segment uterine scar (eg, prior classical cesarean delivery or myomectomy)
Placenta or vasa previa
Advanced cervical dilation
Multiple gestations

CST, contraction stress test.

How to Perform the Test

With the patient in a semi-Fowler's position, left lateral tilt, or lateral recumbent position, external monitors for contraction and fetal heart rate measurement are placed on the patient. In the initial 20 to 30 minutes, fetal heart rate baseline characteristics are established, and tocometry is performed to determine if there are spontaneous contractions. If three contractions lasting at least 40 seconds are noted in a 10-minute epoch, then a spontaneous CST is accomplished and can be evaluated. If there are not adequate contractions, then contractions can be induced with either intravenous oxytocin infusion or nipple stimulation until adequate contractions are noted. Intravenous oxytocin can be implemented using various protocols. A reasonable protocol is initiation of oxytocin infusion at 2 mU/min increasing the infusion rate by 2 mU/min every 15 minutes until adequate contractions are noted.[50] An alternative to intravenous oxytocin infusion is nipple stimulation either manually or with the use of an electric breast pump until adequate contractions are noted.[59,60]

Interpretation

Negative

A negative CST requires no late or significant variable decelerations on the tracing with adequate contraction frequency (3 in 10 minutes) and normal fetal heart rate (Fig. 10.5). Significant variable decelerations can be defined as lasting >60s and reaching a nadir >60 bpm below the baseline or lasting >60s and reaching a baseline of <60 bpm.[61]

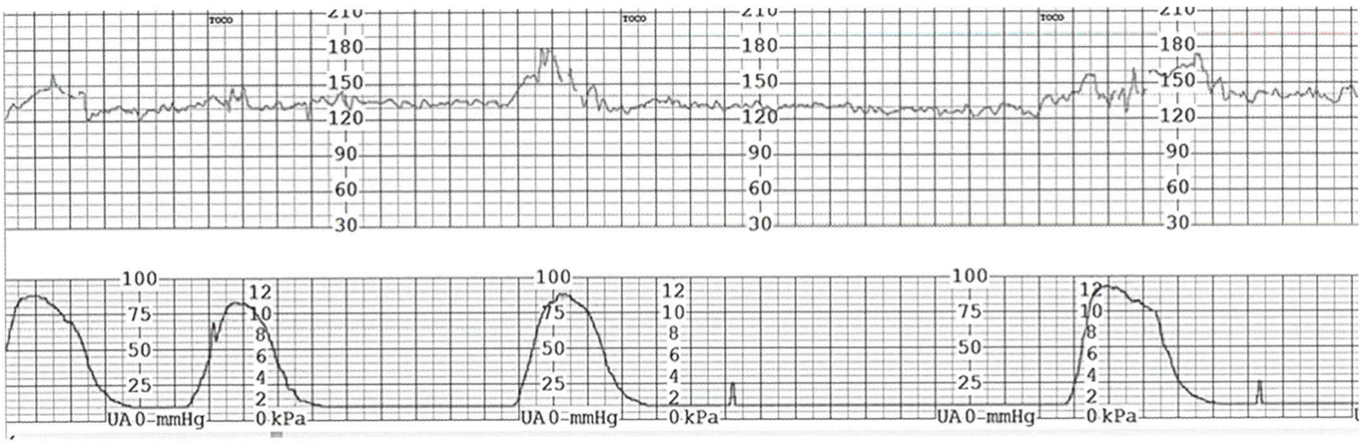

Figure 10.5. Negative contraction stress test induced by nipple stimulation.

Positive

A positive CST requires that late deceleration or significant variable decelerations are present in greater than 50% of contractions without excessive uterine activity (tachysystole) (Fig. 10.6). If recurrent late decelerations are present even in the absence of adequate contractions, this should be considered a positive test. If criteria for a positive CST is met, then contraction stimulation with either oxytocin or nipple stimulation should be discontinued.

Equivocal

Equivocal tests are those tests that do not meet the criteria for positive or negative testing and can be broken down into suspicious, tachysystolic, or unsatisfactory.

- Suspicious: Late decelerations or significant variable decelerations are present with less than 50% of contractions.
- Tachysystolic: Decelerations occur in the setting of contractions that are less than 2 minutes apart or lasting more than 90 seconds. If there are no decelerations in the setting of tachysystole, this can be interpreted as negative testing.
- Unsatisfactory: If adequate contraction frequency (3 in 10 minutes) cannot be induced or fetal heart rate is not of sufficient quality to be interpreted, then test results should be considered unsatisfactory.

Management

A negative CST provides reassurance regarding fetal status, whereas equivocal testing warrants additional evaluation and repeat antenatal testing such as repeating CST or performing other antenatal testing such as NST and BPP. The false positive rate of a CST is 35% to 65%.[25] Positive tests should be managed in the context

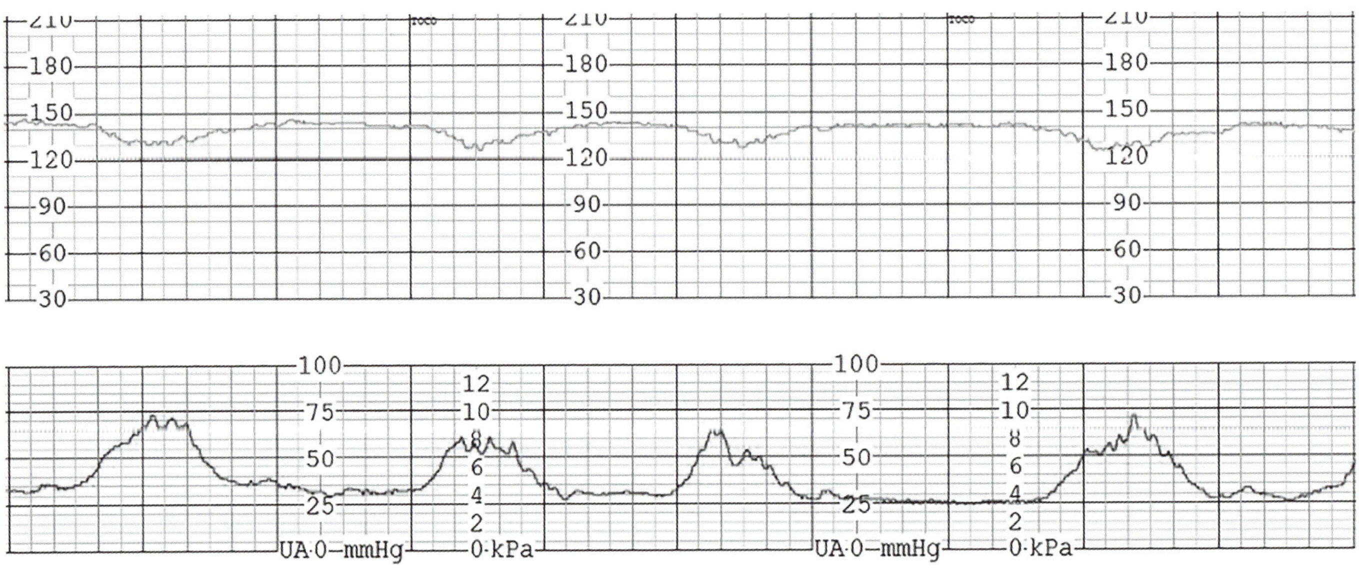

Figure 10.6. Positive contraction stress test with late deceleration seen.

of the clinical condition and gestational age. Management options may include admission for prolonged monitoring, administration of steroids, and delivery. Additionally, the presence of a positive CST may be useful in determining the mode of delivery. Pregnancies with a positive CST suggests increased concerns for fetal intolerance of labor and increased risk for cesarean delivery for nonreassuring fetal status.[62] A positive CST can be used to help decide between induction of labor versus proceeding with cesarean delivery if delivery is indicated. This is especially true if other factors suggesting increased risk for fetal intolerance of labor are present such as fetal growth restriction.[63]

DOPPLER VELOCIMETRY

Assessment of fetal vessels using ultrasound Doppler velocimetry can be an important tool in the assessment of fetal well-being.[64,65] Different fetal vessels have been assessed including the umbilical artery, middle cerebral, umbilical vein, and ductus venosus.

Umbilical Artery Doppler

The placenta represents the vascular tree that allows the perfusion of oxygen and nutrients to fetal blood circulation. Umbilical artery blood flow to the placenta from the fetus is an assessment of the placental resistance. In normal pregnancy, this is a low-resistance system that allows continuous forward flow to the placenta through the passive diastolic phase of fetal cardiac activity. Increasing vascular resistance of the placenta can represent worsening UPI and an increased risk for fetal compromise. In normal umbilical artery flow, there is continuous forward velocity of blood flow from the fetus to the placenta, with higher velocities noted during systole compared to diastole because of the contraction and relaxation of the fetal heart. In states of increasing vascular resistance of the placenta, umbilical artery blood flows show initially an increased ratio of systolic compared to diastolic velocities. If placental resistance increases further, absent end-diastolic flow can be seen as the fetal circulation is not able to overcome the vascular resistance of the placenta during diastole. If resistance further increases, this diastolic flow may even reverse to become retrograde toward the fetus. Umbilical artery Doppler (UA Doppler) alone is a poor indicator of acute fetal compromise. The use of UA Doppler assessment has been shown to identify fetuses at higher risk for perinatal mortality and ultimately reduce the risk of perinatal deaths among pregnancies considered to be high risk.[64] Specifically, risk reduction has been most clearly demonstrated among fetuses with growth restriction. In contrast, a systematic review and meta-analysis published in 2015 did not reveal that the use of UA Doppler assessment in normal pregnancies was beneficial.[65] Thus, current Society of Maternal-Fetal Medicine recommendations advise the use of UA Doppler only for pregnancy complicated by fetal growth restriction.[9] The risk of perinatal mortality is related to the severity of Doppler changes with the highest risk observed in those with reversed end diastolic flow. Guidance on antenatal surveillance and delivery timing is therefore based on UA Doppler findings.

Middle Cerebral Artery Doppler

Assessment of blood flow in the middle cerebral artery (MCA) using Doppler velocimetry has been used in multiple clinical conditions. It is an important assessment tool for fetal anemia related to alloimmunization. There may also be a role for MCA Doppler assessment for fetal anemia from other etiologies, such as including twin-to-twin transfusion syndrome, infection, and hemorrhage.[66] MCA Doppler assessment has also been used in pregnancies with complicated fetal growth restriction, but its routine use for this indication is controversial. In growth-restricted fetuses, there is a preferential brain-sparing effect of blood flow that causes cerebral vasodilation that can be measured with MCA Doppler.[9]

Ductus Venosus Doppler

The fetal ductus venosus shunts oxygenated blood returning from the umbilical vein to the inferior vena cava and central fetal circulation bypassing the liver. Increased shunting of blood flow through the ductus venosus is seen in hypoxic states. Absent or reversed flow in the ductus venosus during fetal atrial contraction (A-wave component) has been shown to be associated with a high risk for fetal compromise and death. An absent A-wave has been associated with a 20% risk of fetal death and a reversed A-wave has been associated with a 46% of fetal death.[9,67] Assessment of the ductus venosus has been proposed as part of the antenatal surveillance of pregnancies complicated by fetal growth restriction with abnormal UA Doppler findings. However, clear evidence that the incorporation of DV monitoring in pregnancies complicated by fetal growth restriction improves clinical outcomes is lacking, and additional research is needed.

Uterine Artery Doppler

Studies have evaluated the use of uterine artery Doppler to identify individuals at higher risk for pregnancy complications such as preeclampsia and fetal growth restriction.[68] There is a theoretical increase in placental vascular resistance that can be seen in these disease conditions, which can be detected by changes in maternal uterine artery blood flow. However, the clinical utility of uterine artery Doppler is limited in the absence of interventions that could improve or prevent adverse pregnancy outcomes.

Umbilical Vein Doppler

The umbilical vein supplies blood from the placenta to fetal circulation. In normal pregnancies, continuous forward nonpulsatile flow is noted in Doppler studies. Pulsatile flow in the umbilical vein has been shown in periods of cord occlusion, fetal heart failure, and fetal asphyxiation, and in fetuses at high risk for perinatal mortality.[69] However, further studies need to be completed before incorporating umbilical vein Doppler evaluation into clinical decision-making.

GENERAL CLINICAL CONSIDERATIONS

Antenatal surveillance is considered an important component in the management of high-risk patients in modern obstetric practice. Despite the clinical utility of these tests to assess fetal status, it is important to recognize all the tests have a residual risk of fetal death. Many of these deaths are attributed to unpredictable events such as massive feto-maternal hemorrhage.[70,71]

Common to each of the antenatal testing methods is a low false negative rate (risk of stillbirth following a normal test) but a much higher false positive risk (refer to Table 10.2). A false positive test result could lead to unnecessary intervention, such as additional monitoring, admission, or even early delivery. The risk of a false positive test result should be a consideration in regard to the timing of initiation of antenatal surveillance. Testing should not be initiated unless there is a plan to proceed with delivery if clinically indicated by the results. The interpretation of the test should take into consideration the maternal and fetal clinical status and indication for surveillance as this affects the positive predictive value of an abnormal test. For example, a fetus with severe growth restriction and abnormal UA Doppler finding at 32 weeks is more likely to have a hypoxic fetus in the setting of a 4/10 BPP than a normally grown fetus with a similar score and no other clinical risk factors. Depending on the clinical situation, the preferred approach to the management of an abnormal antenatal test (eg, NST and modified BPP) is an additional fetal assessment with another antenatal surveillance test rather than immediate delivery, particularly at early gestational ages.[8] This strategy takes advantage of the low false negative rate of each test.

SUMMARY

Antenatal surveillance through NSTs, BPPs, modified BPPs, and less commonly CSTs are useful clinical tools in pregnancies at high risk for complications. These tools can be helpful to identify patients who are at higher risk for stillbirth and warrant further evaluation or delivery. Decisions for delivery should incorporate the viability of the neonate in relationship to factors such as gestational age or the presence of congenital anomalies. Ultimately, each antenatal testing tool should be assessed in relationship to the clinical scenario in which it is being used.

REFERENCES

1. Management of stillbirth: obstetric care consensus no. 10. *Obstet Gynecol.* 2020;135(3):e110-e132. doi: 10.1097/AOG.0000000000003719.
2. Gregory ECW, Valenzuela CP, Hoyert DL. Fetal mortality: United States. *Natl Vital Stat Rep.* 2020;71(4):1-20. Accessed May 12, 2023. https://www.cdc.gov/nchs/products/index.htm.
3. Bukowski R, Carpenter M, Conway D, et al. Causes of death among stillbirths. *JAMA.* 2011;306(22):2459-2468. doi: 10.1001/JAMA.2011.1823.
4. Gibbins KJ, Silver RM, Pinar H, et al. Stillbirth, hypertensive disorders of pregnancy, and placental pathology. *Placenta.* 2016;43:61-68. doi: 10.1016/J.PLACENTA.2016.04.020.
5. Simchen MJ, Ofir K, Moran O, Kedem A, Sivan E, Schiff E. Thrombophilic risk factors for placental stillbirth. *Eur J Obstet Gynecol Reprod Biol.* 2010;153(2):160-164. doi: 10.1016/J.EJOGRB.2010.07.031.
6. Starikov R, Dudley D, Reddy UM. Stillbirth in the pregnancy complicated by diabetes. *Curr Diab Rep.* 2015;15(3):1-9. doi: 10.1007/S11892-015-0580-Y/FIGURES/1.
7. Norton ME, Chauhan SP, Dashe JS. Society for Maternal-Fetal Medicine (SMFM) clinical guideline #7: nonimmune hydrops fetalis. *Am J Obstet Gynecol.* 2015;212(2):127-139. doi: 10.1016/J.AJOG.2014.12.018.

8. Indications for outpatient antenatal fetal surveillance: ACOG committee opinion, number 828. *Obstet Gynecol.* 2021;137(6): e177-e197. doi: 10.1097/AOG.0000000000004407.
9. Martins JG, Biggio JR, Abuhamad A. Society for Maternal-Fetal Medicine Consult Series #52: diagnosis and management of fetal growth restriction. Published online 2020. doi: 10.1016/j.ajog.2020.05.010.
10. Sibai BM. Evaluation and management of severe preeclampsia before 34 weeks' gestation. *Am J Obstet Gynecol.* 2011;205(3): 191-198. doi: 10.1016/j.ajog.2011.07.017.
11. Gillieson M, Dunlap H, Nair R, Pilon M. Placental site, parity, and date of quickening. *Obstet Gynecol.* 1984;64(1):44-45. Accessed May 12, 2023. https://oce-ovid-com.proxy.lib.ohio-state.edu/article/00006250-198407000-00008/HTML.
12. Bocking AD, Harding R. Effects of reduced uterine blood flow on electrocortical activity, breathing, and skeletal muscle activity in fetal sheep. *Am J Obstet Gynecol.* 1986;154(3):655-662. doi: 10.1016/0002-9378(86)90625-3.
13. Natale R, Clewlow F, Dawes GS. Measurement of fetal forelimb movements in the lamb in utero. *Am J Obstet Gynecol.* 1981;140(5):545-551. doi: 10.1016/0002-9378(81)90231-3.
14. Moore TR, Piacquadio K. A prospective evaluation of fetal movement screening to reduce the incidence of antepartum fetal death. *Am J Obstet Gynecol.* 1989;160(5 Pt 1):1075-1080. doi: 10.1016/0002-9378(89)90164-6.
15. Hayes DJL, Dumville JC, Walsh T, et al. Effect of encouraging awareness of reduced fetal movement and subsequent clinical management on pregnancy outcome: a systematic review and meta-analysis. *Am J Obstet Gynecol MFM.* 2023;5(3):100821. doi: 10.1016/j.ajogmf.2022.100821.
16. Norman JE, Heazell AEP, Rodriguez A, et al. Awareness of fetal movements and care package to reduce fetal mortality (AFFIRM): a stepped wedge, cluster-randomised trial. *Lancet.* 2018;392(10158): 1629-1638. doi: 10.1016/S0140-6736(18)31543-5.
17. Galan H, Grobman W. ACOG practice bulletin no. 204: fetal growth restriction. *Obstet Gynecol.* 2019;133(2):E297-E109. doi: 10.1097/AOG.0000000000003070.
18. Pettker CM, Goldberg JD, El Sayed YY, Copel JA. Committee opinion no 700: methods for estimating the due date. *Obstet Gynecol.* 2017;129(5):E150-E154. doi: 10.1097/AOG.0000000000002046.
19. Hadlock FP, Harrist RB, Martinez-Poyer J. In utero analysis of fetal growth: a sonographic weight standard. *Radiology.* 1991; 181(1):129-133. doi: 10.1148/RADIOLOGY.181.1.1887021.
20. Blue NR, Savabi M, Beddow ME, et al. The Hadlock method is superior to newer methods for the prediction of the birth weight percentile. *J Ultrasound Med.* 2019;38(3):587-596. doi: 10.1002/JUM.14725.
21. Kubli FW, Hon EH, Khazin AF, Takemura H. Observations on heart rate and pH in the human fetus during labor. *Am J Obstet Gynecol.* 1969;104(8):1190-1206. doi: 10.1016/S0002-9378(16)34294-6.
22. Hammacher K. Früherkennung intrauteriner Gefahrenzustände durch Elektophonokardiographie und Tokographie. In: Ehlert R, Hüter KA, eds. *Prophylaxe frühkindlicher Hirnschäden.* Thieme; 1966:120.
23. Trierweiler MW, Freeman RK, James J. Baseline fetal heart rate characteristics as an indicator of fetal status during the antepartum period. *Am J Obstet Gynecol.* 1976;125(5):618-623. doi: 10.1016/0002-9378(76)90783-3.
24. Freeman RK, Anderson G, Dorchester W. A prospective multi-institutional study of antepartum fetal heart rate monitoring. II. Contraction stress test versus nonstress test for primary surveillance. *Am J Obstet Gynecol.* 1982;143(7):778-781. doi: 10.1016/0002-9378(82)90009-6.
25. Signore C, Freeman RK, Spong CY. Antenatal testing—a reevaluation: executive summary of a Eunice Kennedy Shriver National Institute of Child Health and Human Development workshop. *Obstet Gynecol.* 2009;113(3):687-701. doi: 10.1097/AOG.0B013E318197BD8A.
26. Natale R, Nasello C, Turliuk R. The relationship between movements and accelerations in fetal heart rate at twenty-four to thirty-two weeks' gestation. *Am J Obstet Gynecol.* 1984; 148(5):591-595. doi: 10.1016/0002-9378(84)90754-3.
27. Castillo RA, Devoe LD, Arthur M, Searle N, Metheny WP, Ruedrich DA. The preterm nonstress test: effects of gestational age and length of study. *Am J Obstet Gynecol.* 1989;160(1):172-175. doi: 10.1016/0002-9378(89)90113-0.
28. Macones GA. ACOG Practice Bulletin No. 106: intrapartum fetal heart rate monitoring: nomenclature, interpretation, and general management principles. *Obstet Gynecol.* 2009;114(1):192-202. doi: 10.1097/AOG.0B013E3181AEF106.
29. Cousins LM, Poeltler DM, Faron S, Catanzarite V, Daneshmand S, Casele H. Nonstress testing at ≤32.0 weeks' gestation: a randomized trial comparing different assessment criteria. *Am J Obstet Gynecol.* 2012;207(4):311.e1-311.e7. doi: 10.1016/J.AJOG.2012.06.032.
30. Glantz JC, Bertoia N. Preterm nonstress testing: 10-beat compared with 15-beat criteria. *Obstet Gynecol.* 2011;118(1):87-93. doi: 10.1097/AOG.0B013E31821D85E5.
31. Meis PJ, Ureda JR, Swain M, Kelly RT, Penry M, Sharp P. Variable decelerations during nonstress tests are not a sign of fetal compromise. *Am J Obstet Gynecol.* 1986;154(3):586-590. doi: 10.1016/0002-9378(86)90606-X.
32. Druzin ML, Gratacós J, Keegan KA, Paul RH. Antepartum fetal heart rate testing. VII. The significance of fetal bradycardia. *Am J Obstet Gynecol.* 1981;139(2):194-198. doi: 10.1016/0002-9378(81)90445-2.
33. Brown R, Patrick J. The nonstress test: how long is enough? *Am J Obstet Gynecol.* 1981;141(6):646-651. doi: 10.1016/S0002-9378(15)33305-6.
34. Tan KH, Smyth RMD, Wei X. Fetal vibroacoustic stimulation for facilitation of tests of fetal wellbeing. *Cochrane Database Syst Rev.* 2013;2013(12):CD002963. doi: 10.1002/14651858.CD002963.PUB2.
35. Tan KH, Sabapathy A. Maternal glucose administration for facilitating tests of fetal wellbeing. *Cochrane Database Syst Rev.* 2012; 2012(9):CD003397. doi: 10.1002/14651858.CD003397.PUB2.
36. Sung S, Abramovitz A. Variable Decelerations—StatPearls—NCBI Bookshelf. StatPearls. Accessed May 13, 2023. https://www.ncbi.nlm.nih.gov/books/NBK546627/.

37. Modanlou HD, Freeman RK. Sinusoidal fetal heart rate pattern: its definition and clinical significance. *Am J Obstet Gynecol.* 1982; 142(8):1033-1038. doi: 10.1016/0002-9378(82)90789-X.
38. Modanlou HD, Murata Y. Sinusoidal heart rate pattern: reappraisal of its definition and clinical significance. *J Obstet Gynaecol Res.* 2004;30(3):169-180. doi: 10.1111/j.1447-0756.2004.00186.x.
39. Manning FA, Platt LD, Sipos L. Antepartum fetal evaluation: development of a fetal biophysical profile. *Am J Obstet Gynecol.* 1980;136(6):787-795. doi: 10.1016/0002-9378(80)90457-3.
40. Gribbin C, James D. Assessing fetal health. *Best Pract Res Clin Obstet Gynaecol.* 2004;18(3):411-424. doi: 10.1016/j.bpobgyn.2004.02.004.
41. Manning FA, Harman CR, Morrison I, Menticoglou SM, Lange IR, Johnson JM. Fetal assessment based on fetal biophysical profile scoring. IV. An analysis of perinatal morbidity and mortality. *Am J Obstet Gynecol.* 1990;162(3):703-709. doi: 10.1016/0002-9378(90)90990-O.
42. Manning FA, Morrison I, Harman CR, Lange IR, Menticoglou S. Fetal assessment based on fetal biophysical profile scoring: experience in 19,221 referred high-risk pregnancies. II. An analysis of false-negative fetal deaths. *Am J Obstet Gynecol.* 1987;157(4 Pt 1): 880-884. doi: 10.1016/S0002-9378(87)80077-7.
43. Baschat AA, Galan HL, Lee W, et al. The role of the fetal biophysical profile in the management of fetal growth restriction. *Am J Obstet Gynecol.* 2022;226(4):475-486. doi: 10.1016/J.AJOG.2022.01.020.
44. Pillai M, James D. Hiccups and breathing in human fetuses. *Arch Dis Child.* 1990;65(10 Spec No):1072. doi: 10.1136/ADC.65.10_SPEC_NO.1072.
45. Salisbury AL, Coyle MG, O'Grady KE, et al. Fetal assessment before and after dosing with buprenorphine or methadone. *Addiction (Abingdon, England).* 2012;107 Suppl 1(0 1):36-44. doi: 10.1111/J.1360-0443.2012.04037.X.
46. Kelly MK, Schneider EP, Petrikovsky BM, Lesser ML. Effect of antenatal steroid administration on the fetal biophysical profile—PubMed. *J Clin Ultrasound.* 2000;28(5):224-226. Accessed May 28, 2023. https://pubmed.ncbi.nlm.nih.gov/10800000/.
47. Vintzileos AM, Campbell WA, Ingardia CJ, Nochimson DJ. The fetal biophysical profile and its predictive value. *Obstet Gynecol.* 1983;62(3):271-278. doi: 10.1097/00006250-198309000-00001.
48. Manning FA, Baskett TF, Morrison I, Lange I. Fetal biophysical profile scoring: a prospective study in 1,184 high-risk patients. *Am J Obstet Gynecol.* 1981;140(3):289-294. doi: 10.1016/0002-9378(81)90275-1.
49. Manning FA, Morrison I, Lange IR, Harman CR, Chamberlain PF. Fetal assessment based on fetal biophysical profile scoring: experience in 12,620 referred high-risk pregnancies. I. Perinatal mortality by frequency and etiology. *Am J Obstet Gynecol.* 1985;151(3):343-350. doi: 10.1016/0002-9378(85)90301-1.
50. Ray M, Freeman R, Pine S, Hesselgesser R. Clinical experience with the oxytocin challenge test. *Am J Obstet Gynecol.* 1972; 114(1):1-9. doi: 10.1016/0002-9378(72)90279-7.
51. Greenberg MB, Druzin ML. Antepartum fetal evaluation. In: *Obstetrics: Normal and Problem Pregnancies.* Published online January 1, 2016:219-243.e1. doi: 10.1016/B978-0-323-32108-2.00011-1.
52. Nageotte MP, Towers CV, Asrat T, Freeman RK, Dorchester W. The value of a negative antepartum test: contraction stress test and modified biophysical profile. *Obstet Gynecol.* 1994; 84(2):231-234. Accessed May 13, 2023. https://pubmed.ncbi.nlm.nih.gov/8041536/.
53. Clark SL, Sabey P, Jolley K. Nonstress testing with acoustic stimulation and amniotic fluid volume assessment: 5973 tests without unexpected fetal death. *Am J Obstet Gynecol.* 1989;160(3): 694-697. doi: 10.1016/S0002-9378(89)80062-6.
54. Kehl S, Schelkle A, Thomas A, et al. Single deepest vertical pocket or amniotic fluid index as evaluation test for predicting adverse pregnancy outcome (SAFE trial): a multicenter, open-label, randomized controlled trial. *Ultrasound Obstet Gynecol.* 2016;47(6):674-679. doi: 10.1002/UOG.14924.
55. Sanchez-Ramos J, Santisimo J, Peman F. La prueba del la oxytocina en el diagnostico del estado fetal anteparto. *Acta Ginecol.* 1971;22:697.
56. Pose S, Escarcena L. The influence of uterine contractions on the partial pressure of oxygen of the human fetus. In: *Effects of Labour on the Foetus and Newborn.* Published online 1967:48.
57. Spurrett B. Stressed cardiotocography in late pregnancy. *J Obstet Gynaecol Br Common.* 1971;78(10):894-900.
58. ACOG Practice Bulletin No. 107: Induction of labor. *Obstet Gynecol.* 2009;114(2 Pt 1):386-397. doi: 10.1097/AOG.0B013E3181B48EF5.
59. Oki EY, Keegan KA, Freeman RK, Dorchester WL. The breast-stimulated contraction stress test. *J Reprod Med.* 1987;32(12): 919-923. Accessed May 13, 2023. https://pubmed.ncbi.nlm.nih.gov/3430501/.
60. Lenke RR, Nemes JM. Use of nipple stimulation to obtain contraction stress test. *Obstet Gynecol.* 1984;63(3):345-348. Accessed May 13, 2023. http://www.ncbi.nlm.nih.gov/pubmed/6700857.
61. Clark SL, Nageotte MP, Garite TJ, et al. Intrapartum management of category II fetal heart rate tracings: towards standardization of care. *Am J Obstet Gynecol.* 2013;209(2):89-97. doi: 10.1016/J.AJOG.2013.04.030.
62. Slomka C, Pheland JP. Pregnancy outcome in the patient with a nonreactive nonstress test and a positive contraction stress test. *Am J Obstet Gynecol.* 1981;139(1):11-15. doi: 10.1016/0002-9378(81)90402-6.
63. Lausman A, Kingdom J. How and when to recommend delivery of a growth-restricted fetus: a review. *Best Pract Res Clin Obstet Gynaecol.* 2021;77:119-128. doi: 10.1016/J.BPOBGYN.2021.09.006.
64. Alfirevic Z, Stampalija T, Dowswell T. Fetal and umbilical Doppler ultrasound in high-risk pregnancies. *Cochrane Database Syst Rev.* 2017;6(6):CD007529. doi: 10.1002/14651858.CD007529.PUB4.
65. Alfirevic Z, Stampalija T, Medley N. Fetal and umbilical Doppler ultrasound in normal pregnancy. *Cochrane Database Syst Rev.* 2015;2015(4):CD001450. doi: 10.1002/14651858.CD001450.PUB4.

66. Moise KJ. The usefulness of middle cerebral artery Doppler assessment in the treatment of the fetus at risk for anemia. *Am J Obstet Gynecol.* 2008;198(2). doi: 10.1016/J.AJOG.2007.10.788.
67. Caradeux J, Martinez-Portilla RJ, Basuki TR, Kiserud T, Figueras F. Risk of fetal death in growth-restricted fetuses with umbilical and/or ductus venosus absent or reversed end-diastolic velocities before 34 weeks of gestation: a systematic review and meta-analysis. *Am J Obstet Gynecol.* 2018;218(2):S774-S782.e21. doi: 10.1016/J.AJOG.2017.11.566.
68. Sciscione AC, Hayes EJ. Uterine artery Doppler flow studies in obstetric practice. *Am J Obstet Gynecol.* 2009;201(2):121-126. doi: 10.1016/j.ajog.2009.03.027.
69. Huisman TWA. Doppler assessment of the fetal venous system. *Semin Perinatol.* 25(1):21-31 Published online 2001. doi: 10.1053/sper.2001.22890.
70. Samadi R, Greenspoon JS, Gviazda I, Settlage RH, Goodwin TM. Massive fetomaternal hemorrhage and fetal death: are they predictable? *J Perinatol.* 1999;19(3):227-229. doi: 10.1038/SJ.JP.7200144.
71. Dayal AK, Manning FA, Berck DJ, et al. Fetal death after normal biophysical profile score: an eighteen-year experience. *Am J Obstet Gynecol.* 1999;181(5 Pt 1):1231-1236. doi: 10.1016/S0002-9378(99)70114-6.

CHAPTER 11

Antepartum Management of the High-Risk Patient

Scott Infusino and Janine Rhoades

The previous chapter described the key components of antepartum fetal surveillance, including fetal heart rate (FHR) testing and biophysical profile (BPP), describing methodology, interpretation, and understanding of the associated limitations and pitfalls. The appropriate application of these methods in various clinical situations is critically important.

The goal of antepartum fetal surveillance is to identify signs of fetal compromise to prevent perinatal morbidity and mortality. Uteroplacental insufficiency, fetal hypoxemia, and acidemia are thought to be the common products of various maternal, fetal, and obstetric conditions leading to stillbirth. The motivation for performing this testing is the evidence-based hypothesis that this deterioration will be represented by changes in the FHR, behavior, and amniotic fluid (AF).

One of the challenges faced by Obstetric providers is the appropriate identification of patients at increased risk of stillbirth and neonatal morbidity. The current expert consensus states that antenatal fetal surveillance should be considered in pregnancies where the risk of stillbirth is greater than the false negative rate of the BPP (0.8 per 1000) or when the risk of stillbirth is twice that of the baseline risk.[1] Common indications for antenatal testing are summarized in Table 11.1. Another consideration in management is the timing and frequency of this testing. Data on prospective fetal mortality rate by gestational week of pregnancy shows a bimodal distribution, with one peak at 20 weeks, followed by a nadir at 29 to 33 weeks, and subsequent rise, remaining low until term.[2] Based on results of retrospective studies and clinical models, initiation of antenatal testing is generally recommended at 32 weeks gestation in pregnancies at higher risk of stillbirth.[1] However, testing can be initiated at an earlier or later gestational age depending on a patient's clinical status or complicating factors. The optimal frequency of antenatal fetal surveillance is unknown as there is a paucity of data addressing this issue. The majority of recommendations call for once- to twice-weekly testing based on expert consensus. The initiation of more frequent surveillance should be individualized.

TABLE 11.1 Indications for antepartum fetal surveillance

Postdate pregnancy
Diabetes Gestational, poorly controlled Gestational, with medication management Pregestational
Preeclampsia
Chronic hypertension
Decreased fetal movement
Previous stillbirth
Fetal growth restriction
Multifetal Gestation Dichorionic gestation Monochorionic-diamniotic gestation Monochorionic-monoamniotic gestation Higher order multifetal gestation
Preterm premature rupture of membranes
Rh isoimmunization
Hemoglobinopathy
Renal disease (Cr greater than 1.4 mg/dL)
Advanced Maternal age

Although antenatal fetal surveillance is the standard of care in high-risk pregnancies, there is a lack of Level A evidence that supports its use.[3] Much of the guidance in this management is based on observational studies and expert opinion. Despite this gap in research, it is important not to overlook the foundation of work that correlates fetal status to these antenatal tests.

The goal of this chapter is to provide an overview of maternal, fetal, and obstetric indications for antenatal surveillance.

WHICH TEST TO USE

Controversy exists as to which form of antepartum surveillance provides optimal results. Issues such as patient population, available facilities, cost, convenience, testing interval, and the specific indication for testing must be considered when selecting a particular means of fetal assessment. As described in the previous chapter, the most frequently used method for primary surveillance is the modified BPP. The nonstress test (NST) is usually performed once or twice weekly. The frequency of the AF volume assessment may also be once or twice weekly. BPP has been compared with a modified biophysical profile (MBPP) in terms of identifying an optimal surveillance method. In a 2008 Cochrane review, there was no significant difference in pregnancy outcomes when comparing these two modalities. It is important to note, however, that most trials included in this review were not of high quality and that the overall incidence of adverse outcomes was low.[4] Specific methods of antenatal surveillance are often determined based on their institutional protocol, preference, and/or clinical context.

MATERNAL INDICATIONS

Hypertensive Disorders of Pregnancy

Gestational Hypertension and Preeclampsia

An increased risk of stillbirth is well documented in hypertensive disorders of pregnancy and is thought to account for 9.2% of cases. There is an estimated 1.2- to 4-fold increased odds of stillbirth in pregnancies complicated by preeclampsia.[5] These pregnancies are more likely to show evidence of placental insufficiency and dysfunction as shown by histopathology studies.[6-8]

For patients with gestational hypertension or preeclampsia, initiation of antenatal fetal surveillance is recommended at the time of diagnosis or at a viable gestational age (Fig. 11.1).[1] The optimal method of fetal testing (NST vs BPP) is not entirely evident, as there is a lack of randomized trials to help guide this aspect of care. It is also important to note that in cases of extreme prematurity, the goal is not necessarily to confirm the presence of fetal heart tracing characteristics such as accelerations but to assess for the presence of a nonreassuring fetal status. For patients without severe preeclampsia, the American College of Obstetricians and Gynecologists (ACOG) recommends twice-weekly fetal surveillance with at least weekly assessment of AF volume until delivery. With the diagnosis of preeclampsia with severe features, ACOG recommends at least daily fetal surveillance. Assessment of fetal growth should take place every 3 to 4 weeks.[1,9]

It is important to consider the following when managing a patient with a hypertensive disorder of pregnancy:

1. A nonreassuring fetal status can occur even in an asymptomatic and normotensive patient.
2. A patient's clinical condition can change rapidly. Should such change occur, a repeat evaluation of the fetus must be performed even when the most recent assessment was reassuring.
3. Fetal condition is one variable to be considered in the broader clinical context of the evaluation and management of these patients.
4. Rapid changes in maternal blood pressure can result in abnormal FHR patterns, and fetal status should be monitored during acute management of severe hypertension.

Chronic Hypertension

Like gestational hypertension and preeclampsia, an increased risk of stillbirth is seen in pregnancies complicated by chronic hypertension. An estimated stillbirth rate of 6 to 25 per 1000 (OR, 1.5-2.7) has been reported in these pregnancies.[10] An increase in adverse perinatal outcomes has been observed as the degree of hypertension worsens.[11] Additionally, the rate of perinatal mortality in patients with chronic hypertension with superimposed preeclampsia is higher than in women diagnosed with preeclampsia without a prior history of hypertension.[12] These pregnancies are also at risk of uteroplacental insufficiency, and pathologic findings in the uterine decidual vessels have been noted in the setting of preexisting hypertension.[13]

In pregnancies complicated by chronic hypertension controlled with medication, ACOG recommends

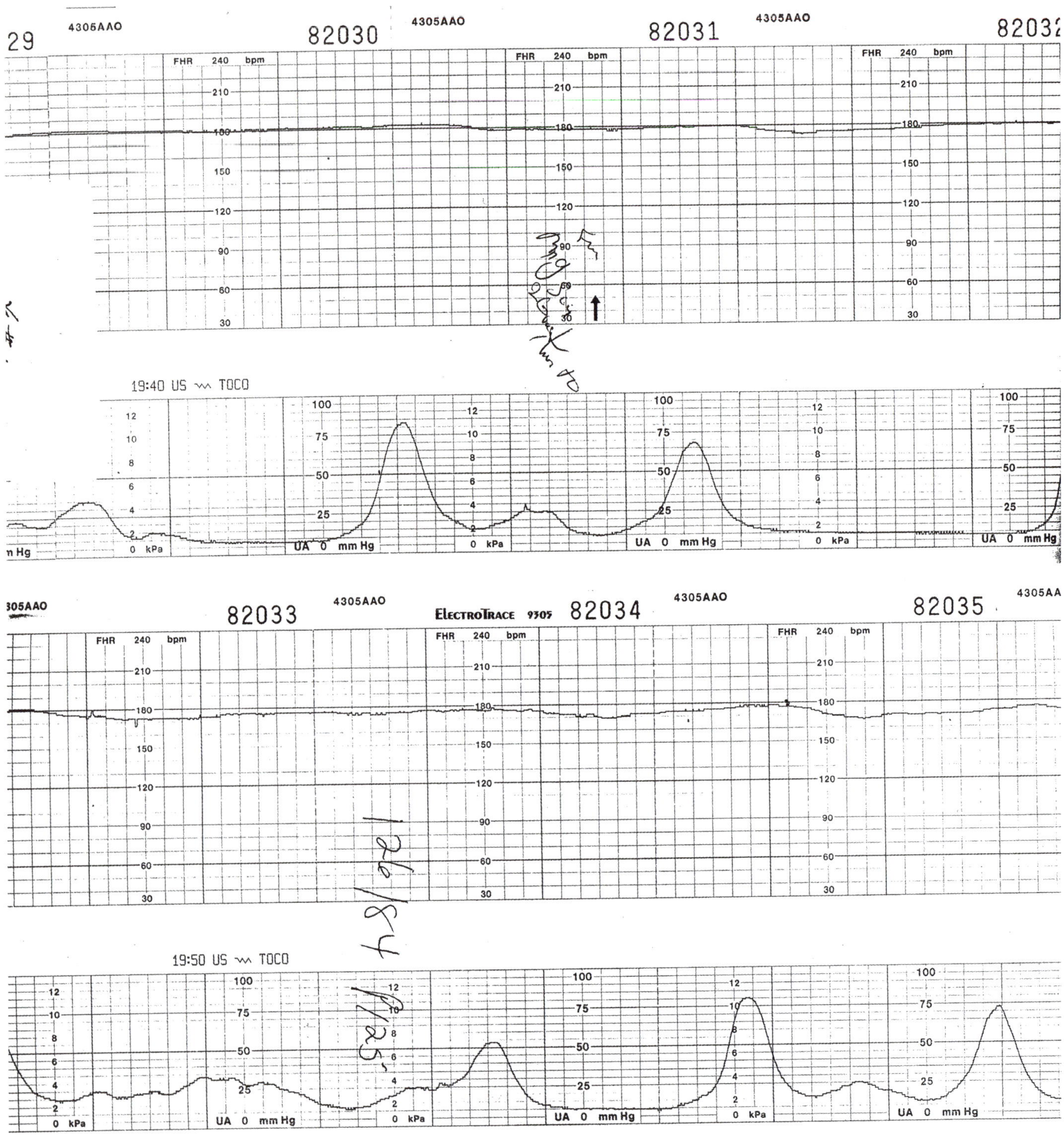

Figure 11.1. This is a 38-year-old gravida 4 para 3 at 29.5 weeks admitted with mild blood pressure elevation, proteinuria, thrombocytopenia, and elevated liver enzyme concentrations. She was seen 2 weeks previously without concern. The external fetal monitor revealed fetal tachycardia, minimal to absent variability, and recurrent late decelerations. After administration of magnesium sulfate, a primary cesarean section was performed. Apgar scores were noted to be 0 at 1 minute, 3 at 5 minutes, and 5 at 10 minutes. Arterial cord pH was 6.90 with BE −22 and venous 7.01 with BE −17. The baby ultimately survived.

initiation of antenatal surveillance at 32 weeks gestation. In pregnancies complicated by poorly controlled hypertension, or with other comorbid medical conditions, surveillance should be individualized.[1] As with other patients, testing can be conducted using the modified BPP.

Patients with chronic hypertension may require changes or adjustments in their medications to control blood pressure during pregnancy. An important point regarding hypertension control and FHR monitoring is that when patients with chronic hypertension develop sudden deterioration of their blood pressure control, or in patients with severe preeclampsia, acute lowering of blood pressure may adversely affect uterine perfusion. Care should be taken to avoid rapid reduction below normal blood pressure because the fetus may exhibit decelerations or decreased variability with too vigorous antihypertensive therapy. Continuous monitoring of FHR while treating severe hypertension is critically important to ensure adequate placental perfusion and identify possible fetal distress. The fetal heart tracing can provide an additional data point to help establish an acceptable blood pressure endpoint for both the fetus and the mother.

Diabetes Mellitus

Pregestational Diabetes

Historically, insulin-dependent diabetes was a significant contributor to stillbirth and neonatal morbidity. Improvement in treatment and initiation of antenatal testing has had a positive impact on improving perinatal outcomes.[14] Perinatal mortality in pregnancies complicated by insulin-dependent diabetes can be reduced to that of nondiabetics.[15,16] Overall, there is still an increased risk of stillbirth with a rate of approximately 13.9 per 1000 pregnancies, which is more prominent in patients with poor glycemic control, polyhydramnios, and fetal macrosomia.[1,17] In patients with pregestational diabetes, antenatal surveillance is usually started at 32 weeks gestation. However, in the setting of other comorbidities or particularly poor glycemic control, earlier monitoring may be warranted.[18] Stillbirth occurring as early as the late second trimester has been reported in patients with concurrent renal disease, hypertension, and/or growth restriction.[17] Frequency of testing is most commonly twice weekly as there is thought to be a higher risk of fetal demise within 7 days of an NST, however it is important to note that the optimal schedule of fetal surveillance has not been ascertained.[18,19]

Gestational Diabetes

Data suggest that gestational diabetes not requiring medications (Class A1) does not increase antenatal fetal mortality in the general population.[20] Thus antenatal surveillance is not routinely recommended in these patients if their pregnancy is otherwise uncomplicated. Gestational diabetes requiring medication management (Class A2) is thought to increase the risk of fetal demise owing to the same principles that affect pregnancies complicated by pregestational diabetes. Therefore, fetal surveillance is recommended once or twice weekly starting at 32 weeks gestation.[21] With appropriate glucose control, appropriate fetal growth, and reassuring fetal surveillance tests, we allow diabetic pregnancies to continue to 39 weeks gestation.

Maternal Autoimmune Disease

Multiple autoimmune diseases can impact pregnancy outcomes, and knowledge of these risks is important for appropriate management. Systemic lupus erythematosus (SLE) is an inflammatory autoimmune disease that can affect multiple systems and is characterized by episodes of flares and periods of remission. Pregnancies are at increased risk of uteroplacental insufficiency, and placental pathology review will often show findings of placentas small for gestational age and signs of vascular lesions.[22] Fetal growth restriction (FGR) is more frequent in pregnancies complicated by SLE with reported rates ranging from 6% to 35%. The risk of stillbirth is also significantly increased and is estimated to be 40 to 150 per 1000 pregnancies.[23] Although there is no data to guide an optimal management strategy for antenatal fetal surveillance, both ACOG and SMFM recommend weekly monitoring starting at 32 weeks gestation.[1,24] SLE with additional complications such as active lupus nephritis, lupus flare, and antiphospholipid antibodies with previous stillbirth should have individualized care with consideration for earlier and more frequent fetal surveillance.

Antiphospholipid syndrome (APS) is an autoimmune condition characterized by a clinical history of vascular thrombosis and/or adverse pregnancy outcomes, as well as the persistence of antiphospholipid antibodies (aPL).[25] There is a well-documented association between stillbirth and placental insufficiency with APS. Data from the Stillbirth Collaborative Research Network showed different odds ratios for stillbirth based on the antibody type present. Anticardiolipin IgG and IgM antibodies were associated with a fivefold and twofold increased odds of stillbirth, respectively, whereas anti-β_2-glycoprotein IgG and antibodies were associated with a threefold increased odds of stillbirth.[26] Higher antibody levels and a history of stillbirth with APS have also been found to increase the risk of stillbirth.[26,27] Given these risks, antenatal surveillance is recommended twice weekly starting at 32 weeks.[1]

Systemic Sclerosis is a disease of vascular dysfunction and fibrosis with a diverse range of clinical manifestations. Data on pregnancy is limited, but there have been reports of increased risk of growth restriction and histologic placenta pathology similar to those found in hypertensive disorders of pregnancy.[28] Given these findings, some providers recommend antenatal testing at 30 to 32 weeks.[29]

The Critically Ill Obstetric Patient

Antepartum management of the critically ill obstetric patient can be a particularly challenging clinical scenario, where the physiologic changes of pregnancy can complicate the diagnosis and treatment of various disease processes. Data on appropriate management is often limited, especially with regard to fetal monitoring. In pregnancies complicated by critical illness that are of a viable gestational age, electronic fetal monitoring (EFM) can be a crucial tool. The FHR can reflect multiple factors such as end-organ perfusion and maternal acid-base status. FHR characteristics such as changes in baseline variability or new onset decelerations should prompt maternal evaluation for a change in status. The following are examples of obstetric critical care scenarios requiring fetal assessment.

Diabetic ketoacidosis (DKA) occurs in 0.5% to 3% of all pregnancies complicated by diabetes. This acute disease process poses significant fetal risk. Maternal hypovolemia resulting in uterine hypoperfusion, placental transfer of ketoacids, and electrolyte imbalance have all been proposed mechanisms that contribute to fetal compromise. Decreased variability, spontaneous decelerations, abnormal BPP, and fetal tachycardia are all findings that can be observed.[30] Historically, studies have reported a fetal loss rate ranging from 9% to 36% of cases, with more recent literature reporting a rate of 5% or less.[31] Given this risk, continuous fetal monitoring at a viable gestational age is essential until metabolic derangements have been corrected. FHR abnormalities should resolve with the improvement of maternal status but may take an additional 4 to 8 hours.[30] Emergency delivery is generally avoided as the fetal status should improve with proper management of DKA (Fig. 11.2).

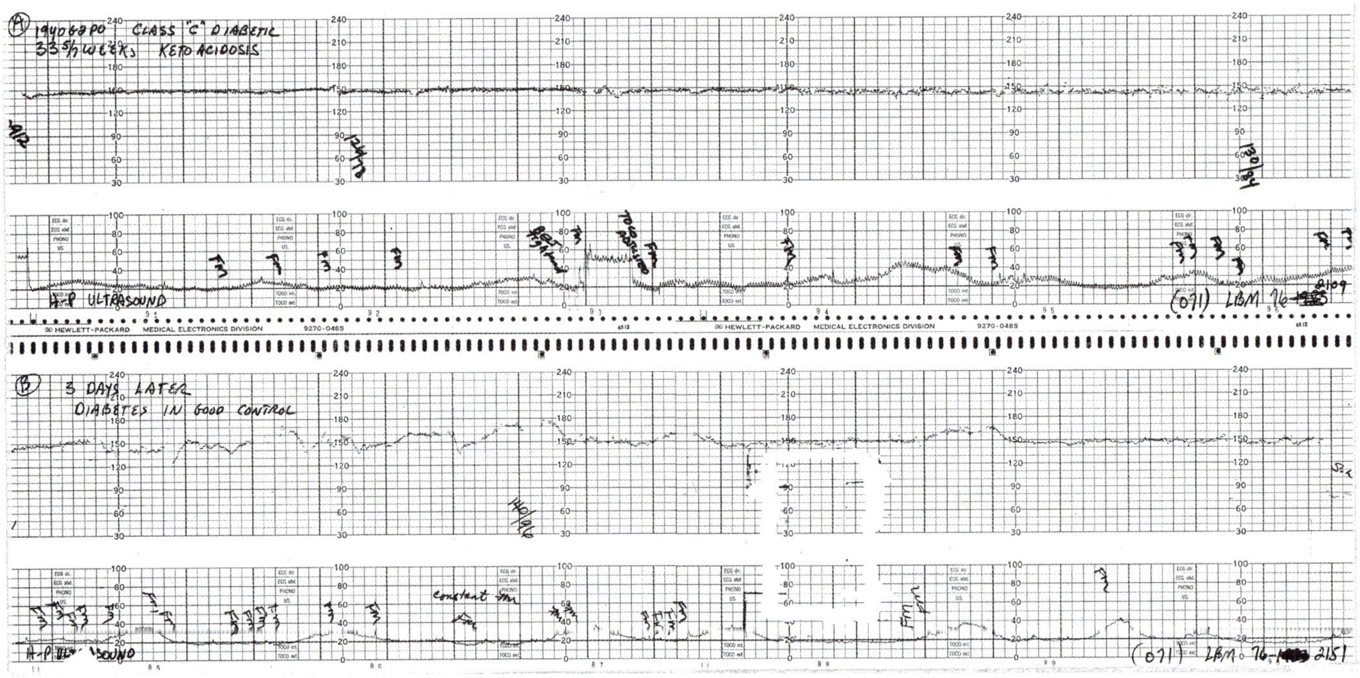

Figure 11.2. This case illustrates the effect of ketoacidosis on the fetus. **Panel A** is the fetal heart rate (FHR) tracing of a diabetic admitted in ketoacidosis at 33.5 weeks. Note the nonreactive pattern. Three days later **(panel B)**, with the patient euglycemic and nonketotic, a normally reactive spontaneous contraction stress test result was seen. This illustrates the potential reversibility of FHR patterns when treatable conditions exist.

Respiratory failure complicates 0.2% of pregnancies and can be secondary to a multitude of disease processes.[32] Fetal monitoring is crucial during this time as hypoxia and maternal acid-base derangements can affect fetal status, and any change in respiratory status should prompt fetal monitoring. Plans for fetal surveillance should be individualized based on clinical status. Extracorporeal membrane oxygenation (ECMO) is rare in pregnancy but saw an increase in use during the H1N1 pandemic in 2009 and the COVID pandemic in 2020. Lankford et al described a fetal monitoring protocol that consisted of continuous EFM for the first 24 hours after ECMO initiation, followed by 1 hour of EFM every 12 hours.[33]

Hemoglobinopathy

Patients with substantially decreased effective oxygen-carrying red blood cells or with other reasons for decreased oxygen delivery to the placenta are at increased risk of uteroplacental insufficiency. Such uteroplacental insufficiency may lead to growth restriction and/or hypoxic compromise. Maternal sickle cell disease has a well-documented association with an increased risk of stillbirth with a rate of 81 per 1000 pregnancies (OR, 4.05).[34] Published data on the efficacy of antenatal surveillance in patients with sickle cell disease is limited but is generally recommended on a once- to twice-weekly basis in uncomplicated patients starting at 32 weeks. In the setting of complications such as frequent vaso-occlusive crises, fetal surveillance should be individualized.[1] Patients with an active vaso-occlusive crisis should undergo fetal monitoring, as abnormal fetal heart tracing and BPP during these episodes have been described in the literature.[35] In the setting of maternal hypoxia or severe anemia, treatment of the maternal condition with oxygen therapy or transfusion may improve ominous FHR patterns. Hemoglobinopathies other than sickle cell disease should have individualized management of fetal surveillance, taking into account a patient's entire clinical picture.[1]

FETAL INDICATIONS

Fetal Growth Restriction

FGR is the failure of the fetus to reach its genetic and biological potential, often secondary to placental dysfunction.[36] Numerous studies have demonstrated an association of FGR with stillbirth and neonatal morbidity. An inverse relationship exists between birthweight percentile and perinatal mortality, as well as with estimated fetal weight and stillbirth.[1,36] Additionally, early-onset FGR (diagnosed <32 weeks) is associated with increased morbidity, mortality, and long-term health risks. The criteria for growth restriction varies between different obstetric societies, but the current definition by the Society for Maternal-Fetal Medicine (SMFM) is an estimated fetal weight or abdominal circumference <10th percentile for gestational age.[37]

Once a diagnosis of growth restriction is made, fetal surveillance should be initiated at a viable gestational age and weight. The cornerstone of antenatal surveillance in this setting consists of fetal Doppler velocimetry, usually supplemented with the BPP or modified BPP.

In early-onset FGR, a worsening of fetal status is often preceded by a progressive deterioration of fetal Doppler studies. This pattern of decline has been well described in the literature.[38] Currently in the United States, the SMFM recommends routine use of the umbilical artery (UA) Doppler in the management of FGR. The characteristic changes in this Doppler waveform start with an increase in systolic-to-diastolic ratio, followed by absent-end diastolic flow (AEDF), and subsequently reversed-end diastolic flow (REDF) that reflects an increase in placental vascular resistance and compromise of the fetoplacental vascular tree. There is an abundance of data on the utility of UA Doppler in FGR, and its use in surveillance is associated with a 29% reduction in perinatal death.[39] SMFM recommends that once FGR is diagnosed, serial UA Doppler evaluation should be performed. Assessment 2 to 3 times per week is recommended with deterioration to AEDF, and hospitalization with administration of betamethasone and frequent FHR monitoring is recommended with REDF.[37] The nuance of clinical management of these Doppler findings as well as the utility of other Doppler studies such as the ductus venosus, middle cerebral artery, and uterine artery are beyond the scope of this chapter.

Initiation of FHR monitoring (NST) is recommended on a weekly basis at minimum upon diagnosis of FGR with a viable gestational and estimated fetal weight where intervention would be recommended.[37] Frequency should increase with deterioration of fetal UA Doppler. The rationale of FHR monitoring is that a nonreactive or abnormal NST will be associated with fetal hypoxia, acidemia, or a worsening of fetal status. Although the utility of cardiotocography on outcomes in FGR is inconclusive, it can help guide management in instances of fetal deterioration at extreme prematurity. Ominous changes in fetal heart tracing can dictate

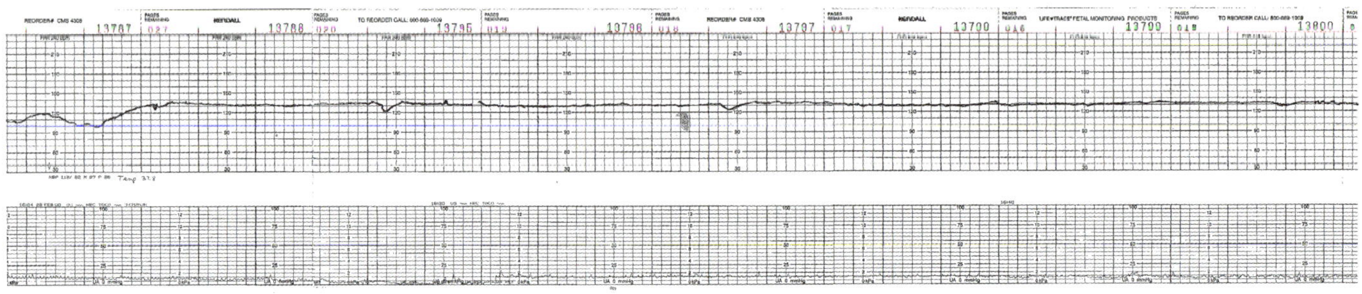

Figure 11.3. This patient was a 19-year-old gravida 1 para 0 at 26 weeks' gestation. She had a history of arthritis and laboratory abnormalities suggestive of possible systemic lupus erythematosus. An ultrasound done at the time of the initial consultation revealed fetal growth restriction with reversed-end diastolic flow of the umbilical artery. She was sent immediately to labor and delivery for fetal monitoring. The tracing was flat with spontaneous decelerations. The biophysical profile was 2 of 10 for fluid only. She underwent immediate cesarean section delivering a 526-g male with Apgar scores 6 at 1 minute and 6 at 5 minutes and cord gases of arterial 7.06 BE −12, venous 7.18, and BE −8. The baby ultimately survived and is developing normally at age 2.

delivery at earlier gestational ages outside the recommendations of standard guidelines (Fig. 11.3).

AF assessment and BPP are additional tools used to assess fetal well-being in pregnancies complicated by FGR. Regular assessment of AF volume is generally performed and the diagnosis of concurrent oligohydramnios with FGR is associated with fetal compromise.[40,41] BPP or modified BPP are also performed in conjunction with these surveillance tools, with the goal of improving outcomes and excluding acidemia.[1]

Multifetal Gestation

Dichorionic Diamniotic Twin Gestation

The optimal timing of antenatal fetal surveillance of uncomplicated dichorionic twins is unknown. An increasing risk of stillbirth has been noted with increasing gestational age beyond 34 weeks to a rate of 10.6 per 1000 pregnancies at 38 weeks.[1] Expert consensus states that in uncomplicated dichorionic diamniotic pregnancies, weekly fetal surveillance can be considered starting at 36 weeks gestation.[42] Dichorionic pregnancies complicated by selective fetal growth restriction (sFGR) are at a higher risk of perinatal morbidity and mortality, and initiation of antenatal surveillance is recommended at the time of diagnosis (Fig. 11.4).[42,43]

Monochorionic Diamniotic Twin Gestation

Monochorionic diamniotic pregnancies have a higher complication and stillbirth rate, with a risk of severe consequences to the surviving co-twin because of shared placental vasculature. The stillbirth rate is as high as 9.6 per 1000 at 37 weeks. Antenatal surveillance is typically recommended starting at 32 weeks gestation, with screening for complications such as twin-to-twin transfusion syndrome (TTTS) starting at 16 weeks.[1] Monochorionic pregnancies have a higher rate of sFGR than in dichorionic pregnancies, with a reported prevalence of 19.7% and 10.5%, respectively. This is likely because of unequal placental sharing and blood flow.[43]

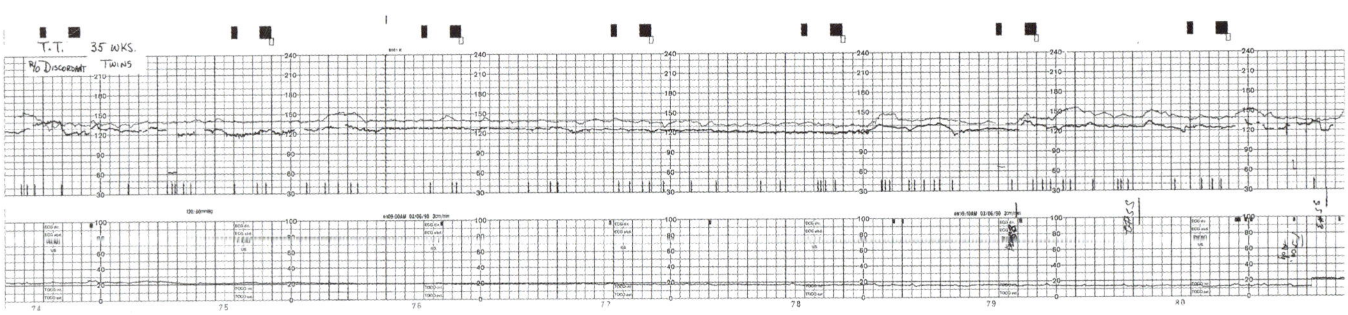

Figure 11.4. This patient had a twin gestation at 35 weeks with suspected growth discordance. Twice-weekly nonstress tests were performed. It is interesting to observe the degree of concordance of accelerations between the twins as well as similar changes in baseline.

Gratacos et al published a classification system of sFGR in monochorionic pregnancies, separating the condition into three types based on the UA Doppler flow of the smaller twin.[44] This model has become the standard in guiding the management of this particularly high-risk complication of monochorionic pregnancies. Antenatal fetal surveillance should be initiated at diagnosis of sFGR and be individualized based on severity.

Monochorionic Monoamniotic Twin Gestation

Monochorionic monoamniotic twin pregnancy has an even higher perinatal mortality rate, ranging from 12% to 23%.[1] Although such complications as TTTS and sFGR can also occur in these pregnancies, cord entanglement may potentially contribute to this higher mortality rate. Cord entanglement occurs in most monoamniotic pregnancies, and it is thought that intermittent umbilical cord occlusion can be associated with neurologic morbidity.[45,46] The optimal management of these pregnancies is unknown, but the majority of maternal-fetal medicine specialists will initiate inpatient surveillance at 24 to 28 weeks gestation, administer betamethasone, and perform intermittent fetal monitoring 2 to 3 times per day.[47]

Decreased Fetal Movement

Maternal perception of decreased fetal movement has been associated with an increased risk of stillbirth.[48,49] Although usually not a cause for true alarm, decreased fetal movement may be the only sign of impending fetal death in an otherwise normal pregnancy. This change in perceived fetal behavior could potentially be secondary to uteroplacental insufficiency. An NST and assessment of AF should not be delayed in the setting of decreased fetal movement. If the NST is reactive with normal AF, no further testing is necessary if the patient has no other risk factors and the test does not need repeating unless there is a recurrence or persistence of symptoms. If decelerations are present and/or the tracing is nonreactive, further assessment is indicated. A rare but very serious etiology for loss of fetal movement is fetal to maternal hemorrhage. Such a diagnosis should be considered in patients with a complaint of loss of fetal movement when there is a nonreactive or suspicious NST with spontaneous decelerations.

It is also important for high-risk patients to be instructed to monitor fetal movement. Should a high-risk patient report decreased fetal movement, the same policy as described earlier is followed, regardless of when the last fetal surveillance was performed. It is of interest to note that the only type of prospective study employing some form of fetal surveillance that has been shown to be of significant value in decreasing antepartum stillbirth is one comparing patients instructed in monitoring fetal movements daily with a group not noting daily movements.[50]

OBSTETRIC INDICATIONS

Second- and Third-Trimester Bleeding

Patients with second- and third-trimester bleeding are a difficult challenge in antepartum management, and care must be individualized. Management depends on maternal and fetal statuses, as well as gestational age. Initial assessment should include the evaluation of the patient's hemodynamic status, coagulation profile, and fetal well-being. With, and subsequent to, any bleeding episode, continuous fetal monitoring is indicated if the pregnancy is at a viable gestational age. Occasionally, even with only minimal uterine activity, late decelerations can alert the physician to a significant placental abruption (Fig. 11.5). In premature gestations, especially those with contractions, even a small amount of bleeding is abnormal and should alert the clinician to the possibility of an underlying etiology. The characteristic picture of placental abruption on the fetal monitor are late decelerations and a tachysystolic uterine contraction pattern. One, both, or neither may be present and may or may not correlate with the apparent size of the abruption. With a major bleeding episode, normal FHR tracing is an essential variable in the decision to prolong pregnancy or allow a trial of labor.

Once the acute episode is resolved and a reasonable time (usually at least 24 hours) of continuous fetal monitoring has provided reassurance, the patients can revert to intermittent antepartum testing. In patients with suspected chronic placental abruption deemed appropriate for outpatient management, strong consideration should be given to once- or twice-weekly antenatal fetal surveillance and regular assessment of fetal growth. Patients undergoing expectant management are at increased risk of developing FGR.[1,51] Chronic abruption oligohydramnios sequence (CAOS) is a complication that has also been described in the literature, further highlighting the importance of regular fetal surveillance.[52]

Oligohydramnios and Polyhydramnios

The AF volume represents a well-regulated balance of production and absorption. This fluid volume can be

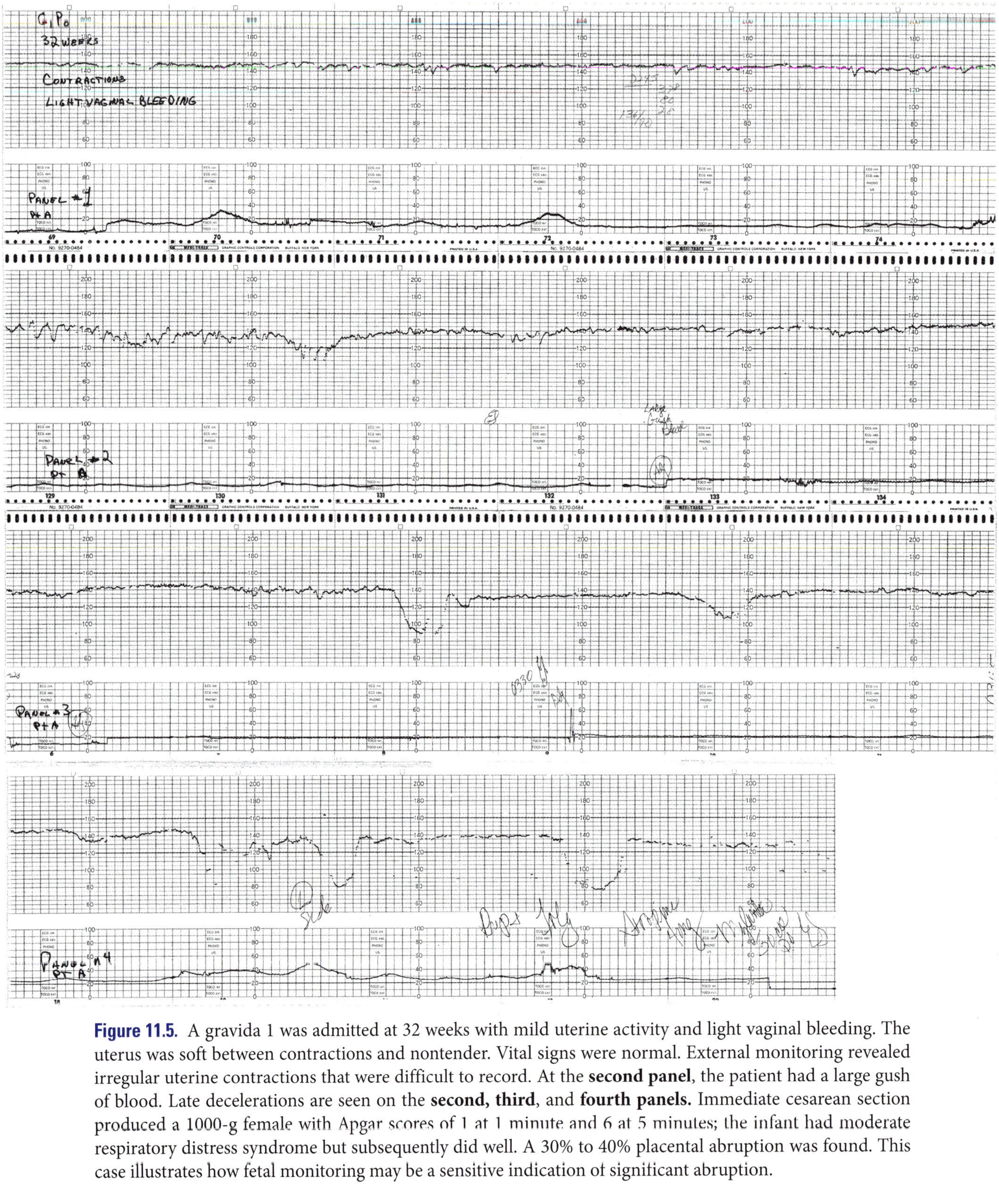

Figure 11.5. A gravida 1 was admitted at 32 weeks with mild uterine activity and light vaginal bleeding. The uterus was soft between contractions and nontender. Vital signs were normal. External monitoring revealed irregular uterine contractions that were difficult to record. At the **second panel**, the patient had a large gush of blood. Late decelerations are seen on the **second, third**, and **fourth panels.** Immediate cesarean section produced a 1000-g female with Apgar scores of 1 at 1 minute and 6 at 5 minutes; the infant had moderate respiratory distress syndrome but subsequently did well. A 30% to 40% placental abruption was found. This case illustrates how fetal monitoring may be a sensitive indication of significant abruption.

quantified with ultrasound by the amniotic fluid index (AFI) or the maximum vertical pocket (MVP). Upon diagnosis of oligohydramnios, a thorough investigation should be undertaken to rule out potential causes such as rupture of membranes, FGR, or congenital malformation. Without a pathologic cause identified, this is termed isolated oligohydramnios. An MVP <2 cm, as opposed to AFI, should be used to diagnose oligohydramnios as this is associated with a lower rate of intervention without a significant difference in adverse pregnancy outcome.[53] Current recommendations for the management of isolated oligohydramnios include once- to twice-weekly fetal surveillance initiated at the time of diagnosis with delivery at 36 0/7 to 37 6/7 weeks.[1,16]

As with oligohydramnios, a diagnosis of polyhydramnios should come with an investigation to evaluate for a potential etiology. It is often categorized as mild (AFI 24.0-29.9 cm, DVP 8-11 cm), moderate (AFI 30.0-34.9 cm, MVP 12-15 cm), and severe (AFI ≥ 35 cm, DVP ≥ 16 cm). There is currently no evidence that isolated polyhydramnios are associated with uteroplacental insufficiency. Current recommendations call for once- to twice-weekly antenatal testing for moderate-to-severe polyhydramnios starting at 32 to 34 weeks gestation.[1,54]

Preterm Prelabor Rupture of Membranes

Approximately, 3% of pregnancies are complicated by preterm prelabor rupture of the membranes (PPROM).[55] There is no consensus on the optimal form of antenatal surveillance. Most schemes of expectant management include the use of daily or twice-daily NSTs. Concern regarding infection, cord accidents, and abruption justifies the efforts to use frequent fetal monitoring in women with this complication. In pregnancies complicated by PPROM that are being managed expectantly, the authors perform twice-daily NST. The FHR baseline and the presence or absence of accelerations and decelerations are specifically noted. Variable decelerations, suggesting possible cord compression secondary to decreased AF volume, are not uncommon and may indicate early labor or fetal distress.[56]

A randomized trial comparing daily NST with daily BPP by Lewis et al concluded that the NST was equivalent to the BPP in this situation and significantly less time-consuming and cost-effective except in pregnancies <28 weeks where nonreactivity was common because of early gestational age.[57] Thus, the NST is an appropriate screen for cord compression and fetal compromise. Because of the significant maternal and fetal risks in patients with preterm PROM, careful and frequent determination of fetal well-being is critically important with expectant management.

Late-Term Gestation and Postdate Pregnancy

Although there has been a recent trend toward induction of labor at 39 weeks gestation, it is still important to consider management of the late-term gestation and postdate pregnancy.[58,59] Unfortunately, limited data exists on the optimal timing of fetal surveillance in these otherwise uncomplicated pregnancies. Retrospective studies have shown an increased frequency of oligohydramnios and FHR abnormalities after 41 weeks.[60,61] Increased risk of fetal, maternal, and neonatal complications have been noted beyond 41 weeks gestation, and the prevalence of stillbirth only rises with this increasing gestational age. Given these findings, ACOG recommends initiation of once- or twice-weekly antenatal surveillance for late-term gestation at 41 weeks.[1] It is important to note, however, that several studies examining antenatal testing in this population have done so on a twice-weekly basis with both NST and AF assessment.[60,62,63] One case series noted an abrupt decrease in AF in the postdate population.[61] Multiple randomized trials have evaluated induction versus expectant management of late-term gestation with results suggesting a potential decrease in perinatal mortality and cesarean section with induction.[64,65] A 2018 Cochrane review of 30 randomized control trials including 12,479 women compared induction of labor versus expectant management at or beyond term, and found that induction was associated with a decreased rate of cesarean section, NICU admission, low Apgar score, and a small reduction in perinatal death.[66] The most recent recommendation by ACOG states that induction can be considered at 41 weeks gestation and is recommended starting at 42 weeks.[67] However, it is important to note that in otherwise uncomplicated pregnancies, delivery can be considered starting at 39 weeks.[68]

MANAGEMENT OF PATIENTS WITH NONREASSURING TESTS

Nonreactive Nonstress Test

The NST should be viewed as a screening test when used as the primary means of antepartum testing. Nonreactive patterns may be caused by fetal hypoxia, previous central nervous system (CNS) injury, anomalies, sleep states, or CNS-depressant drugs. While performing the NST, if there are not two or more 15 beats per minute (bpm) accelerations above the baseline FHR within the initial 20 to 30 minutes, stimulation of the fetus with vibroacoustic stimulation can be considered. Another 20-minute period is then monitored, and if the fetus is still nonreactive, a BPP should be performed. An NST that remains nonreactive and is followed by a normal BPP may be repeated in 1 week.

ABNORMAL BIOPHYSICAL PROFILE

When using the BPP, either as primary surveillance or as backup to the nonreactive NST, the response should be based on the entire clinical situation. A BPP of 8 or 10 is normal and requires repeat evaluation as dictated by the clinical context. A BPP of 6 is equivocal and requires repeat evaluation within 24 hours. If a part of the reduction in BPP score is caused by decreased AF volume, the management will often be dictated by the presence of comorbid conditions and gestational age. A BPP of 4 warrants delivery for the term fetus and possibly for the preterm fetus depending on gestational age. Finally, a BPP of 0 to 2 is almost always an indication of delivery in the viable fetus (Table 11.2). The only exception may be cases of extreme prematurity where the decision for delivery should never be undertaken unless all tests indicate an absolute need. Unnecessary delivery may result in prematurity that may have dire neonatal and long-term consequences. One other point to make is that no matter what means of surveillance is chosen, negative tests are associated with a very low likelihood of adverse outcomes. Positive test results should be thoroughly evaluated to avoid unnecessary premature intervention. Therefore, multimodal fetal testing should be used in making the decision to deliver, rather than relying on one test, particularly in very premature gestations.

TABLE 11.2 Biophysical profile scoring, management protocol

Score	Interpretation management
10	Normal infant, low risk. Repeat testing at weekly intervals.
8	Normal infant, low risk. Repeat testing at standard scheduled intervals. If oligohydramnios is diagnosed, evaluate for causes.
6	Equivocal test, suspect fetal asphyxia. Repeat testing within 24 h. If 6/10 BPP persists, delivery may be indicated depending on gestational age. A 6/8 BPP should always be followed by a nonstress test to assign a final score.
4	Suspect chronic asphyxia. Delivery is usually indicated depending on gestational age.
0-2	Delivery, if gestational viability determined, is almost always indicated for 0/10 or 2/10 BPP, with a strong suspicion of fetal asphyxia.

Adapted from Manning FA, Baskett TF, Morrison I, Lange I. Fetal biophysical profile scoring: a prospective study in 1,184 high-risk patients. *Am J Obstet Gynecol.* 1981;140(3):289-294.

SUMMARY

Managing the high-risk antepartum patient is a difficult and challenging problem. Decisions regarding intervention have potentially grave consequences and should not be made on one parameter alone without knowledge of gestational age and risk related to the underlying maternal, fetal, or obstetric conditions. The goal should be to deliver a healthy neonate as near term as possible by the safest route for the mother and the fetus. Antepartum fetal surveillance can contribute significantly toward this goal if understood well and used appropriately.

REFERENCES

1. Indications for outpatient antenatal fetal surveillance: ACOG committee opinion, number 828. *Obstet Gynecol.* 2021;137(6): e177-e197.
2. MacDorman MF, Gregory ECW. Fetal and perinatal mortality: United States, 2013. *Natl Vital Stat Rep.* 2015;64(8):1-24.
3. Devoe LD. Antenatal fetal assessment: contraction stress test, nonstress test, vibroacoustic stimulation, amniotic fluid volume, biophysical profile, and modified biophysical profile—an overview. *Semin Perinatol.* 2008;32(4):247-252.
4. Lalor JG, Fawole B, Alfirevic Z, Devane D. Biophysical profile for fetal assessment in high risk pregnancies. *Cochrane Database Syst Rev.* 2008;2008(1):CD000038.
5. Gibbins KJ, Silver RM, Pinar H, et al. Stillbirth, hypertensive disorders of pregnancy, and placental pathology. *Placenta.* 2016; 43:61-68.
6. Jones CJ, Fox H. An ultrastructural and ultrahistochemical study of the human placenta in maternal pre-eclampsia. *Placenta.* 1980;1(1):61-76.
7. Allaire AD, Ballenger KA, Wells SR, et al. Placental apoptosis in preeclampsia. *Obstet Gynecol.* 2000;96(2):271-276.
8. Huppertz B, Kingdom J, Caniggia I, et al. Hypoxia favours necrotic versus apoptotic shedding of placental syncytiotrophoblast into maternal circulation. *Placenta.* 2003;24(2-3):181-190.

9. Gestational hypertension and preeclampsia: ACOG practice bulletin, number 222. *Obstet Gynecol.* 2020;135(6):e237-e260.
10. Fretts RC. Etiology and prevention of stillbirth. *Am J Obstet Gynecol.* 2005;193(6):1923-1935.
11. Harper LM, Tita A, Karumanchi SA. Pregnancy-related hypertension. In: Lockwood CJ, Copel JA, Dugoff L, et al., eds. *Creasy and Resnik's Maternal-Fetal Medicine: Principles and Practice.* 9th rev. ed. Saunders Elsevier; 2023:849-850.
12. Linn CC, Lindheimer MD, River P, Moawad AH. Fetal outcome in hypertensive disorders of pregnancy. *Am J Obstet Gynecol.* 1982;142(3):255-260.
13. Robertson WB, Brosens I, Dixon HG. The pathological response of the vessels of the placental bed to hypertensive pregnancy. *J Pathol Bacteriol.* 1967;93(2):581-591.
14. Signore C, Freeman RK, Spong CY. Antenatal testing: a reevaluation—executive summary of a Eunice Kennedy Shriver National Institute of Child Health and Human Development workshop. *Obstet Gynecol.* 2009;113(3):687-701.
15. Gabbe SG, Mestman JH, Freeman RK, et al. Management and outcome of pregnancy in diabetes mellitus, classes B to R. *Am J Obstet Gynecol.* 1977;129:723-732.
16. Goldstein AI, Cronk DA, Garite TJ, Amile RN. Perinatal outcome in the diabetic pregnancy: a retrospective analysis. *J Reprod Med.* 1978;20:61-66.
17. ACOG practice bulletin no. 201: pregestational diabetes mellitus. *Obstet Gynecol.* 2018;132(6):e228-e248.
18. Lagrew DC, Pircon RA, Tower CV, Dorchester W, Freeman RK. Antepartum fetal surveillance in patients with diabetes: when to start? *Am J Obstet Gynecol.* 1993;168(6 Pt 1):1820-1825.
19. Grundy H, Freeman RL, Lederman S, Dorchester W. Nonreactive contraction stress test: clinical significance. *Obstet Gynecol.* 1984;64:337-342.
20. Gabbe SG, Freeman RK, Mestman JH, Anderson GV, Lowensohn RI. Management and outcome of class A diabetes mellitus. *Am J Obstet Gynecol.* 1977;127:465-469.
21. Practice bulletin no. 180: gestational diabetes. *Obstet Gynecol.* 2017;130(1):e17-e37.
22. Magid MS, Kaplan C, Sammaritano LR, Peterson M, Druzin ML, Lockshin MD. Placental pathology in systemic lupus erythematosus: a prospective study. *Am J Obstet Gynecol.* 1998;179(1):226-234.
23. ACOG, SMFM, Metz TD, et al. Obstetric care consensus #10: management of stillbirth. *Am J Obstet Gynecol.* 2020;222(3): B2-B20.
24. SMFM, Silver R, Craigo S, et al. Society for Maternal-Fetal Medicine consult series #64: systemic lupus erythematosus in pregnancy. *Am J Obstet Gynecol.* 2023;228(3):B41-B60.
25. Committee on Practice Bulletins—Obstetrics, American College of Obstetricians and Gynecologists. Practice bulletin no. 132: antiphospholipid syndrome. 2012;120(6):1514-1521.
26. Silver RM, Parker CB, Reddy UM, et al. Antiphospholipid antibodies and stillbirth. *Obstet Gynecol.* 2013;122(3):641-657.
27. Bouvier S, Cochery-Nouvellon E, Lavigne-Lissalde G, et al. Comparative incidence of pregnancy outcomes in treated obstetric antiphospholipid syndrome: the NOH-APS observational study. *Blood.* 2014;123(3):404-413.
28. Betelli M, Breda S, Ramoni V, et al. Pregnancy in systemic sclerosis. *J Scleroderma Relat Disord.* 2018;3(1):21-29.
29. Sammaritano LR, Salmon J, Branch DW. Pregnancy and rheumatic diseases. In: Lockwood CJ, Copel JA, Dugoff L, et al., eds. *Creasy and Resnik's Maternal-Fetal Medicine: Principles and Practice.* 9th rev. ed. Saunders Elsevier; 2023:1289-1290.
30. Sibai B, Viteri OA. Diabetic ketoacidosis in pregnancy. *Obstet Gynecol.* 2014;123(1):167-178.
31. Bryant SN, Herrera CL, Nelson DB. Diabetic ketoacidosis complicating pregnancy. *J Neonatal Perinatal Med.* 2017;10(1): 17-23.
32. Lapinsky SE. Acute respiratory failure in pregnancy. *Obstet Med.* 2015;8(3):126-132.
33. Lankford AS, Chow JH, Jackson AM, et al. Clinical outcomes of pregnant and postpartum extracorporeal membrane oxygenation patients. *Anesth Analg.* 2021;132(3):777-787.
34. Boafor TK, Olayemi E, Galadanci N, et al. Pregnancy outcomes in women with sickle-cell disease in low and high income countries: a systematic review and meta-analysis. *BJOG.* 2016;123(5):691-698.
35. Anyaegbunam A, Morel MI, Merkatz IR. Antepartum fetal surveillance tests during sickle cell crisis. *Am J Obstet Gynecol.* 1991;165(4 Pt 1):1081-1083.
36. Lees CC, Romero R, Stampalija T, et al. Clinical opinion: the diagnosis and management of suspected fetal growth restriction: an evidence-based approach. *Am J Obstet Gynecol.* 2022; 226(3):366-378.
37. SMFM, Martins JG, Biggio JR, et al. Society for Maternal-Fetal Medicine Consult Series #52: diagnosis and management of fetal growth restriction. *Am J Obstet Gynecol.* 2020;223(4): B2-B17.
38. Turan OM, Turan S, Gungor S, et al. Progression of Doppler abnormalities in intrauterine growth restriction. *Ultrasound Obstet Gynecol.* 2008;32(2):160-167.
39. Sebire NJ. Umbilical artery Doppler revisited: pathophysiology of changes in intrauterine growth restriction revealed. *Ultrasound Obstet Gynecol.* 2003;21(5):419-422.
40. Bastide A, Manning F, Harman C. Ultrasound evaluation of amniotic fluid: outcome of pregnancies with severe oligohydramnios. *Am J Obstet Gynecol.* 1986;154(4):895-900.
41. Mari G, Hanif F, Treadwell MC, Kruger M. Gestational age at delivery and Doppler waveforms in very preterm intrauterine growth-restricted fetuses as predictors of perinatal mortality. *J Ultrasound Med.* 2007;26(5):555-559.
42. Multifetal gestations: twin, triplet, and higher-order multifetal pregnancies: ACOG Practice Bulletin, Number 231. *Obstet Gynecol.* 2021;137(6):e145-e162.
43. Antonakopoulos N, Pateisky P, Liu B, Kalafat E, Thilaganathan B, Khalil A. Selective fetal growth restriction in dichorionic twin pregnancies: diagnosis, natural history, and perinatal outcome. *J Clin Med.* 2020;9(5):1404.
44. Gratacos E, Lewi L, Munoz B, et al. A classification system for selective intrauterine growth restriction in monochorionic pregnancies according to umbilical artery Doppler flow in the smaller twin. *Ultrasound Obstet Gynecol.* 2007;30(1):28-34.

45. Dias T, Mahsud-Dornan S, Bhide A, Papageorghiou AT, Thilaganathan B. Cord entanglement and perinatal outcome in monoamniotic twin pregnancies. *Ultrasound Obstet Gynecol.* 2010;35(2):201-204.
46. Ishii K. Prenatal diagnosis and management of monoamniotic twins. *Curr Opin Obstet Gynecol.* 2015;27(2):159-164.
47. Desai N, Lewis D, Sunday S, Rochelson B. Current antenatal management of monoamniotic twins: a survey of maternal-fetal medicine specialists. *J Matern Fetal Neonatal Med.* 2012; 25(10):1913-1916.
48. Levy M, Michal K, Barda G, et al. Reduced fetal movements at term, low-risk pregnancies: is it associated with adverse pregnancy outcomes? Ten years of experience from a single tertiary center. *Arch Gynecol Obstet.* 2020;301(4):987-993.
49. Stacey T, Thompson JMD, Mitchell EA, Ekeroma A, Zuccollo J, McCowan LME. Maternal perception of fetal activity and late stillbirth risk: findings from the Auckland stillbirth study. *Birth.* 2011;38(4):311-316.
50. Kaltreider DF, Kohl F. Epidemiology of preterm delivery. *Clin Obstet Gynecol.* 1980;23:17-31.
51. Hull AD, Resnik R, Silver RM. Placenta previa and accreta, vasa previa, subchorionic hemorrhage, and abruptio placentae. In: Lockwood CJ, Copel JA, Dugoff L, et al., eds. *Creasy and Resnik's Maternal-Fetal Medicine: Principles and Practice.* 9th rev. ed. Saunders Elsevier; 2023:806-809.
52. Elliot JP, Gilpin B, Strong TH, Finberg HJ. Chronic abruption-oligohydramnios sequence. *J Reprod Med.* 1998;43(5):418-422.
53. Sekhon S, Rosenbloom J, Doering M, et al. Diagnostic utility of maximum vertical pocket versus amniotic fluid index in assessing amniotic fluid volume for the prediction of adverse maternal and fetal outcomes: a systematic review and meta-analysis. *J Matern Fetal Neonatal Med.* 2021;34(22):3730-3739.
54. SMFM, Dashe J, Pressman E, et al. SMFM consult series #46: evaluation and management of polyhydramnios. *Am J Obstet Gynecol.* 2018;219(4):B2-B8.
55. Mercer BM. Preterm premature rupture of membranes: current approaches to evaluation and management. *Obstet Gynecol Clin North Am.* 2005;32(3):411-428.
56. Moberg LJ, Garite TJ, Freeman RK. Fetal heart rate patterns and fetal distress in patients with preterm premature rupture of membranes. *Obstet Gynecol.* 1984;64:60-64.
57. Lewis DF, Adair CD, Weeks JM, Barrilleaux PS, Edwards MS, Garite TJ. A randomized clinical trial of daily nonstress testing versus biophysical profile in the management of preterm premature rupture of membranes. *Am J Obstet Gynecol.* 1999;181:1495-1499.
58. Gilroy LC, Al-Kouatly HB, Minkoff HL, McLaren RA Jr. Changes in obstetrical practices and pregnancy outcomes following the ARRIVE trial. *Am J Obstet Gynecol.* 2022;226(5):716.e1-716.e12.
59. Wood R, Freret TS, Clapp MA, Little S. Changes in induction of labor and cesarean delivery post arrive trial: a quasi experimental analysis [Conference presentation]. 2023, February 9; SMFM 2023 Annual Pregnancy Meeting, San Francisco, CA, United States.
60. Guidetti DA, Divon MY, Langer O. Postdate fetal surveillance: is 41 weeks too early? *Am J Obstet Gynecol.* 1989;161(1):91-93.
61. Clement D, Schifrin BS, Kates RB. Acute oligohydramnios in postdate pregnancy. *Am J Obstet Gynecol.* 1987;157(4 Pt 1):884-886.
62. Bochner CJ, Williams J, Castro L, Medearis A, Hobel CJ, Wade M. The efficacy of starting postterm antenatal testing at 41 weeks as compared with 42 weeks of gestational age. *Am J Obstet Gynecol.* 1988;159(3):550-554.
63. Boehm FH, Salyer S, Shah DM, Vaughn WK. Improved outcome of twice weekly nonstress testing. *Obstet Gynecol.* 1986; 67(4):566-568.
64. Wennerholm UB, Saltvedt S, Wessberg A, et al. Induction of labour at 41 weeks versus expectant management and induction of labour at 42 weeks (SWEdish Post-term Induction Study, SWEPIS): multicentre, open label, randomized, superiority trial. *BMJ* 2019;367:l6131.
65. Hannah ME, Hannah WJ, Hellmann J, Hewson S, Milner R, Willan A. Induction of labor as compared with serial antenatal monitoring in post-term pregnancy. A randomized controlled trial. The Canadian multicenter post-term pregnancy trial group. *N Engl J Med.* 1992;326(24):1587-1592.
66. Middleton, P, Shepherd E, Crowther CA. Induction of labor for improving birth outcomes for women at or beyond term. *Cochrane Database Syst Rev.* 2018;5(5):CD004945.
67. Practice bulletin no. 146: management of late-term and post-term pregnancies. *Obstet Gynecol.* 2014;124(2 Pt 1):390-396.
68. Grobman WA, Rice MM, Reddy UM, et al. Labor induction versus expectant management in low-risk nulliparous women. *N Engl J Med.* 2018;379(6):513-523.

CHAPTER 12

Fetal Heart Rate Patterns Associated with Fetal Central Nervous System Dysfunction

Joshua I. Rosenbloom

Fetal heart rate (FHR) patterns are under the control of the autonomic nervous system with input from the central nervous system (CNS). Therefore, hypoxemia and acidosis are capable of altering CNS responsiveness which is then reflected in the FHR pattern, as is often seen during labor. In addition, however, fetuses with severe nonhypoxic CNS abnormalities may have FHR patterns that differ from those in fetuses with intact CNSs.[4-8] When a fetus demonstrates evidence of CNS dysfunction on the FHR tracing, possible explanations include the following:

1. A preexisting abnormality of CNS function with no hypoxia at any time
2. A previous hypoxic CNS injury with resolution and no current hypoxia
3. Ongoing chronic hypoxia but normal acid-base balance because of placental exchange
4. Chronic hypoxia with superimposed acute hypoxia from labor and, therefore, fetal metabolic acidosis
5. No chronic hypoxia and only acute intrapartum fetal hypoxia with metabolic acidosis

For both medical and medicolegal reasons, differentiating between evolving intrapartum neurological damage (asphyxia) and preexisting nervous system dysfunction is of the utmost importance. The focus of this chapter is on the FHR patterns in fetuses with a preexisting CNS condition with either a hypoxic or nonhypoxic cause, that is, Scenarios 1 or 2 discussed earlier. When these patterns are identified upon presentation to labor and delivery or antepartum monitoring, there is a high likelihood of a preexisting CNS condition.

As more experience is gained with FHR pattern observation in fetuses that subsequently show CNS damage as neonates, it is increasingly clear that the patterns preceding birth are often more characteristic of a lack of CNS control than of ongoing hypoxia. Certainly, these same characteristics are seen in fetuses with CNS dysfunction resulting from acute ongoing hypoxia, and fetuses with chronic oxygen deprivation may also show evidence of CNS dysfunction in the FHR prior to labor. Therefore, although preexisting CNS insults or abnormalities may produce changes in the FHR indicating CNS dysfunction, these same changes may accompany FHR patterns indicating ongoing hypoxia; it is not possible to determine the degree of CNS dysfunction that is preexisting and the degree of dysfunction that is caused by an ongoing hypoxic process. It should also be pointed out that not all fetuses with CNS abnormalities will have signs of CNS dysfunction on the FHR monitor strip.

FHR PATTERNS IN SEVERE CNS ABNORMALITIES

It is well established that fetuses with severe nonhypoxic CNS abnormalities may have FHR patterns that differ from those in babies with intact CNSs.[4-8] When the modulatory function of the CNS is impaired, a lack of variability is the most common effect seen in the FHR pattern.[6] However, other changes are observed when CNS control is impaired.[9] Many of these changes are also seen in very premature fetuses in which, presumably, the brain is less well developed. They can also occur when the mother has taken drugs that affect the fetal brain.[10-15]

Interestingly, FHR evidence of CNS dysfunction in anencephalic fetuses varies with the level of the defect, from normal to severely abnormal.[4,16] It would appear that when a sufficient amount of cerebral cortex and midbrain are present in anencephalic fetuses, FHR variability may be normal and accelerations may be present. However, with no midbrain or cortex present, variability is absent. When the fetus has a complete heart block or when there is a supraventricular fetal tachycardia caused by an ectopic pacemaker, not under CNS control, there will also be a complete lack of variability.[6] Furthermore, recent research shows that maternal infection with chorioamnionitis and funisitis may result in cytokine-mediated CNS dysfunction and damage, and FHR patterns found in this condition may also reflect CNS dysfunction without preceding FHR patterns known to be associated with fetal hypoxia.

FHR monitoring cannot truly determine whether preexisting brain damage was present at the time fetal monitoring was initiated. The patterns described in this chapter, fortunately, are not common and have not been studied in a systematic fashion, and we therefore depend on somewhat anecdotal accounts.

The following FHR patterns are often evidence of fetal CNS dysfunction:

1. Flat FHR[2,3]
2. Blunted patterns[2,3,17,18]
3. Unstable baseline[1]
4. Overshoot[19]
5. Sinusoidal patterns[1,20]
6. "Check mark" pattern[21]

FLAT FETAL HEART RATE

When CNS dysfunction is present, there may be virtually no fluctuation in the FHR pattern (Figs. 12.1-12.6). This change does not occur in cycles lasting 20 to 40 minutes, as is observed in cases of fetal state change. We are often restricted to external FHR recordings and, as a result, cannot be absolutely sure that short-term variability is absent; however, with the newer autocorrelation method (see Chapter 4), we can get a better idea of short-term variability. Long-term variability (3-5 cycles per minute) is reduced or absent, and if present, takes on a very smooth shape (Fig. 12.4).

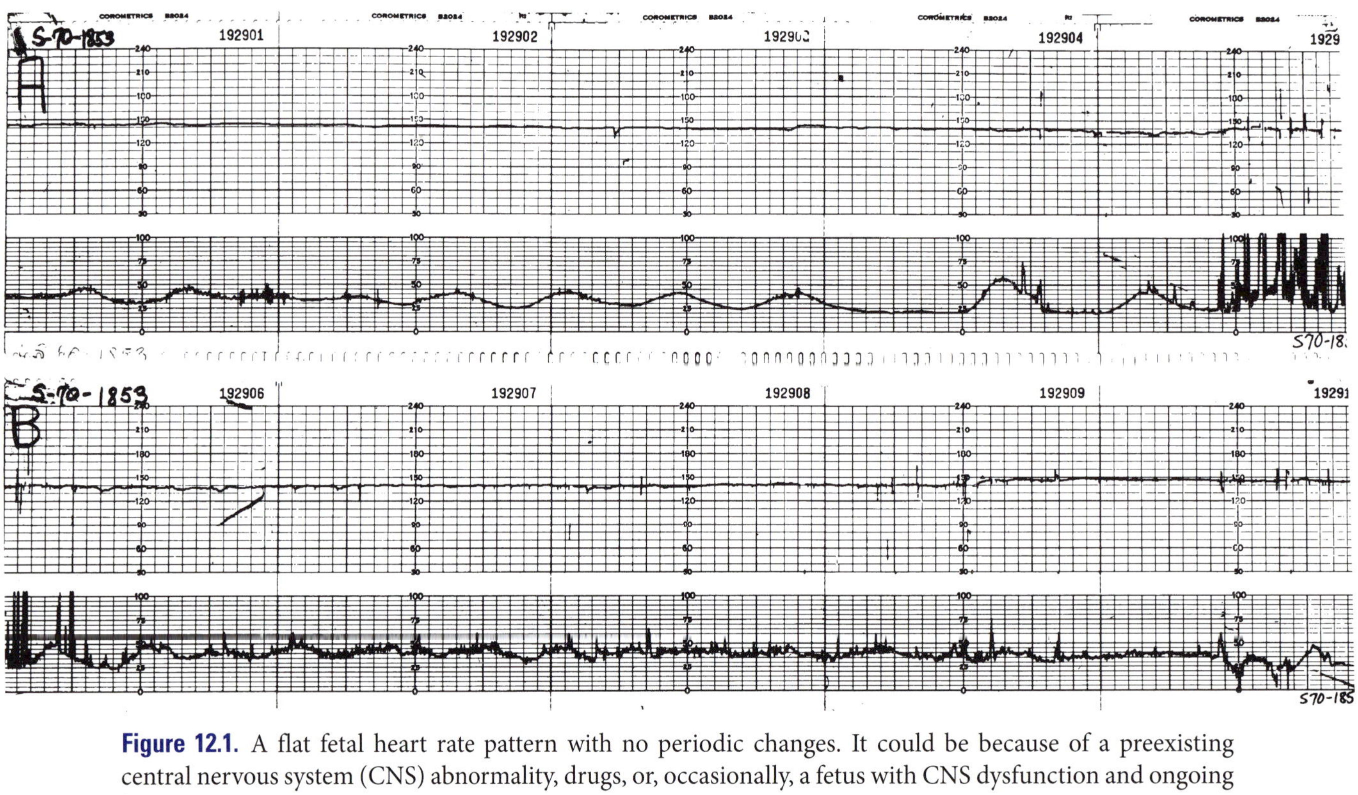

Figure 12.1. A flat fetal heart rate pattern with no periodic changes. It could be because of a preexisting central nervous system (CNS) abnormality, drugs, or, occasionally, a fetus with CNS dysfunction and ongoing hypoxia.

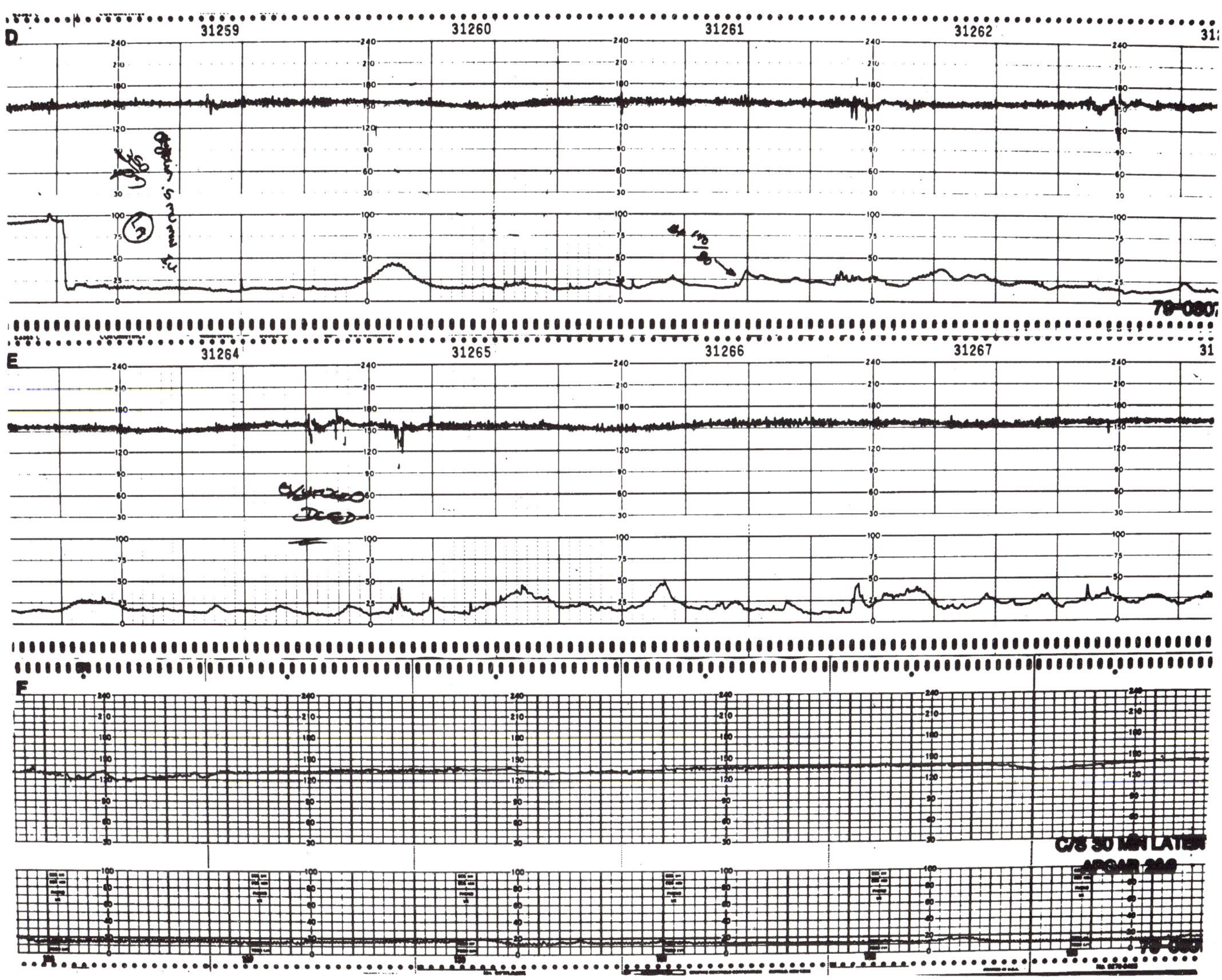

Figure 12.2. A flat fetal heart rate tracing with associated subtle late decelerations, indicating the probability of ongoing hypoxia. This fetus was found to have metabolic acidosis, a low Apgar score, neonatal seizures, and subsequent evidence of cerebral palsy.

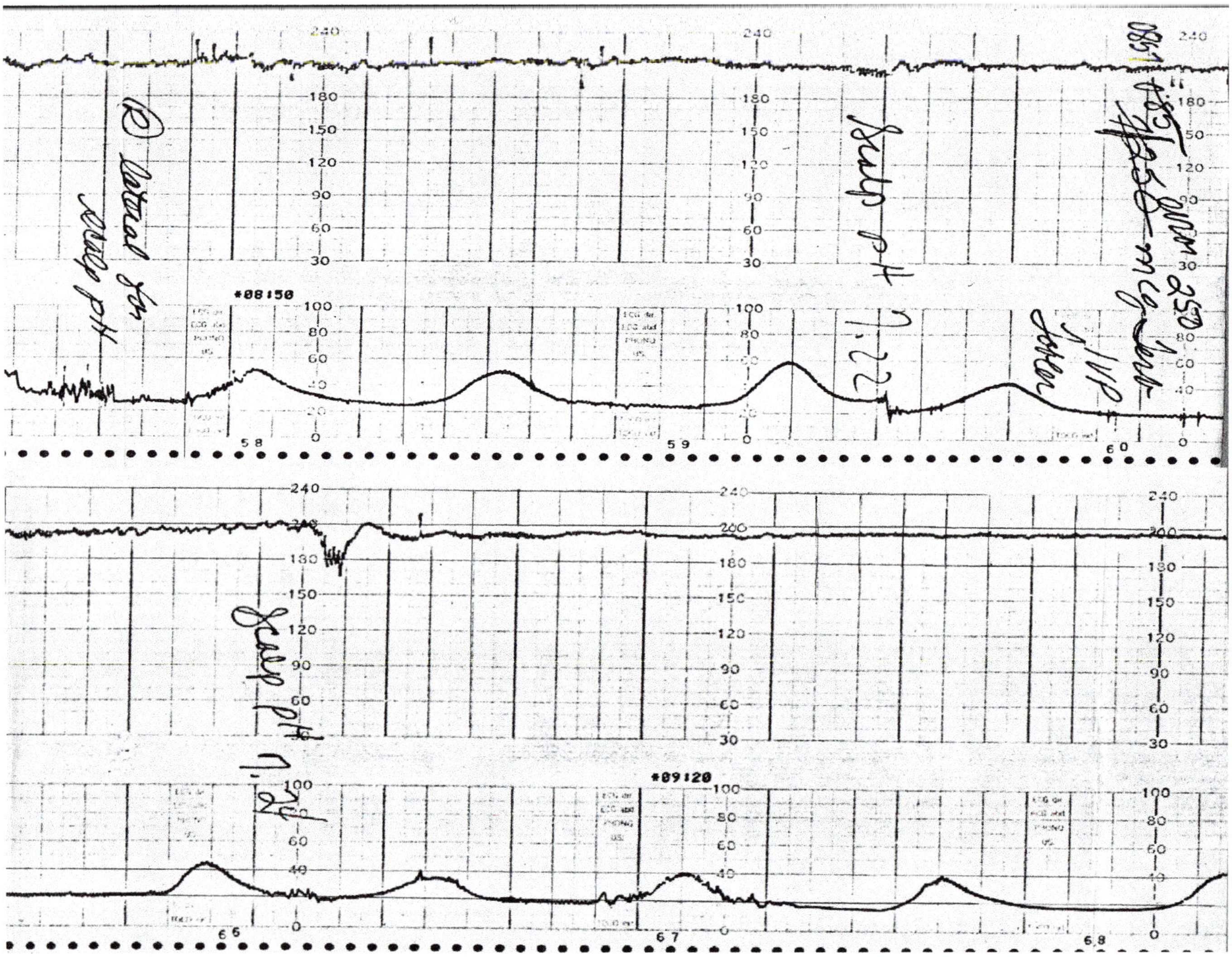

Figure 12.3. This tracing shows fetal tachycardia associated with maternal chorioamnionitis. Note the scalp pH of 7.22 and the cord pH were in the same range. The neonate developed encephalopathy and now has cerebral palsy. This may be an example of the fetal inflammatory response to maternal chorioamnionitis mediated by cytokines, with neonatal encephalopathy not distinguishable from hypoxic-ischemic encephalopathy.

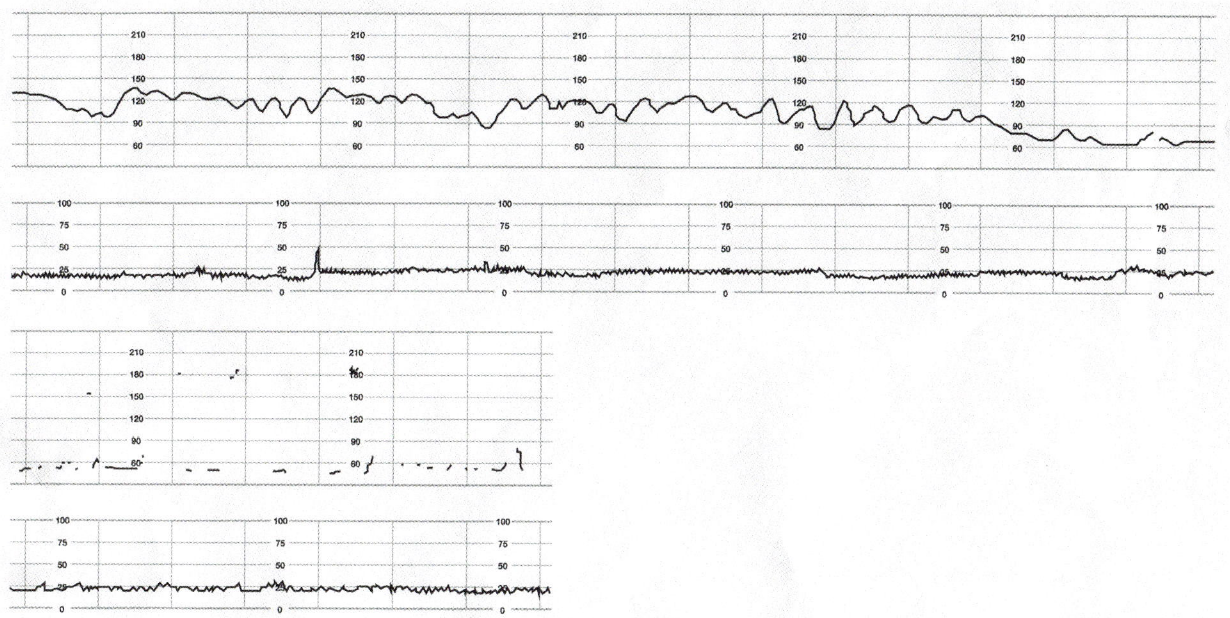

Figure 12.4. An example of a tracing from a fetus who died on the monitor with a blunted pattern leading to terminal bradycardia. The placenta showed acute chorioamnionitis and funisitis, indicating a fetal inflammatory response as the cause of death.

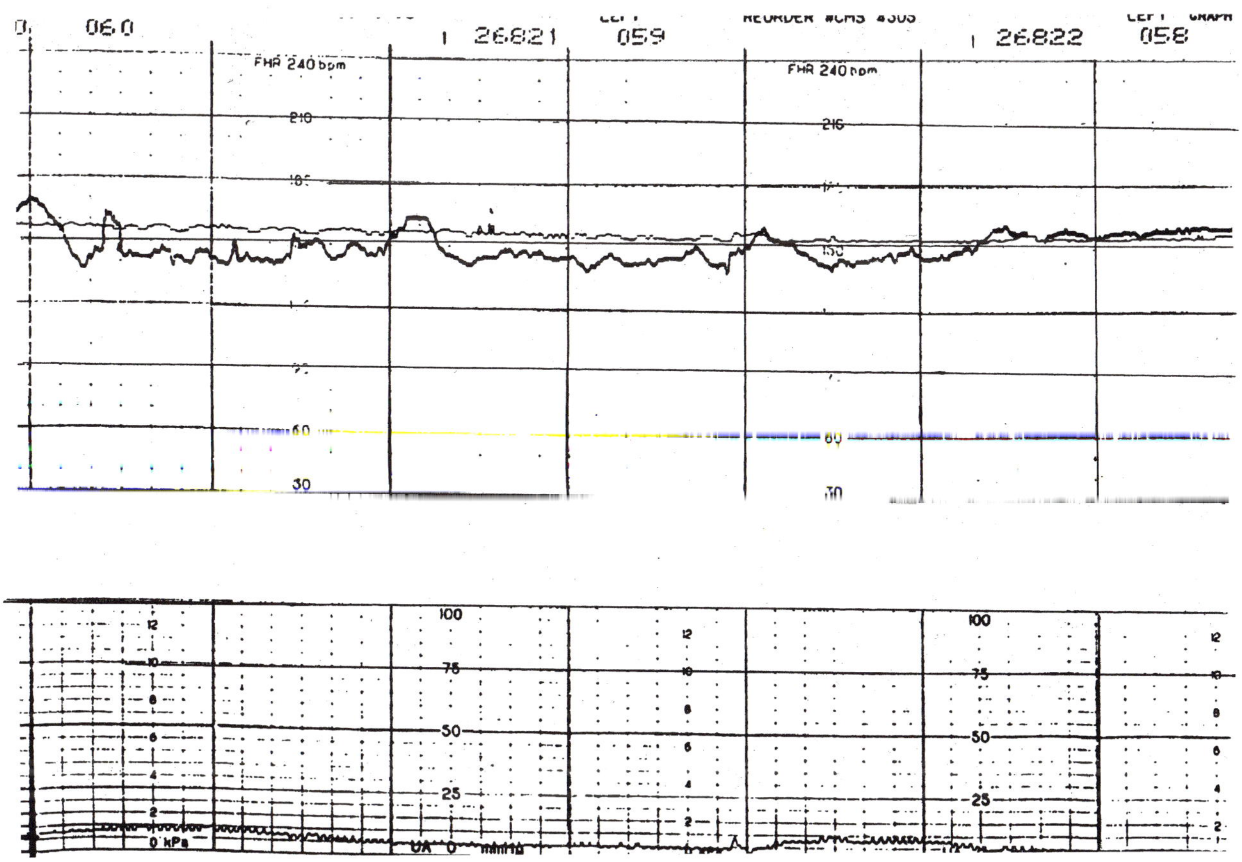

Figure 12.5. Twins at 32 weeks. Twin B is the light tracing showing a flat fetal heart rate. Twin A is the dark tracing showing average variability and reactivity. Twin B had a biophysical profile of 2 for fluid and delivered with low Apgar scores and decreased pH. Twin B now has cerebral palsy.

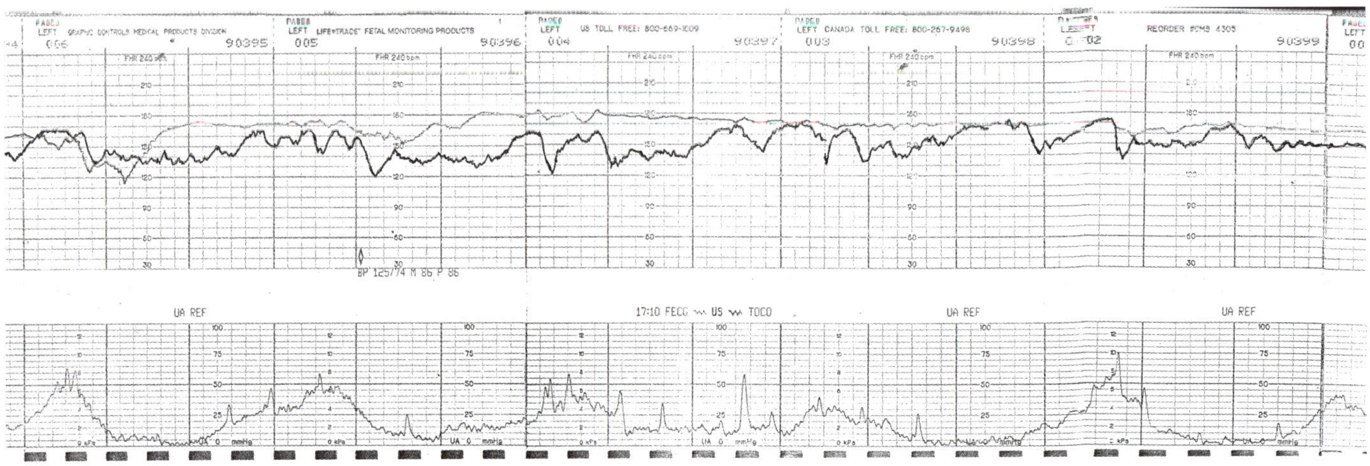

Figure 12.6. Twin pregnancy at 35 weeks. Twin A is the light tracing showing a flat blunted fetal heart rate pattern. Twin B is the dark tracing showing normal variability and reactivity. Twin A had a pH of 6.96 and Apgar scores of 0 at 1 minute, 2 at 5 minutes, and 4 at 10 minutes. Twin B had a normal pH and Apgar scores. Twin A now has spastic diplegia and magnetic resonance imaging findings of periventricular leukomalacia.

BLUNTED PATTERNS

When periodic changes do occur in patients with fetal CNS dysfunction, the changes are usually smooth and take on a "blunted" characteristic (Figs. 12.7-12.9). This is especially evident with variable decelerations. There is a loss of the angular components of FHR change that is seen with intact fetuses. Blunted variable decelerations may be of low magnitude and, as a result, may not be noticed easily.

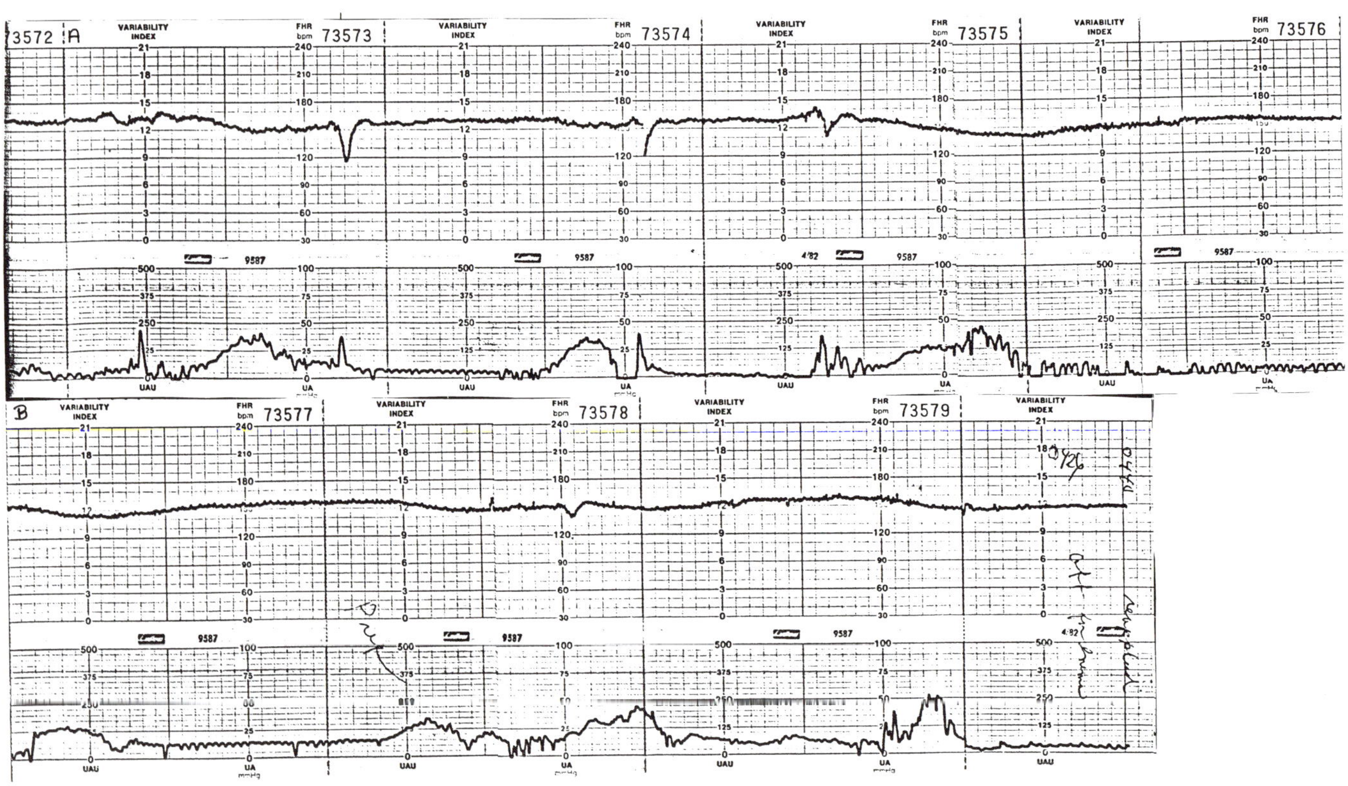

Figure 12.7. An example of blunted, rounded variable decelerations associated with a flat fetal heart rate. There is also an unstable baseline. This tracing was observed for several hours before delivery of a neonate with a normal neonatal pH but low Apgar scores. The neonate began convulsing soon after birth and now has cerebral palsy. This represents an example of preexisting central nervous system damage.

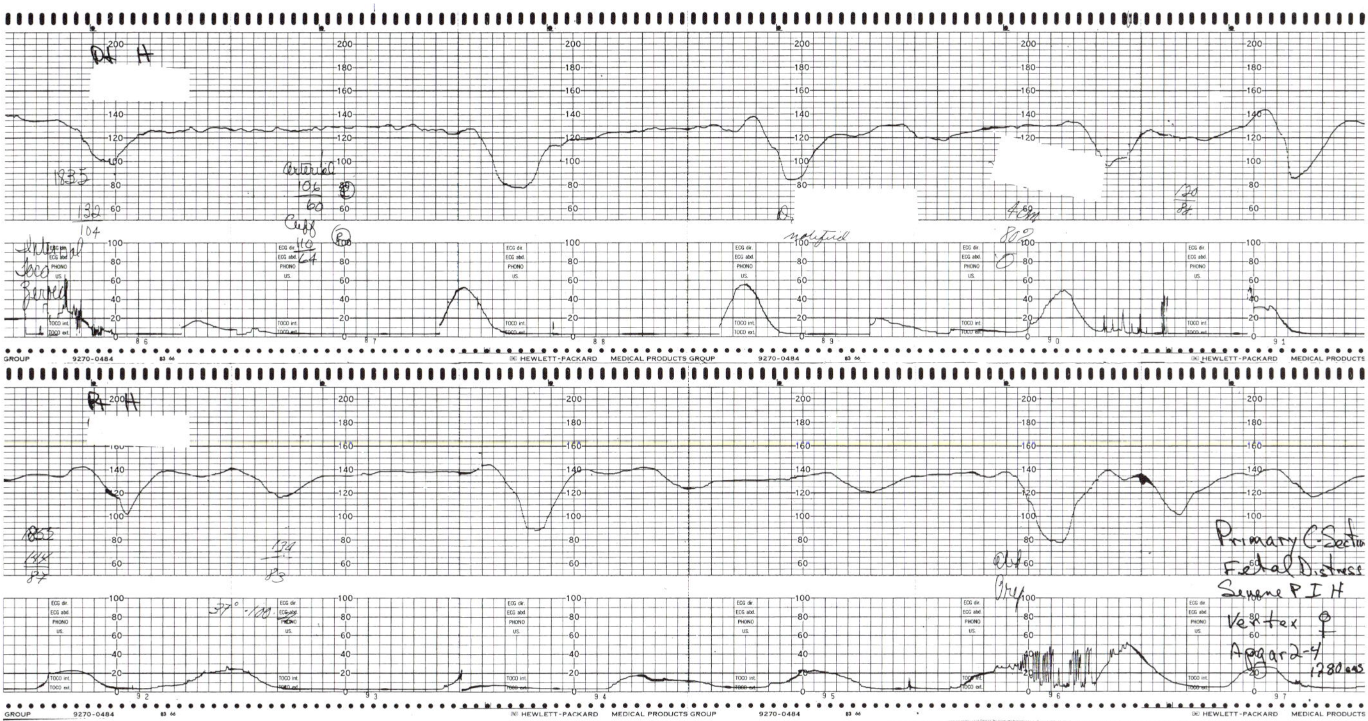

Figure 12.8. A flat fetal heart rate pattern and blunted variable decelerations representing central nervous system dysfunction. Note, however, the associated late decelerations indicating ongoing hypoxia. This fetus was born with fetal acidosis and began convulsing soon after birth. The child now has cerebral palsy.

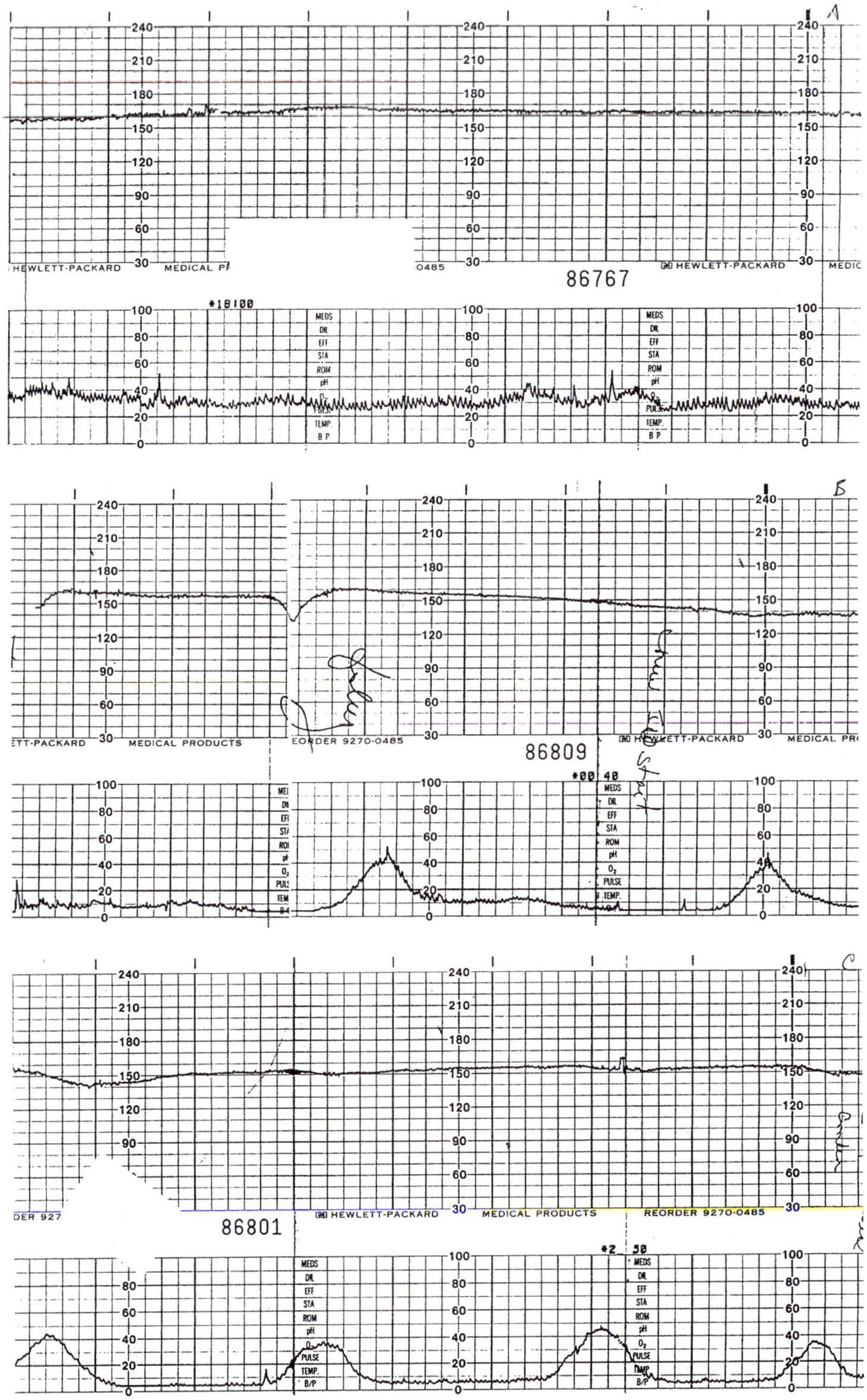

Figure 12.9. Decreased fetal movements at 34 weeks lead to this antepartum tracing. There is an unstable baseline associated with blunted variable decelerations. The neonate had a pH of 6.9 and a base deficit of 18. The neonate had seizures and an intraventricular hemorrhage.

UNSTABLE BASELINE

The baseline FHR characteristically remains constant for intact fetuses, although it can change over a long period or in response to maternal fever, acute hypoxia, or certain drugs. However, with the CNS dysfunctional fetus, the baseline may appear to wander, and it may be difficult to establish exactly where the baseline is (Figs. 12.10 and 12.11).

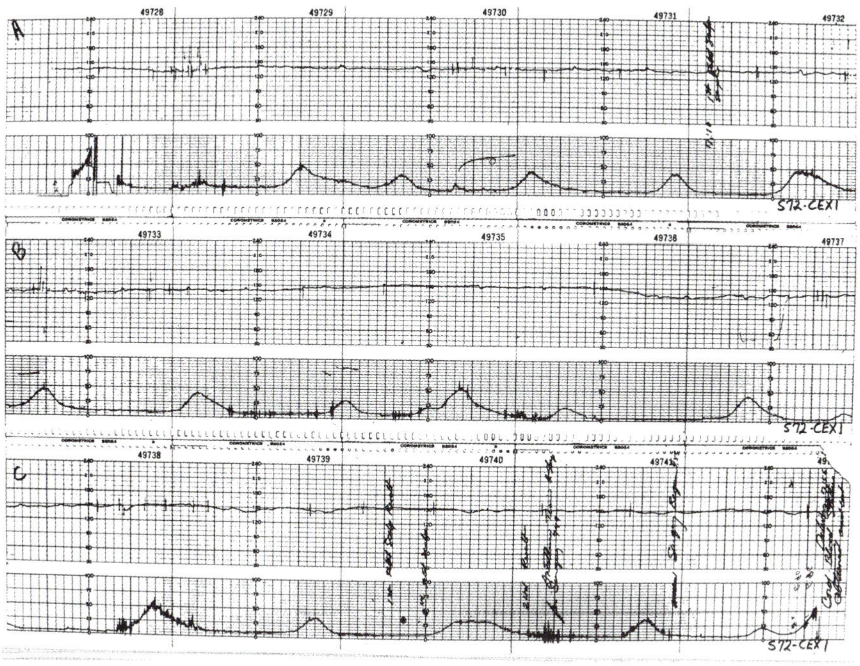

Figure 12.10. A flat fetal heart rate pattern with a wandering or unstable baseline. Note there are no late decelerations or other periodic changes suggesting fetal distress. The fetal scalp pH, however, was 7.01, and the neonate was born with low Apgar scores and subsequently died with evidence of central nervous system dysfunction.

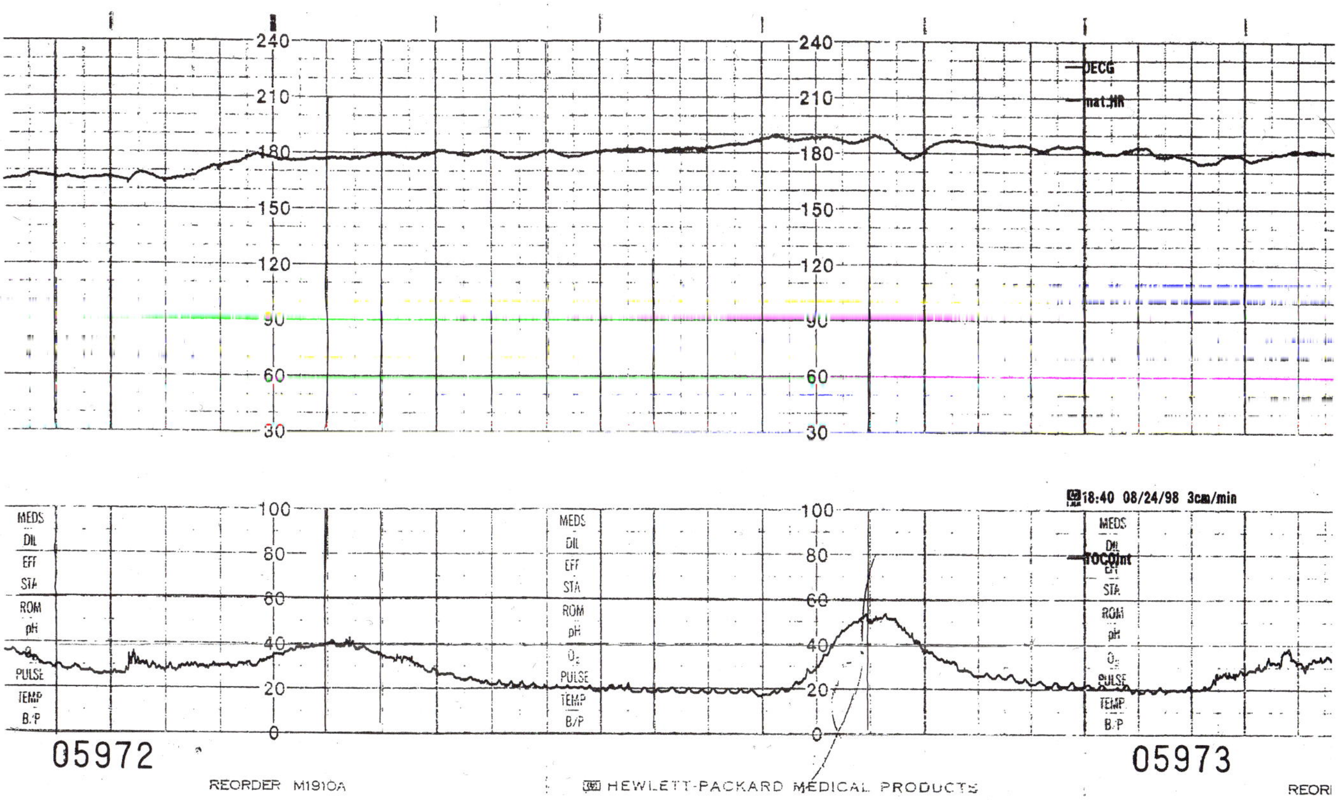

Figure 12.11. Unstable baseline with fetal central nervous system dysfunction.

OVERSHOOT

Rarely, in fetuses with CNS dysfunction, a prolonged smooth acceleration occurs following a variable deceleration that may take several minutes to return to baseline. The accelerations that may precede and follow reassuring variable decelerations are often referred to as shoulders and should not be confused with overshoot. The variable deceleration may not be of large magnitude. It is always associated with a smooth baseline FHR. This "overshoot" has the shape of a rapid but rounded rise followed by a very gradual return to baseline (Figs. 12.12 and 12.13).

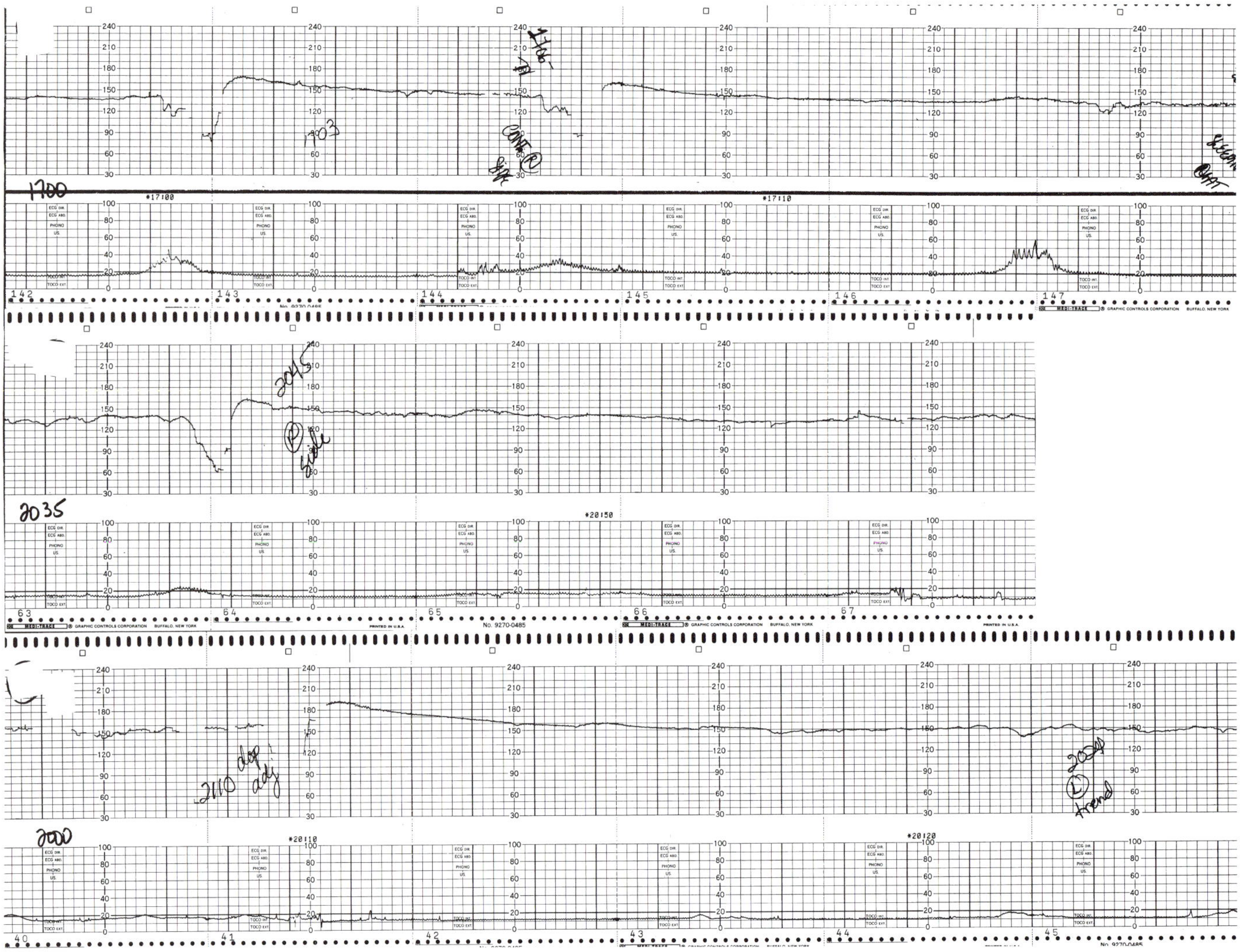

Figure 12.12. The **upper tracing** is an example of overshoot following variable decelerations in a fetus who delivered with a subsequent umbilical arterial pH of 7.10. Note the very slow return to baseline and the associated flat fetal heart rate (FHR). The **lower tracing** is from an anencephalic fetus. Note the flat FHR, blunted variable decelerations, and overshoot. This fetus died during labor, and it is not possible to determine whether this FHR change was all because of the central nervous system (CNS) anomaly or was partially related to hypoxic CNS dysfunction.

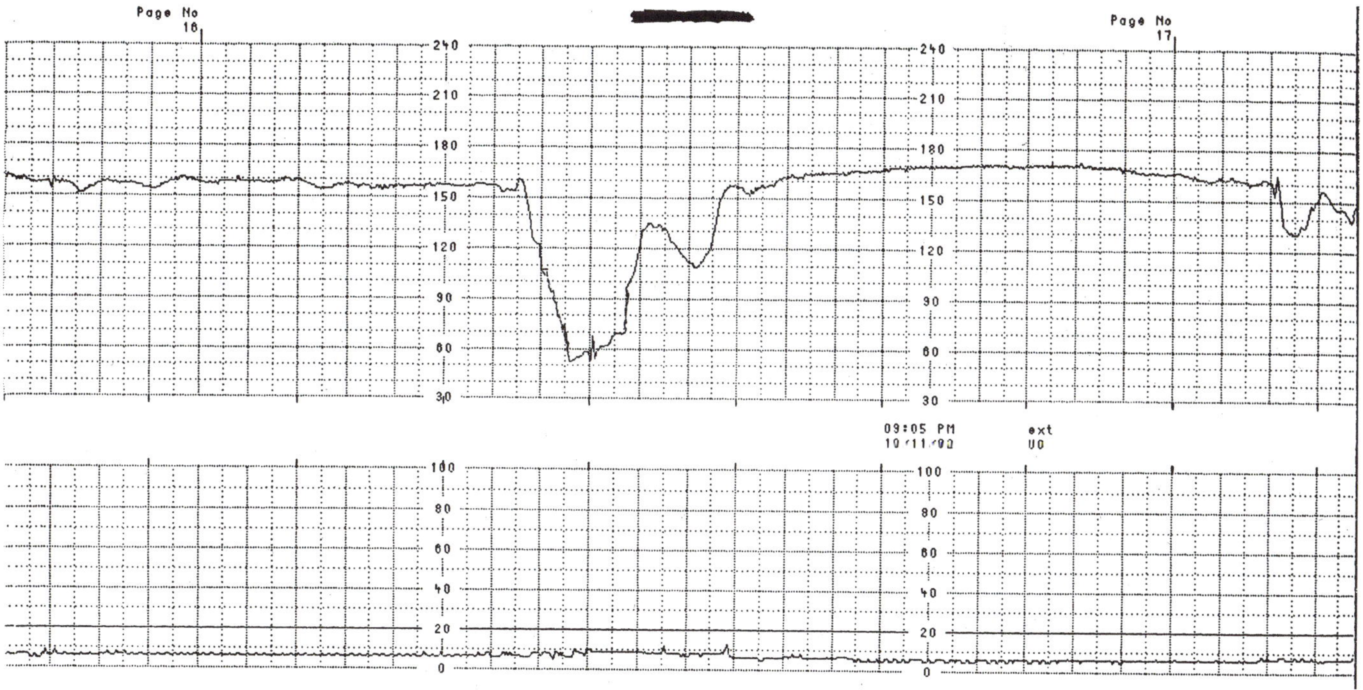

Figure 12.13. This tracing shows blunted variable decelerations with overshoot.

SINUSOIDAL PATTERNS

Sinusoidal patterns are described elsewhere in this book. They are very rare and are characterized by a complete lack of reactivity and by a basically smooth FHR, with the exception of the sinusoidal aspect (Fig. 12.14). There is no short-term variability, and the long-term variability is uniform, going above and below the baseline, with a smooth character and a frequency of three to five cycles per minute with an amplitude that may vary from 10 to 40 beats per minute. There are often areas of completely flat FHR, and late decelerations may also occur. This pattern has been classically associated with fetal anemia, but it can also occur with fetal hypoxia without fetal anemia (Fig. 12.15A,B). It does not indicate irreversible damage in all cases.

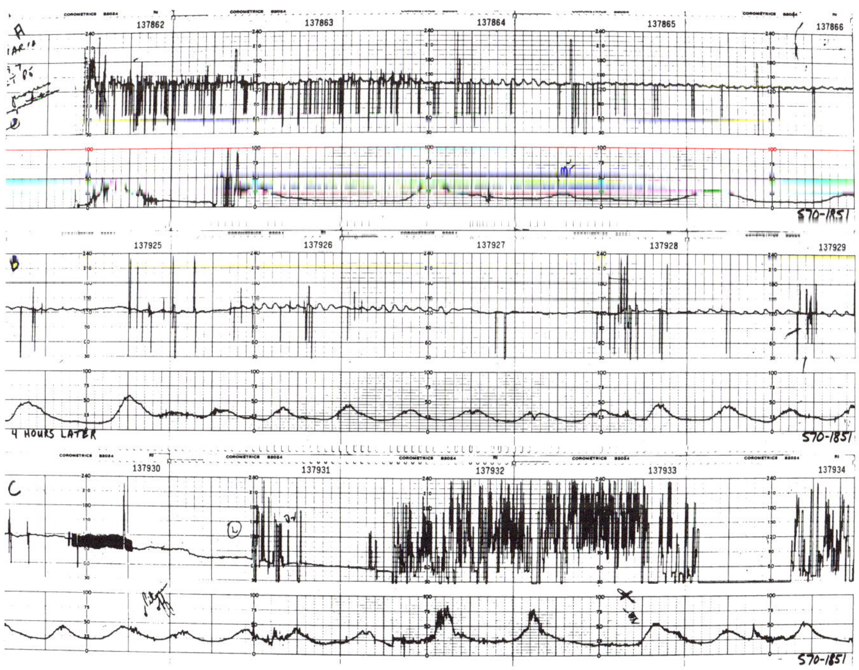

Figure 12.14. A flat fetal heart rate (FHR) pattern with intermittent bursts of sinusoidal heart rate. This fetus was severely hypoxic and died during labor. Note that there are no late decelerations or other periodic FHR changes suggesting fetal distress

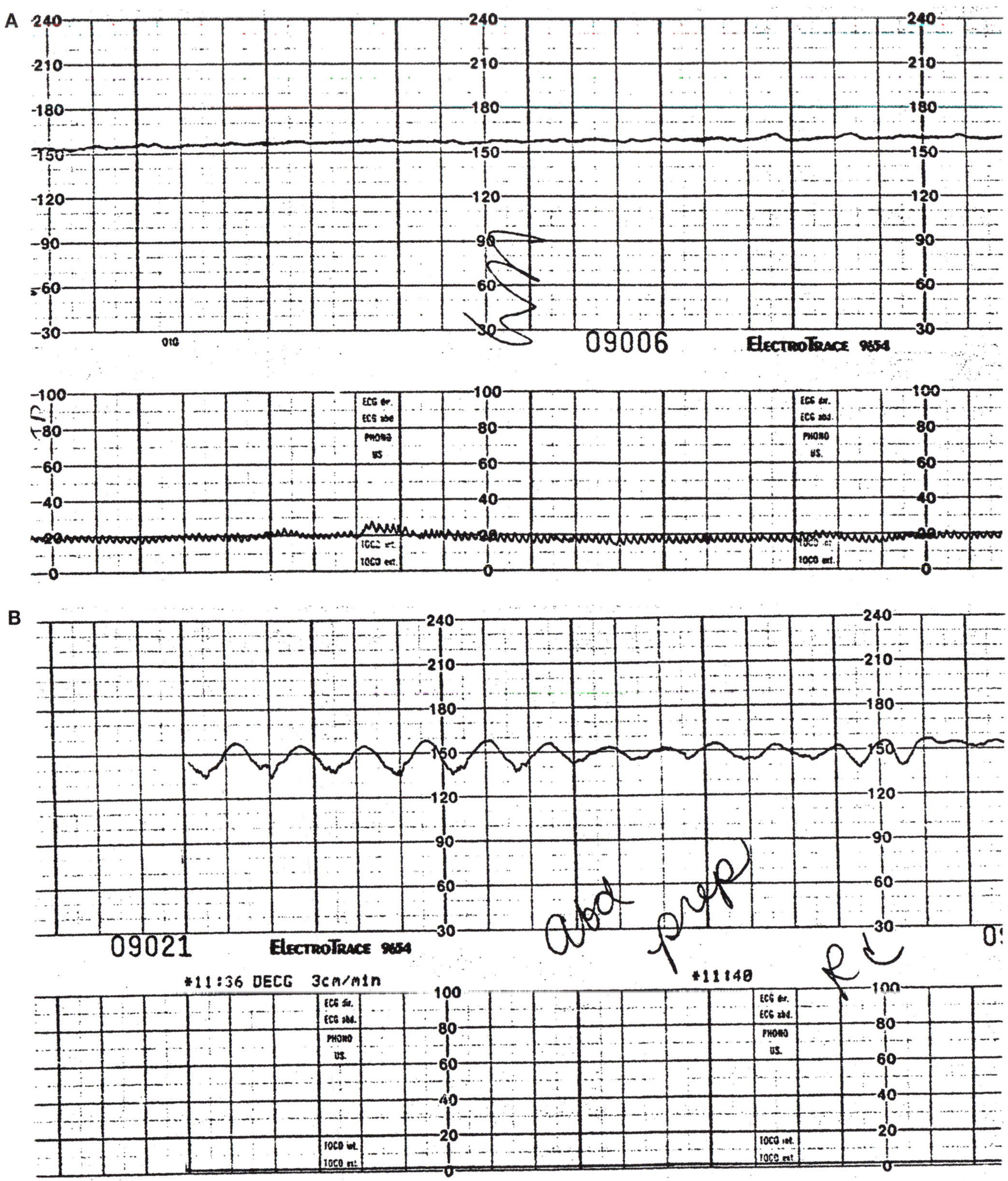

Figure 12.15. This tracing was from a patient with gestational diabetes mellitus at term found at the time of a routine nonstress test done at 0830 in **panel A**. The patient was sent to the hospital for a contraction stress test and when first observed at 1200 had the sinusoidal pattern seen in **panel B**. The neonate was delivered by cesarean section and had Apgar scores of 2 at 1 minute and 8 at 5 minutes. The cord arterial pH was 7.06, and the cord hemoglobin was 19.8 gm%. The neonate developed neonatal seizures with cerebral edema seen on a computed tomography scan in the first 24 hours. Now the child has spastic quadriplegia. The sinusoidal pattern appears to be associated with chronic hypoxia without fetal anemia.

"CHECK MARK" PATTERN

This is an extremely rare pattern that was first described by Cruikshank[21] in a case where the mother had had a previous cardiorespiratory arrest. The neonate began convulsing immediately after birth. This pattern has been seen with both normal pH and low fetal pH. Interestingly, there is normal short-term variability, and the check mark pattern occurs approximately every 20 seconds (Figs. 12.16-12.18). The check mark pattern may represent intrauterine fetal convulsions.

It is possible to see some elements of one or all of these patterns in any given fetus with CNS dysfunction. With the exception of the check mark pattern, FHR variability is characteristically absent. It is never possible to tell from the FHR pattern whether the CNS dysfunction is reversible or not.

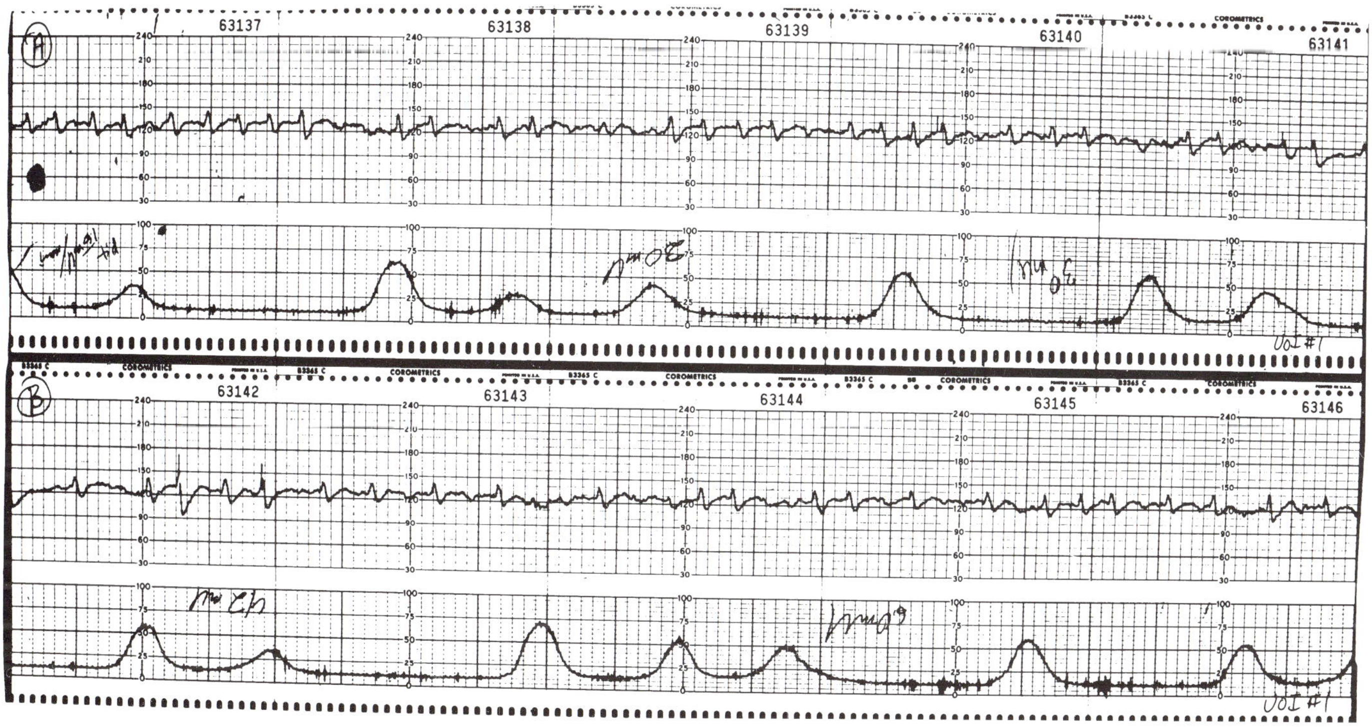

Figure 12.16. A pattern with characteristic "check mark" fetal heart rate changes. Note the normal variability between the check mark changes. This fetus was born following maternal recovery from a severe hypoxic episode and had an umbilical arterial pH of 7.25 but Apgar scores of 1 and 5. The child never breathed spontaneously and had a flat electroencephalograph until its death on the fifth day of life.

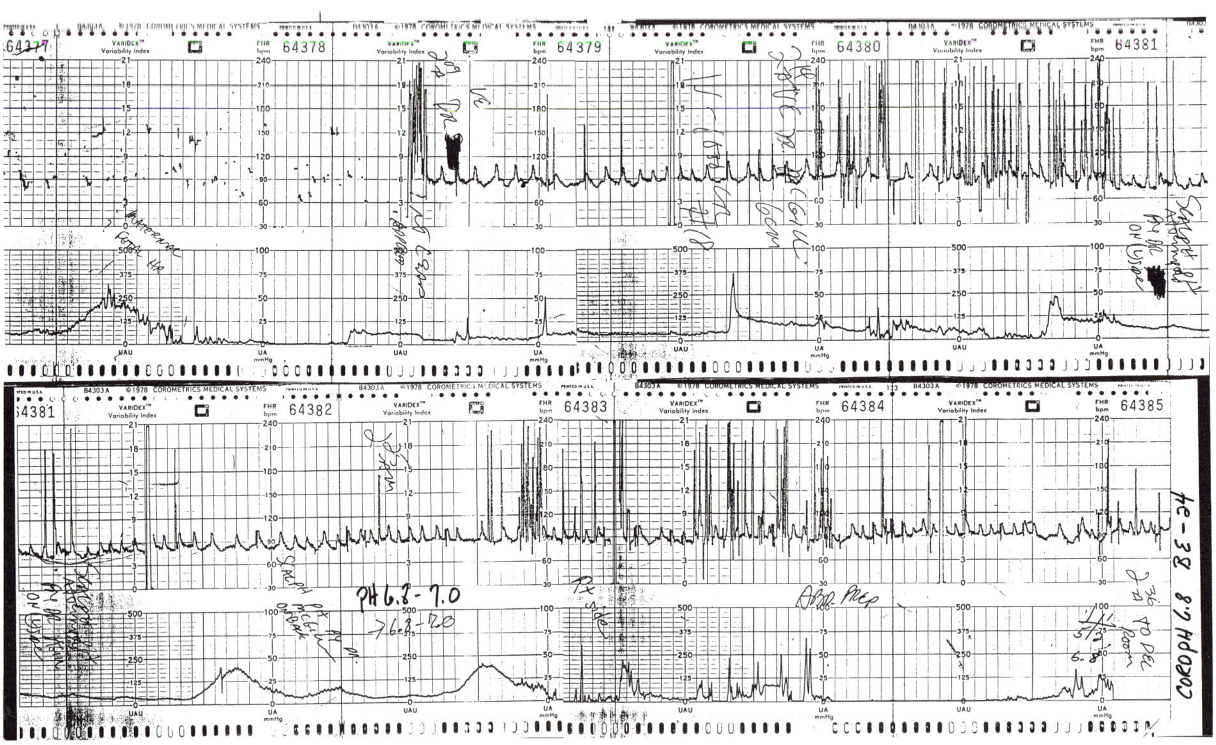

Figure 12.17. Check mark pattern in a fetus with ongoing hypoxia.

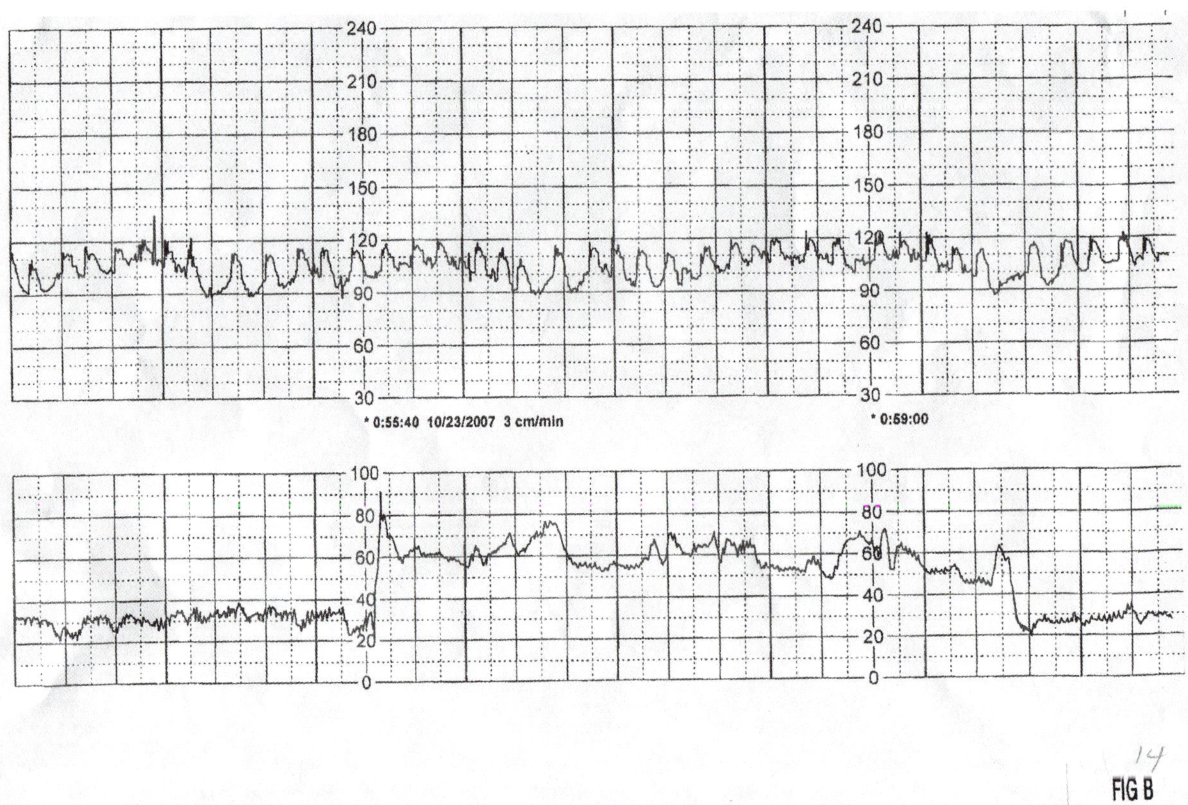

Figure 12.18. This pattern was seen in a patient who had had a very abnormal pattern on admission and was then not monitored for over an hour. Delivery resulted in a neonate with low Apgar scores and severe umbilical arterial metabolic acidosis. The neonate developed neonatal encephalopathy and now has cerebral palsy. The pattern is probably a variant of the check mark pattern.

ETIOLOGIES OF FETAL CENTRAL NERVOUS SYSTEM DYSFUNCTION

The following are examples of clinical situations in which CNS abnormalities may be evident on the FHR tracing as a result of a preexisting condition with a hypoxic or nonhypoxic cause:

1. CNS malformation, for example, anencephaly, hydrocephaly (Fig. 12.19)
2. CNS destruction, for example, tumor (Fig. 12.20)
3. CNS infection, for example, rubella, cytomegalovirus, syphilis, and toxoplasmosis (TORCH)
4. Fetal inflammatory response from maternal chorioamnionitis
5. CNS anoxic insult, for example, maternal cardiac arrest (Fig. 12.21)
6. CNS physical trauma, for example, cerebral contusion
7. Toxic fetal encephalopathy, for example, mercury poisoning
8. Fetal cerebral irradiation with resulting microcephaly
9. Intrauterine fetal CNS hemorrhage
10. Developmental abnormalities, for example, chromosomal (Fig. 12.22)
11. Drugs (Fig. 12.23).

Medicolegally, in cases with evidence of CNS dysfunction on the FHR pattern, it would be desirable to be able to assess when CNS dysfunction became irreversible. Unfortunately, the current state of knowledge does not allow us to make this determination. We can only say that the FHR pattern is consistent or not consistent with CNS dysfunction. The observations described in this chapter have usually been made from a retrospective analysis of FHR patterns from babies with CNS damage. For this reason, we are unable to determine how often fetuses with evidence of CNS dysfunction in their FHR patterns develop normally, but it certainly does happen. Therefore, we know that these patterns do not always mean that damage has occurred,

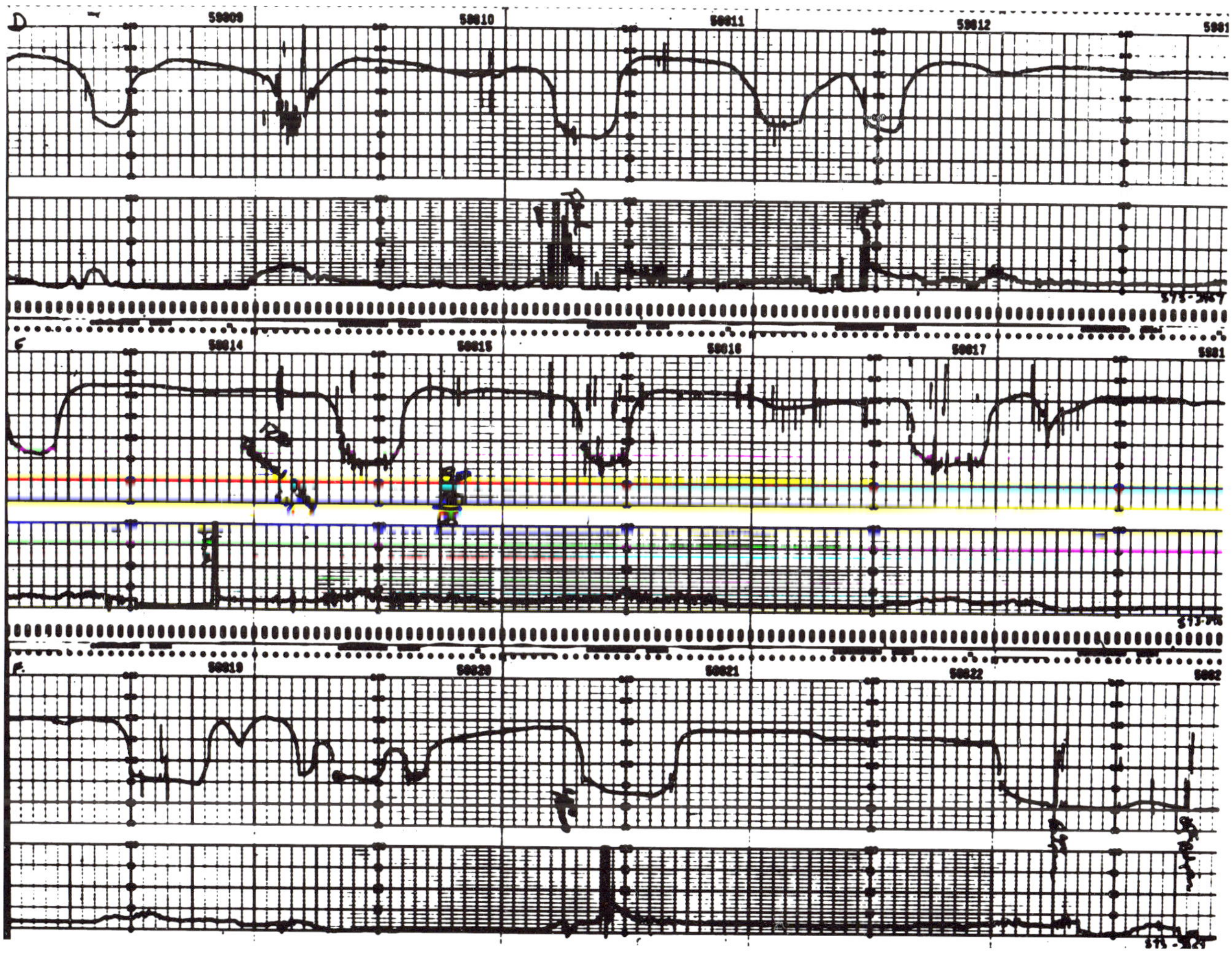

Figure 12.19. A tracing from an internal fetal scalp electrode on an anencephalic fetus. Note the blunted character of the variable decelerations and the flat fetal heart rate baseline.

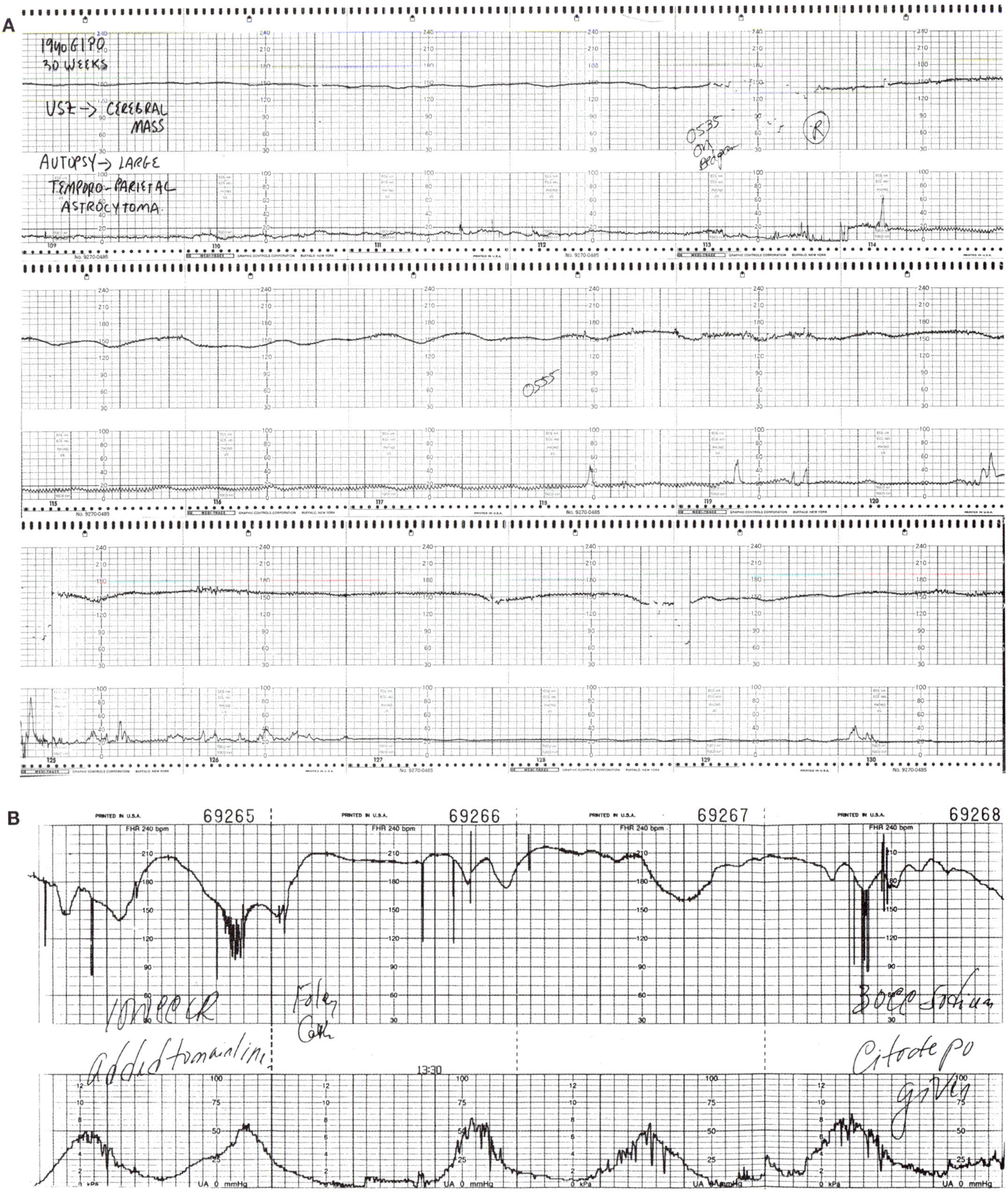

Figure 12.20. **A.** An external monitor recording of a fetus with an intracranial lesion detected on ultrasound that was diagnosed as a parietal astrocytoma in the neonate. Note the flat, blunted character of the pattern. **B.** An internal tracing taken during labor. The outcome was a cesarean section for fetal distress. The fetus had a brain tumor.

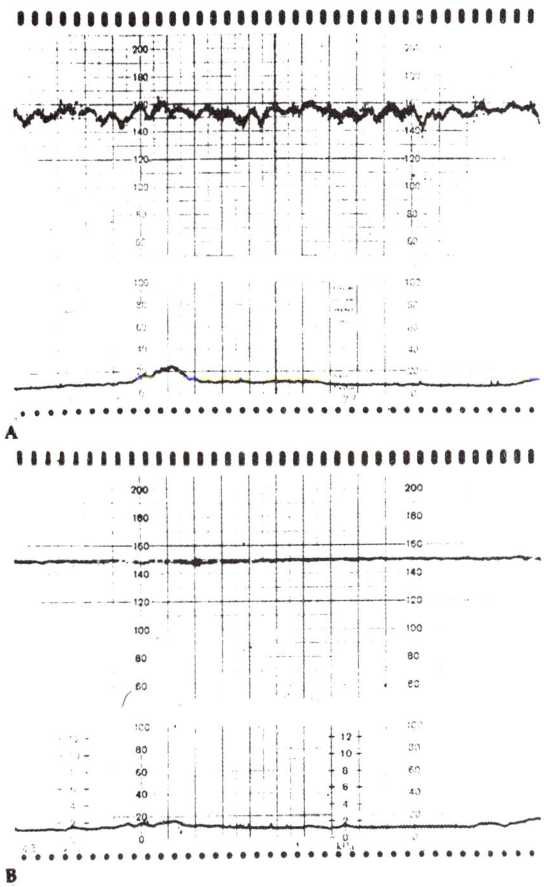

Figure 12.21. The **upper tracing** is an example of a 2-cm-per-minute (20 beats/minute/cm vertical scale) external Doppler tracing taken prior to a maternal cardiorespiratory arrest. Note the normal variability. The **lower panel** represents a tracing from the same fetus following resuscitation of the mother with no ongoing hypoxia. Note the flat fetal heart rate that represents central nervous system (CNS) damage from the prior CNS hypoxic insult. (From van der Moer PE, Gerretsen G, Visser GH. Fixed fetal heart rate pattern after intrauterine accidental decerebration. *Obstet Gynecol.* 1985; 65:125-127, with permission.)

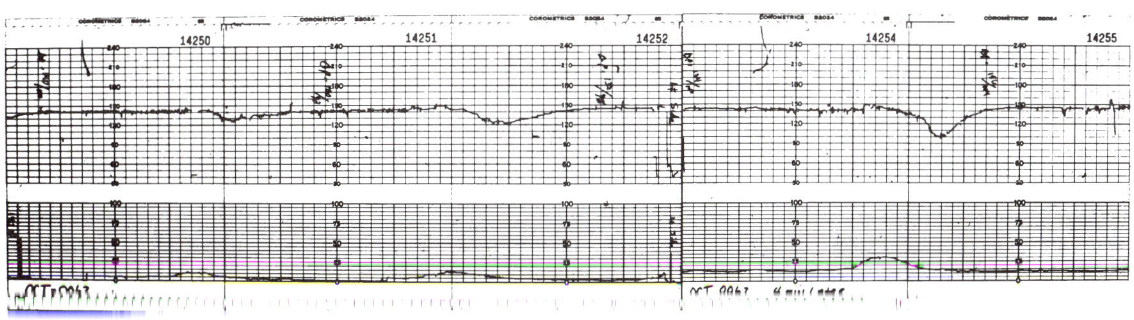

Figure 12.22. Tracing from a fetus with trisomy 18.

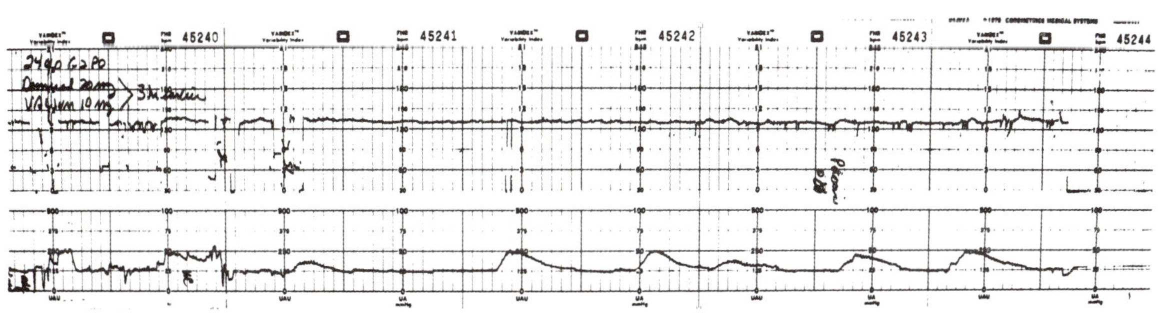

Figure 12.23. An external Doppler tracing from a fetus whose mother received meperidine (Demerol) and diazepam (Valium). Note the flat fetal heart rate pattern without any decelerations, representing central nervous depression caused by drugs.

TABLE 12.1 Relationship between fetal heart rate changes, hypoxia, and CNS dysfunction

Pattern	Group 1[a]	Group 2[a]	Group 3[a]
Late deceleration	Yes	No	Yes
Variable deceleration	Yes	Yes	Yes
Decreased variability	No	Yes	Yes
Blunted patterns	No	Yes	Yes
Acidosis	No	No	Yes
Scalp acceleration	Yes	No	No
Unstable baseline	No	Yes	Yes
Sinusoidal patterns	No	Yes	Yes

CNS, central nervous system.
[a]Group 1, hypoxia without CNS dysfunction; Group 2, CNS dysfunction without current hypoxia; Group 3, CNS dysfunction with ongoing hypoxia.

and an element of reversibility is clearly possible at least in some cases. In addition, we now know that neonates and children demonstrate improvement with time in many instances of initial developmental delay.

How we attempt to differentiate these situations is important both for patient management and from a medicolegal causation standpoint (Table 12.1).

In summary, there are a number of characteristic FHR patterns in fetuses with CNS dysfunction. Some of these patterns are associated with likely preexisting brain damage, whereas others demonstrate evolving dysfunction. However, differentiating between these patterns can be difficult.

REFERENCES

1. Cetrulo CL, Schifrin B. Fetal heart rate patterns preceding death in utero. *Obstet Gynecol.* 1976;48:521-527.
2. Gaziano EP, Freeman DW. Analysis of heart rate patterns preceding fetal death. *Obstet Gynecol.* 1977;50:578-582.
3. Serafini PC, Amisial PA, Murgalo JA, Skipton R. Unusual fetal heart rate pattern associated with severe neonatal asphyxia and death. *Am J Obstet Gynecol.* 1981;140:715-718.
4. Terao T, Kawashima Y, Noto H, et al. Neurological control of fetal heart rate in 20 cases of anencephalic fetuses. *Am J Obstet Gynecol.* 1984;149:201-208.
5. Garite TJ, Linzey EM, Freeman RK, Dorchester W. Fetal heart rate patterns and fetal distress with congenital anomalies. *Obstet Gynecol.* 1979;53:716-720.
6. Navot D, Mor-Yosef S, Granat M, Sadovsky E. Antepartum fetal heart rate pattern associated with major congenital malformations. *Obstet Gynecol.* 1984;63:414-417.
7. Karp LE, Meis PJ. Trisomy-18 and antepartal fetal distress. *J Reprod Med.* 1977;19:345-347.
8. Powell Phillips WD, Towell ME. Abnormal fetal heart rate associated with congenital abnormalities. *Br J Obstet Gynaecol.* 1980;87:270-274.
9. Kodama Y, Sameshima H, Ikeda T, Ikenoue T. Intrapartum fetal heart rate patterns in infants (≥34 weeks) with poor neurological outcome. *Early Hum Dev.* 2009;85:235-238.
10. Baxi LV, Gindoff PR, Pregenzer GJ, Parras MK. Fetal heart rate changes following maternal administration of a nasal decongestant. *Am J Obstet Gynecol.* 1985;153:799-800.
11. Keegan KA, Paul RH, Broussard PM, McCart D, Smith MA. Antepartum fetal heart rate testing. III. The effect of phenobarbital on the nonstress test. *Am J Obstet Gynecol.* 1979;138:579-580.
12. Rayburn WF, Motley MF, Zuspan FP. Conditions affecting nonstress test results. *Obstet Gynecol.* 1982;59:490-493.
13. Ayromlooi J, Tobias M, Berg P. The effects of scopolamine and ancillary analgesics upon the fetal heart recording. *J Reprod Med.* 1980;25:323-326.
14. Petrie R. How intrapartum drugs affect the FHR. *Contemp Obstet Gynecol.* 1980;16:61.
15. Westgren M, Holmquist P, Svenningsen NW, Ingemarsson I. Intrapartum fetal monitoring in preterm deliveries: prospective study. *Obstet Gynecol.* 1982;60:99-106.
16. Pelig D, Goldman J. Fetal heart patterns: a study of the anencephalic fetus. *Obstet Gynecol.* 1979;53(4):530-533.
17. Baskett TF, Sandy EA. The oxytocin challenge test: an ominous pattern associated with severe fetal growth retardation. *Obstet Gynecol.* 1979;54:365-366.
18. Krebs HB, Petres RE, Dunn LJ. Intrapartum fetal heart rate monitoring. VIII. Atypical variable decelerations. *Am J Obstet Gynecol.* 1983;145:297-305.
19. Goodlin RC, Lowe EW. A functional umbilical cord occlusion heart rate pattern: the significance of overshoot. *Obstet Gynecol.* 1974;43:22-30.
20. Baskett TF, Ko KS. Sinusoidal fetal heart rate pattern: a sign of fetal hypoxia. *Obstet Gynecol.* 1974;44:379-382.
21. Cruikshank DP. An unusual fetal heart rate pattern. *Am J Obstet Gynecol.* 1978; 130:101-102.

CHAPTER 13

Quality Assurance and Risk Mitigation in Fetal Monitoring

Katherine H. Campbell and Christian M. Pettker

INTRODUCTION

An obstetric unit that provides safe, high-quality, and reliable maternal and fetal care can only be achieved with careful strategic planning. Unit leadership must engage in purposeful implementation of pragmatic tools that support patients and healthcare workers (HCWs) and use an iterative process to drive an effective, team-based culture. Obstetrics is a high-reward, yet high-risk, specialty that may result in adverse patient outcomes even when hospital policy is followed, best professional practices are applied, disrupting events are caught on time, and the best is done to mitigate the impact of a medical event on patients. Creating a desired safe and high-quality environment requires breaking down the traditional clinical boundaries and culture of blame and building a transparent, just culture of safety. A just culture promotes disclosure and learning in the aftermath of an unanticipated adverse clinical event, and these events can be used as learning opportunities for systems improvement but also for workers to understand their capabilities and limits. This framework was introduced in the Institute of Medicine's 2000 report "To Err Is Human" and described in stark detail the dire need to improve the quality and safety in U.S. health care.[1]

Malpractice litigation is prevalent in obstetrics, and the associated stress exerts a heavy toll on all healthcare providers.[2,3] Over half of the liability cases in obstetrics and gynecology are related to the obstetrics process, with birth asphyxia being the most frequent case type.[4] As a result, how, why, and when fetal monitoring is performed as well as the systems we create to respond to fetal monitoring abnormalities are critical to building a safe, high-quality obstetric unit environment with optimal risk mitigation.

Some of the most common allegations leveled against obstetric teams related to fetal monitoring include failure to correctly interpret and/or manage fetal heart rate (FHR) tracings, failure to follow policy (especially related to oxytocin administration), failures related to team communication, failure of appropriate provider response to nursing notification of FHR findings, and failure to initiate the chain of escalation when there is clinical disagreement.[5] The most common contributing factors behind those failures are described in Figure 13.1; substandard clinical judgment is involved in 77% of cases. Fetal monitoring will not achieve the promise of reducing neonatal adverse outcomes unless these contributing factors are reduced to a minimum. Several centers have successfully instituted safety approaches to reduce adverse obstetric outcomes and improve teamwork, with overlapping similarities among these initiatives.[6-8] These include communication and teamwork training, standardized approaches to common clinical practices, improvements in situational awareness, and rapid response teams for emergency situations.

This chapter presents tools and processes to build an obstetric unit that will provide safe, high-quality, and reliable maternal and fetal care, specifically related to fetal monitoring, with the underlying tenets of just culture and systems-based improvement. Hypothetical cases will be integrated into the chapter to provide clinical scenarios and real-world application of the presented tools and processes. We will highlight the creation of supporting infrastructure to maintain a high functioning obstetric unit as well and discuss the use of event reporting systems that can provide the foundation for the use of iterative processes to drive an effective team-based culture.

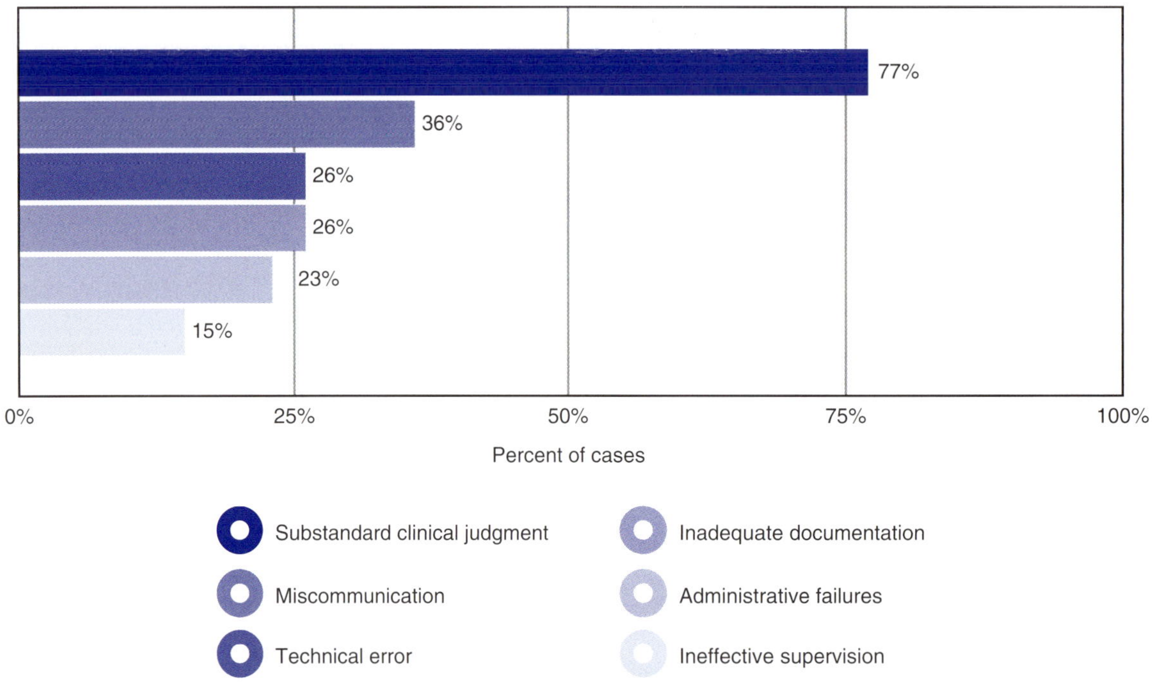

Figure 13.1. Factors with highest contributions to OB claims. (Reproduced with permission from CRICO Candello. 2010: Annual Benchmarking Report: Malpractice Risks in Obstetrics. Copyright © 2011 CRICO.)

CASE PRESENTATIONS

Case 1

The patient is a G4P2012 at 38 weeks of gestation presenting for the induction of labor because of preeclampsia. The patient has a history of two prior uncomplicated spontaneous vaginal deliveries. The fetal tracing is reactive and of category I at the time of cervical ripening with a transcervical balloon catheter (Fig. 13.2A). Overnight, the patient develops irregular contractions, the transcervical balloon catheter falls out, and cervical exam is 3 cm, 50% effaced, with a ballotable fetal station. Oxytocin is initiated, and 3 hours later, the patient requests and receives an epidural for painful, regular contractions at 4 cm dilation with high fetal station. The covering obstetric (OB) provider is currently managing two other laboring patients, and the labor floor is busy with occupancy of all labor rooms. The fetal tracing is now of category II with minimal to moderate variability and intermittent variable and late decelerations (Fig. 13.2B). The bedside nurse provides intrauterine resuscitation with maternal position change, and oxytocin is continued. The FHR tracing remains of category II, and the nurse asks the covering resident to review the tracing. The decision is made to continue the current plan of care as there is moderate FHR variability (Fig. 13.2C). Over the course of the next several hours, spontaneous rupture of the membranes occurs, notable for light meconium. The plan is to continue oxytocin and provide ongoing bedside support. The patient enters the second stage of labor and is encouraged to push and expedite the birth of the baby because of the persistent fetal tracing of category II and repetitive decelerations (Fig. 13.2D). The attending obstetrician is called to the bedside to assist in the direct care of the patient. The second stage lasts 2 hours; there are recurrent FHR decelerations and progressive loss of FHR variability (Fig. 13.2E, F). The baby is delivered via vacuum-assisted vaginal delivery; prior to delivery, FHR variability is absent (Fig. 13.2G). The newborn's Apgar scores are 1, 2, and 7, and the baby is admitted to the neonatal intensive care unit (NICU) for ongoing support, including the initiation of therapeutic hypothermia and management of a subgaleal hematoma.

Case 2

The patient is a G2P1001 at 40 weeks of gestation who presents overnight for labor support in the setting of trial of labor after cesarean delivery; she is noted to be 6 cm dilated (Fig. 13.3A). She has a history of low transverse cesarean delivery performed because of breech presentation. In the current pregnancy, the first stage of labor progresses normally with a category I FHR tracing (Fig. 13.3B); neuraxial anesthesia with epidural is placed. A prolonged FHR deceleration occurs when the patient is lying supine and a low blood pressure is noted (Fig. 13.3C). Intrauterine resuscitation is performed with maternal position change and a bolus of

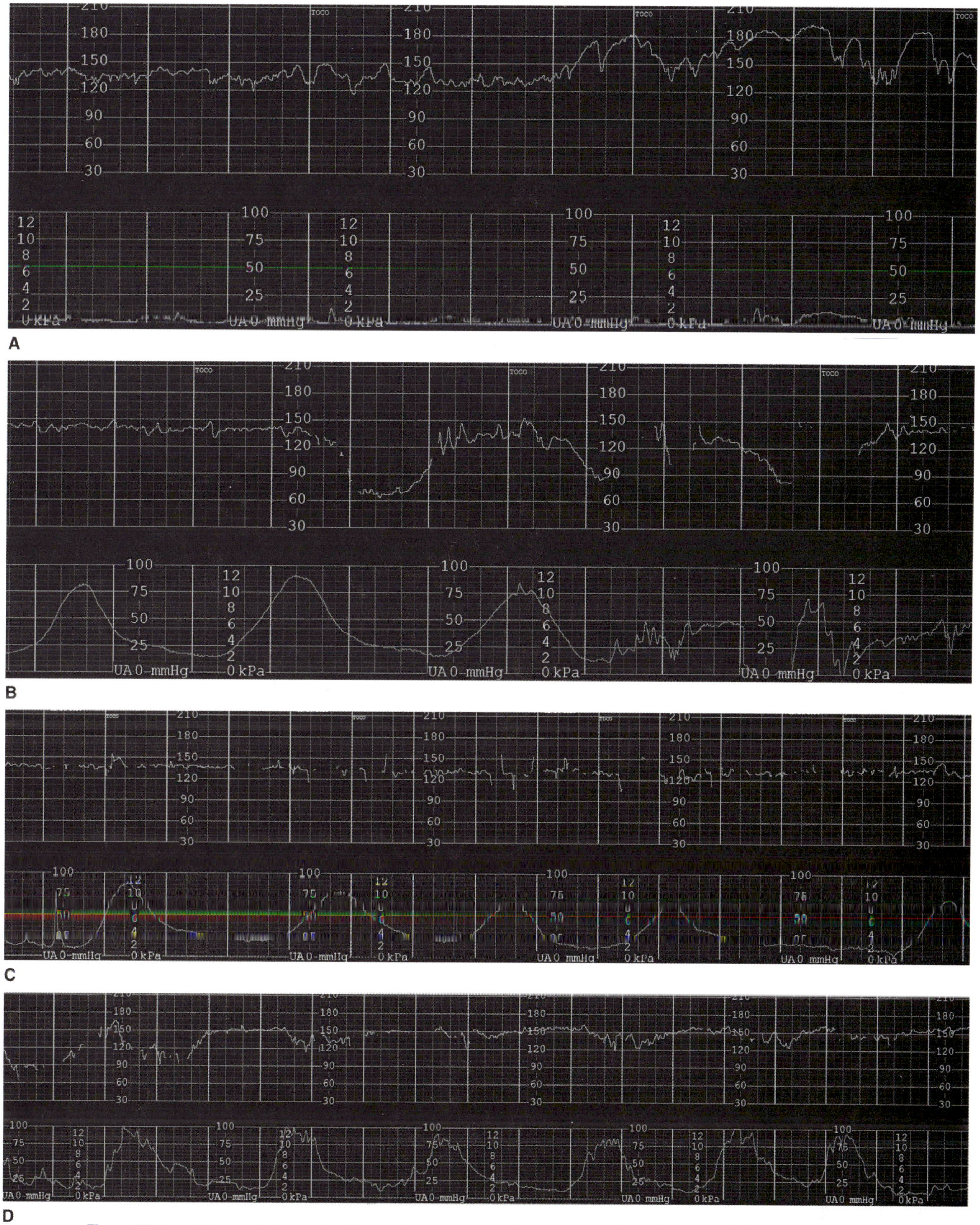

Figure 13.2. **A.** Thirty-eight weeks of gestation, preeclampsia, presenting for induction of labor. **B.** Thirty-eight weeks of gestation, preeclampsia, induction of labor with oxytocin. **C.** Thirty-eight weeks of gestation, preeclampsia, ongoing induction of first stage of labor with oxytocin. **D.** Thirty-eight weeks of gestation, preeclampsia, second stage of labor with oxytocin. *(Continued)*

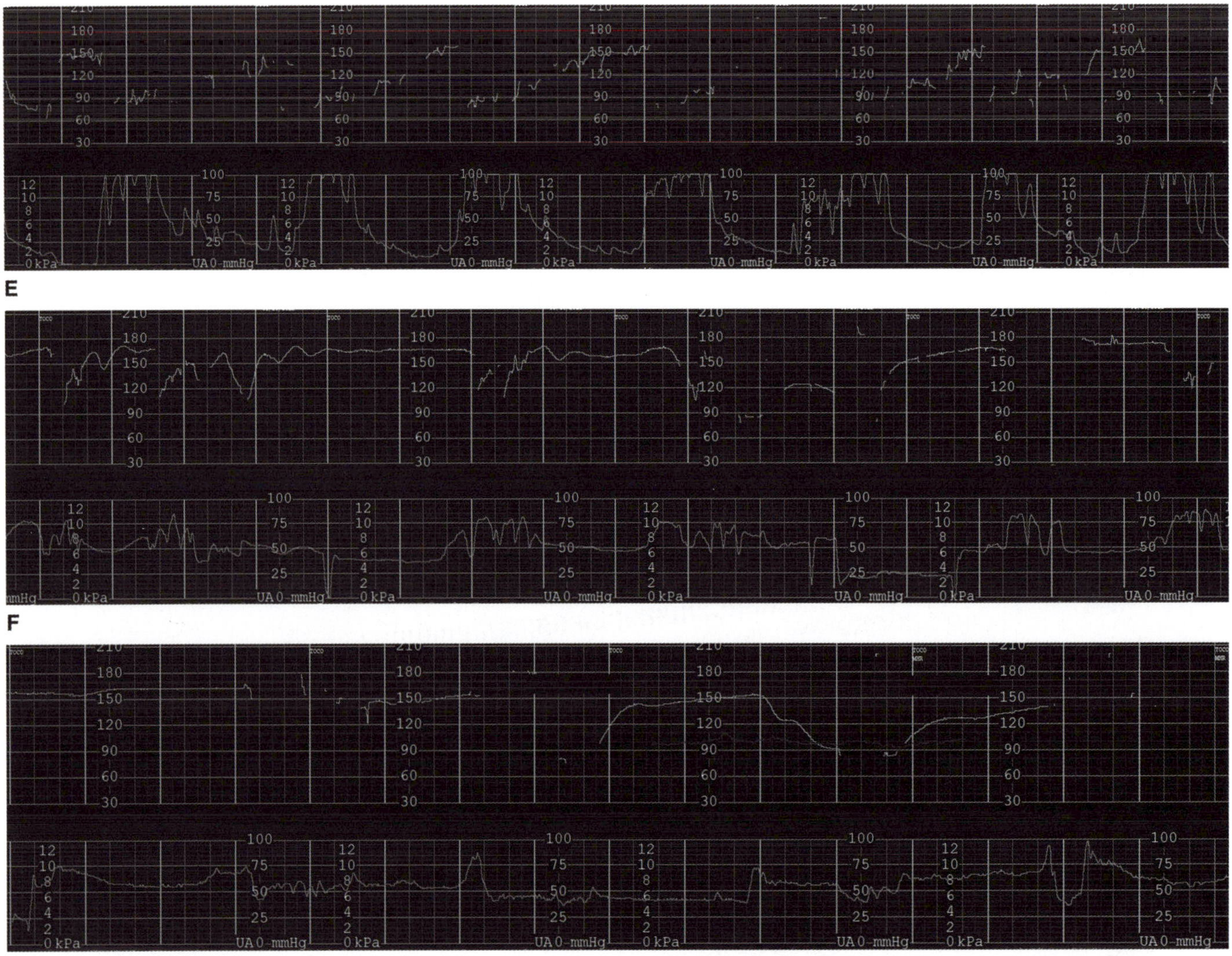

E F G

Figure 13.2. *(Continued)* **E.** Thirty-eight weeks of gestation, preeclampsia, second stage of labor with oxytocin, pushing. **F.** Thirty-eight weeks of gestation, preeclampsia, second stage of labor with oxytocin, continued pushing. **G.** Thirty-eight weeks of gestation, preeclampsia, second stage of labor with oxytocin, decelerations, absent variability and delivery.

intravenous fluid, and the FHR is now of category II (Fig. 13.3D). The patient enters the second stage of labor, and variable FHR decelerations are noted (Fig. 13.3E). The patient then begins pushing and subsequently experiences nausea and presyncope with simultaneous loss of FHR tracing. A fetal scalp electrode is placed, and FHR decelerations to 70 occur, lasting several minutes (Fig. 13.3F). An emergent laparotomy is performed, and uterine rupture at the site of the previous hysterotomy is diagnosed. The fetal head is seen coming through the hysterotomy. The newborn's Apgar scores are 1, 2, and 3 at 1, 5, and 10 minutes respectively. Arterial umbilical cord gas shows the pH value of 6.98 and the base excess of –14. The newborn is admitted to the NICU for ongoing support, including the initiation of therapeutic hypothermia.

Figure 13.3. **A.** Forty weeks of gestation, spontaneous labor, trial of labor after prior cesarean, initial presentation. **B.** Forty weeks of gestation, spontaneous labor, trial of labor after prior cesarean, first stage of labor. **C.** Forty weeks of gestation, spontaneous labor, trial of labor after prior cesarean, prolonged fetal heart rate deceleration, resolved with maternal position change and blood pressure support. **D.** Forty weeks of gestation, spontaneous labor, trial of labor after prior cesarean, first stage of labor. **E.** Forty weeks of gestation, spontaneous labor, trial of labor after prior cesarean, entering second stage of labor. **F.** Forty weeks of gestation, spontaneous labor, trial of labor after prior cesarean, second stage of labor.

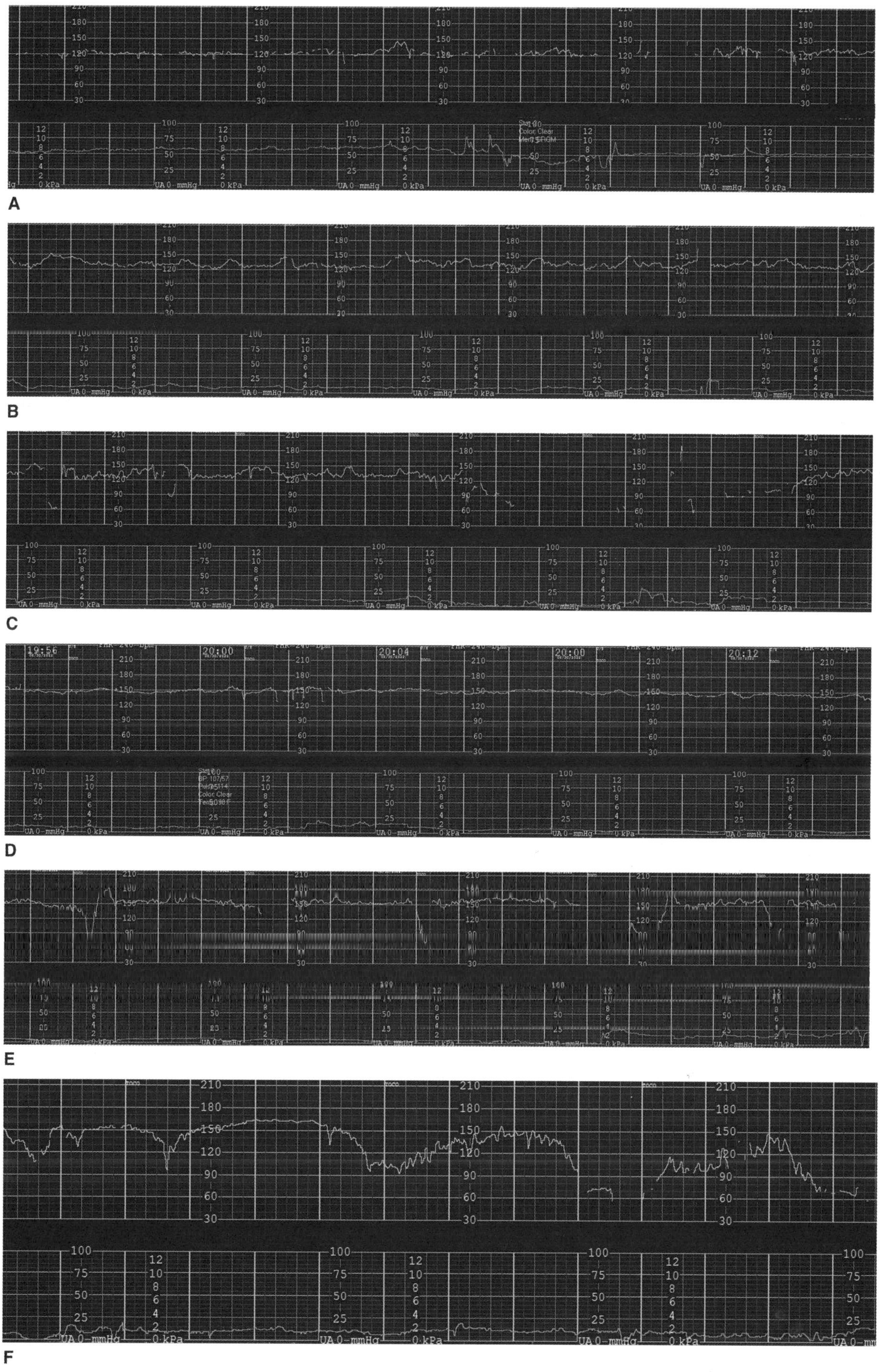

Case 3

The patient is a G2P0010 at 37 weeks of gestation who has complaints of decreased fetal movement; she is invited into the outpatient office for evaluation. With normal range maternal vitals and positive FHR, the recommendation is for fetal testing and ongoing assessment at the inpatient obstetric unit. Upon arrival, the patient is placed on the fetal monitor, and minimal fetal variability is noted (Fig. 13.4A). The patient is admitted for continuous fetal monitoring owing to nonreactive fetal tracing (Fig. 13.4B). The labor floor is busy, and the obstetric team is in the operating room (OR). The FHR tracing continues to be nonreactive with minimal variability, a biophysical profile is 6/10 (−2 for nonreactive NST and −2 for fetal movement) (Fig. 13.4C). The patient strongly desires vaginal delivery, and the induction of labor is started for abnormal fetal testing at term. Fetal monitoring continues to show minimal FHR variability. The bedside obstetric nurse escalates concerns to the obstetrician (Fig. 13.4D). A huddle is called by the unit charge registered nurse (RN) to review the tracing as a team, and a sinusoidal FHR pattern is diagnosed. The patient's delivery plan is changed to urgent cesarean

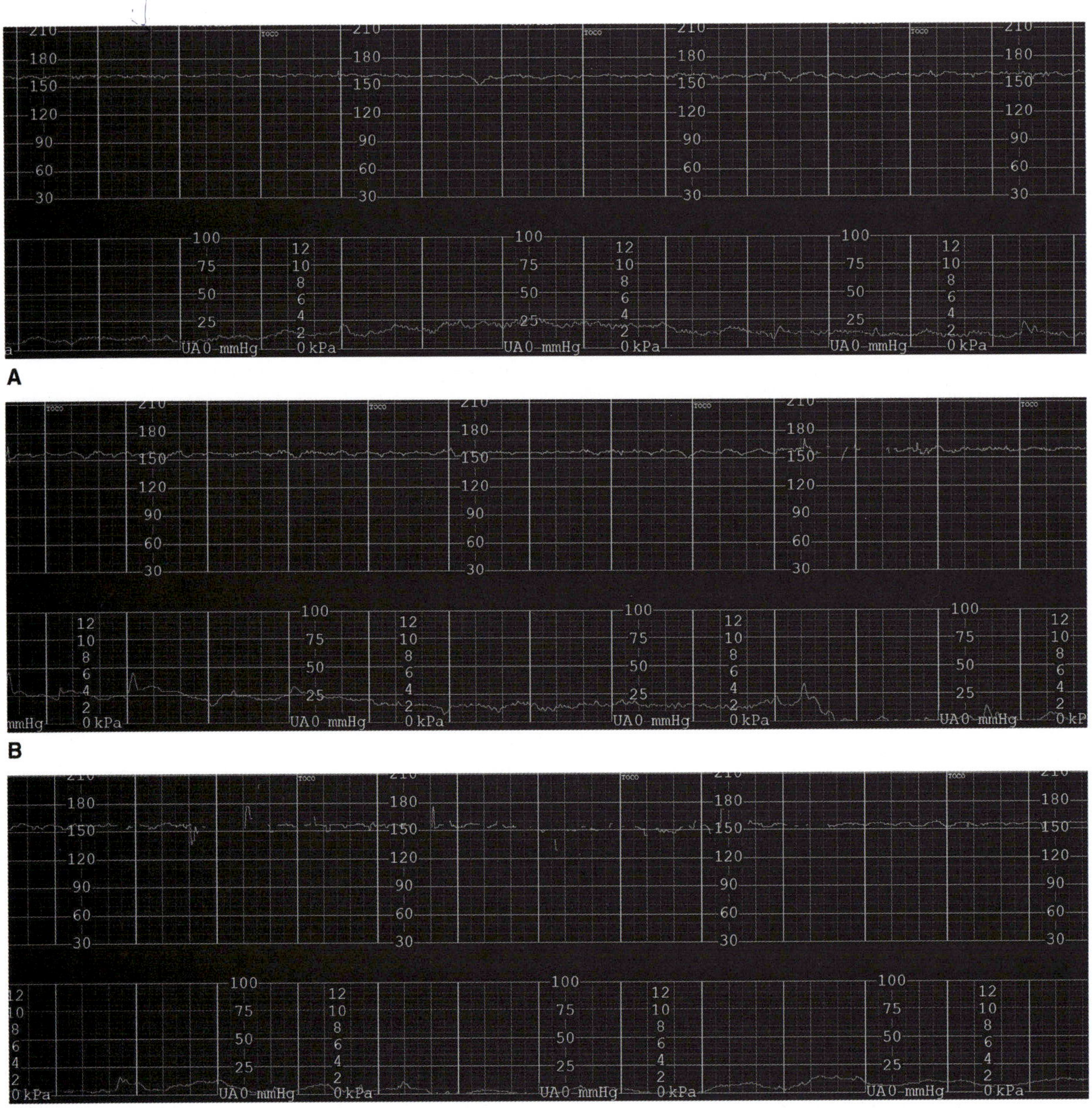

Figure 13.4. **A.** Thirty-seven weeks of gestation, decreased fetal movement, transferred to the inpatient obstetric unit. **B.** Thirty-seven weeks of gestation, decreased fetal movement, admitted to the inpatient unit for observation. **C.** Thirty-seven weeks of gestation, decreased fetal movement, admitted to the inpatient unit, induction of labor started. *(Continued)*

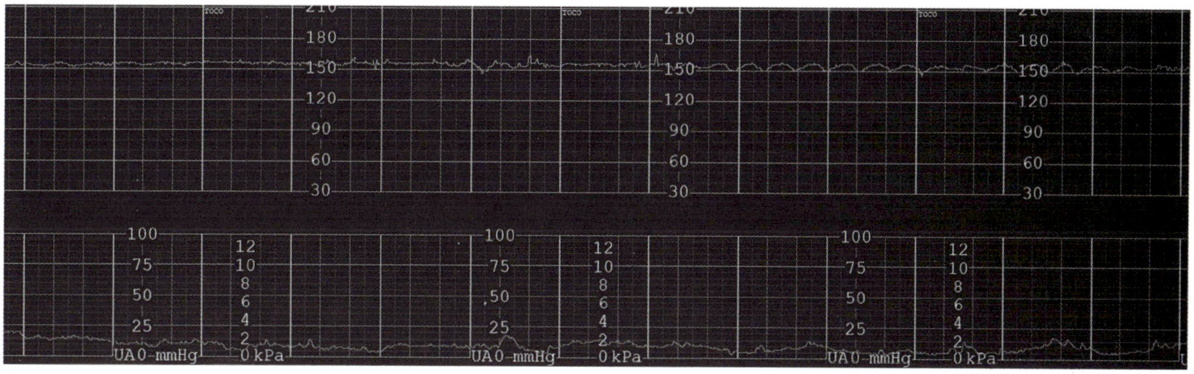

D

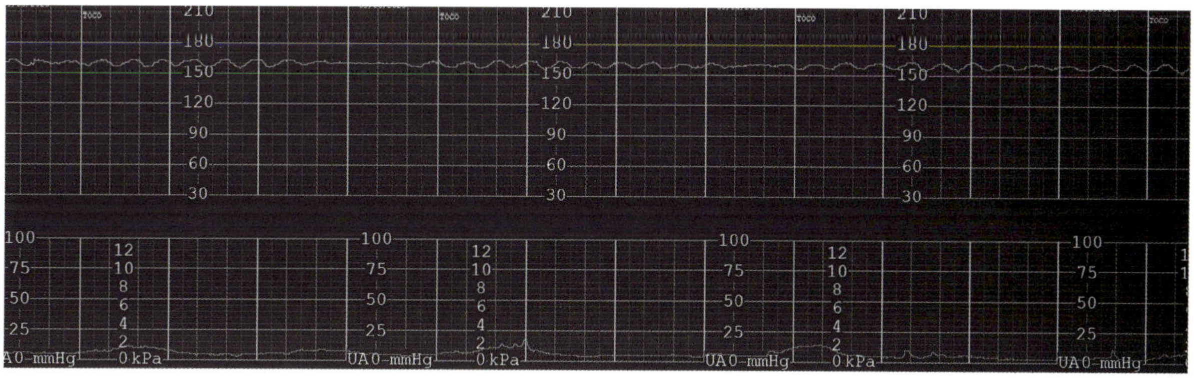

E

Figure 13.4. *(Continued)* **D.** Thirty-seven weeks of gestation, decreased fetal movement, admitted to the inpatient unit, nursing concern with the fetal tracing is elevated to the obstetric care team. **E.** Thirty-seven weeks of gestation, decreased fetal movement, admitted to the inpatient unit, sinusoidal tracing. Urgent cesarean delivery for category III tracing.

delivery (Fig. 13.4E). A cesarean delivery is performed, and the newborn emerges pale and bradycardic with the Apgar scores 2, 6, and 7. The newborn is admitted to the NICU for the ongoing workup of suspected anemia. The newborn hematocrit is recorded as 13.6%, and the newborn requires blood transfusions. A maternal fetal flow cytometry is positive for a significant amount of fetal blood in the maternal circulation, and the working cause of the abnormal fetal testing with sinusoidal pattern and fetal/neonatal anemia is idiopathic fetal-maternal hemorrhage.

Summary of Cases

As you continue to read this chapter, reflect on these cases and the infrastructure that is necessary to provide a safe labor environment for the patient and the fetus. Figures 13.9 to 13.11 attempt to integrate the discussion that follows into how specific measures are designed to mitigate risk in common obstetric scenarios. How can we optimize the use of fetal monitoring – an imperfect, but ciritcal tool in modern-day obstetric care? Where on the obstetric timelines are the opportunities for alternative decision-making? Where are the opportunities to avoid or be relieved from the "tunnel vision" that can develop when working closely and intensely with patients and other care providers on an obstetric unit? How can communication be enhanced? Importantly, how can clinical judgment and technical skills be optimized?

ORGANIZING A SAFE AND HIGH-QUALITY INPATIENT OBSTETRIC UNIT

Personnel and Culture

The collection of individual people working on an obstetric unit is the most important variable and critical foundation to the creation of a successful unit.[9] It is also the hardest element to control and improve. The obstetric unit team consists of individuals working to support the unit and include the following: direct bedside care (nurses, obstetricians, midwives, anesthesiologists, medical residents, and medical assistants), learners (medical, midwifery, and nursing students), clinical support roles (surgical technologists and blood bank staff), unit support roles (schedulers, environmental services, front desk staff, patient transport, and food services), as well as hospital and unit leadership. The functioning of the obstetric team is a direct result of the cultural milieu of the larger healthcare organization, though a unit can create and optimize safety culture for itself. Psychological safety, defined as feeling safe to take interpersonal risks, to speak up, to disagree openly, and to surface concerns without fear of negative repercussions, is a prerequisite for people to be at their best and a ubiquitous element of all high functioning teams. Concepts and processes of a high reliability organization can be integrated into the hospital culture and serve as the driver of psychological safety and creation of high functioning teams.

A high reliability organization is an organization that operates in complex, high-hazard domains for long periods without serious accidents or catastrophic failures.[10] This concept aligns with the needs of an obstetric unit as the operations are complex, and there is risk of significant or catastrophic harm when failures occur. High reliability organizations cultivate a culture of persistent mindfulness of team members and work to develop an environment where potential problems are anticipated, identified early, and responded to early enough to prevent catastrophic consequences. This mindset is defined by five ways of thinking: preoccupation with failure, reluctance to simplify explanations for operational successes and failures, sensitivity to situational awareness, deference to frontline expertise, and commitment to resilience (Table 13.1).

Creating and maintaining the high reliability organization culture require a strong foundation and leadership commitment. Five components of safety culture are identified to promote the necessary organizational foundation, including trust, accountability, identifying unsafe conditions, strengthening systems, and assessment.[11] To develop a these five components and reach high reliability, individuals have to (1) trust the reports of others and be willing to base beliefs and actions on them, (2) report honestly so that others can use the observations to help

TABLE 13.1 Characteristics of high reliability organizations

Characteristic	Description
Preoccupation with failure	■ Awareness of and thinking about potential for failure ■ New threats emerge regularly from situations no one imagined ■ Teams are alert to small signs of potential problems ■ Absence of errors does not lead to complacency but to a heightened sense of vigilance ■ Near misses viewed as opportunities to learn and improve
Reluctance to simplify	■ Resist simplifying understanding of work processes and why things succeed or fail ■ Work is complex and dynamic ■ Seek underlying rather than surface explanations ■ There is value in standardization to reduce variation, but complexity is inherent to daily operations and real-time operational adjustments need to occur
Sensitivity to operations	■ Strive to maintain high awareness of operational conditions: "situation awareness" ■ Teams cultivate the understanding of the context of the current state of their work in relation to the unit or organizational state
Deference to expertise	■ Those closest to the work are the most knowledgeable about the work ■ In an emergency, the person with the greatest knowledge of the situation might not be the person with the most seniority ■ Deference to local and situational expertise creates a spirit of inquiry and de-emphasizes hierarchy in favor of learning as much as possible ■ Everyone is expected to share concerns with others ■ Organizational climate supports all staff members to speak up about potential safety concerns
Commitment to resilience	■ Fundamental understanding of the frequently unpredictable nature of system failures ■ Assuming that the system is at risk for failure and practice performed rapid assessment of and response to challenging situations (simulation) ■ Teams cultivate situation assessment and cross monitoring to quickly identify potential safety threats and respond before safety problems cause harm

Adapted from https://psnet.ahrq.gov/primer/high-reliability. Accessed October 14, 2023.

form valid beliefs, and (3) maintain self-respect, which is done by respecting personal perceptions and beliefs and integrating them with the reports of others without belittling either them or ourselves.[9] Implementing these elements can help promote a high level of psychological safety for team members.

One approach to developing the desired culture is to implement unit- or hospital-wide team training or crew resource management training.[12] TeamSTEPPS is an evidence-based curriculum designed to optimize the performance of healthcare teams.[7,12] The program is guided by research related to teams, team performance, communication, and adult learning, based on training used effectively in the military and commercial aviation. Skills learned in team training helps trainees improve communication, leadership, situation monitoring, and provide mutual support to their team members. An important detail in team training implementation is that all individuals on a unit, not just the clinicians, should be required to participate. The skills learned in crew resource management training directly translate to the improved use of, interpretation of, and response to all types of scenarios related to fetal monitoring by creating more reliable systems of communication and cross checks that systems are working correctly. Hospital and unit safety culture can and should be measured. Structured and validated tools are available, with the most common being the Hospital Survey on Patient Safety Culture hosted by the Agency for Healthcare Research and Quality (AHRQ).[13] This survey places particular emphasis on teamwork practices and event reporting and response. An obstetric unit leadership team should always interpret the results of a survey in the context of how they fit with electronic fetal monitoring (EFM) use.

Physical Infrastructure

The built environment connects birth outcomes with building occupant experiences, behaviors, and satisfaction. Thus, the physical infrastructure of an obstetric unit has direct and indirect effects on childbirth outcomes.[14,15] Areas for consideration include unit layout configuration, provider hub(s), social room, configuration of the birth room, size and shape of the birth room, filter, and sensory elements. When there is opportunity, the optimization of the physical infrastructure of the obstetric unit can improve quality assurance and provide risk mitigation. The principles that guide high reliability organization culture should be considered, including how the physical space will impact intra- and interprofessional communication, collaboration, teamwork, case discussion, and note writing.[16] Labor support persons should feel welcome on the unit, and spaces should be created to promote ideal, emotional, psychological, physiological, and neurobiological responses of the birthing person to optimize obstetric outcomes.[17,18] Strategic use of centralized fetal monitoring can be very helpful for risk mitigation. Traditionally, central monitors that display an entire unit's tracings are placed in nursing stations and charting rooms. However, unit leaders should not underestimate how clinicians with strong high reliability organization skills will also use their surveillance skills in other areas even when they are resting (lounges) or performing other tasks (the OR). The placement of central monitoring throughout a unit helps support a surveillance culture that is seen in top-performing high reliability organizations.

Policies, Guidelines, and Procedures

Standardization with policies, guidelines, and procedures related to fetal monitoring interpretation and management provides a solid foundation to develop safe, high-quality obstetric care.[19] The need of a unit can be understood by asking about how to initiate timely care, how to provide fetal testing, how to interpret and respond to fetal monitoring, how to safely give high risk medications, and how excellent care can be provided equitably with avoidance/minimization of bias and discrimination. Table 13.2 identifies the challenges, suggests opportunities, and elaborates who and what is involved to develop the unit's standards and which standards should be considered standard for a high-quality obstetric unit. Incorporating standard guidelines and policies—in particular for oxytocin administration, intermittent auscultation, fetal monitoring interpretation and management, and OR triage (in the setting of abnormal FHR patterns)—provides a shared mental model for how individuals should provide care. The importance of uniformity in EFM training, interpretation, and management for nurses, physicians, and midwives cannot be overemphasized and has been shown to decrease liability and improve outcomes.[7,20]

Communication Strategies

Communication may be the singular rate-limiting step to ensuring a safe, high-quality obstetric unit. Root cause analyses reviewed by the Joint Commission have demonstrated that communication failures account for approximately 60% of sentinel events, 51% of reportable maternal events, and 68% of reportable perinatal deaths.[21] The communication around interpretation and management of abnormal FHR tracings

TABLE 13.2 Standardization of policies, guidelines, and procedures on the obstetric unit

Identify the challenge	Opportunities	Who/What is involved?
How do we help patients be where they need to be?	■ Provide simple, easy to follow guidelines for how patients contact their obstetrician or midwife and access the obstetric unit ■ Guidelines (with drills/simulations) to urgently transfer patients from ambulatory settings to the inpatient obstetric unit ■ Guidelines for operating room triage and timing of cesarean delivery based on indications ■ Guidelines for recognizing, triaging, and initiating obstetric emergencies in other hospital departments	Community obstetrician and midwife offices, local ambulance company, hospital leadership, including representation from obstetrics, anesthesia, operating room, emergency department
How do we provide fetal monitoring at the right time?	■ Guidelines for outpatient antepartum fetal testing (indications, timing, type) ■ Guidelines for inpatient antepartum fetal testing (indications, timing, type) ■ Guidelines for intrapartum electronic fetal monitoring interpretation and management ■ Guidelines for intermittent auscultation	Best practice guidelines from national and international organizations such as ACOG, RCOG, WHO, NICHD, AWHONN
How do we interpret and respond to all type of fetal heart rate patterns?	■ Certification in electronic fetal monitoring for all inpatient obstetricians, midwives, and OB nurses ■ Ongoing maintenance of competency in electronic fetal monitoring with training or testing ■ Establish competency norms for inpatient obstetricians, midwives, and OB nurses ■ Provide coaching and learning strategies at the individual level	Hospital and obstetric leadership, hospital credentialing office, EFM testing platforms like PQF (Perinatal Quality Foundation) and NCC (National Certification Corporation)
How do we safely give high risk obstetric medications?	■ Hospital cervical ripening policy ■ Hospital oxytocin policy/guideline ■ Hospital magnesium sulfate policy	Hospital and obstetric leadership. Guidance from regulatory and accreditation bodies (state department of health, The Joint Commission)
How do we provide equitable care and minimize unnecessary variability in the care provided?	■ Create standardized approaches to clinical care from the perspective of diversity, equity, inclusion, and belonging ■ Create standardized approaches to building and enhancing the work environment and teamwork from the perspective of diversity, equity, inclusion, and belonging ■ Create standardized, uniform, approaches to diagnose, manage and treat various clinical diagnoses with emphasis on evidence-driven best practices	Unit-based interdisciplinary Diversity, Equity, Inclusion, and Belonging Committee, software to integrate standardized clinical care pathways into the electronic health record (eg, Agile MD)

ACOG Practice Bulletin No. 106: Intrapartum fetal heart rate monitoring: nomenclature, interpretation, and general management principles. *Obstet Gynecol.* 2009;114(1):192-202; Macones GA, Hankins GD, Spong CY, Hauth J, Moore T. The 2008 National Institute of Child Health and Human Development workshop report on electronic fetal monitoring: update on definitions, interpretation, and research guidelines. *Obstet Gynecol.* 2008;112(3):661-666; ACOG Practice Bulletin No. 116: Management of intrapartum fetal heart rate tracings. *Obstet Gynecol.* 2010;116(5):1232-1240; Indications for outpatient antenatal fetal surveillance: ACOG Committee Opinion, Number 828. *Obstet Gynecol.* 2021;137(6):e177-e197; Antepartum Fetal Surveillance: ACOG Practice Bulletin No. 229. *Obstet Gynecol.* 2021;137(6):e116-e127; Committee on Obstetric Practice. Committee Opinion No. 687: Approaches to limit intervention during labor and birth. *Obstet Gynecol.* 2017;129(2):e20-e28.

TABLE 13.3 Communication strategies

Communication type	Examples of best practices	Who/What is involved?
Continuous	■ Electronic fetal monitoring broadcast in designated areas of the unit ■ Welcome board to indicate who is present and working on the unit that day	■ Software to broadcast the fetal heart rate tracing into critical hubs of the unit

Timed	■ Nursing and provider sign-out is scheduled and occurs for every change of shift
	■ Patient safety huddles occur at regular intervals throughout the day
	  ■ Review all patients admitted to the unit
	  ■ Review all fetal tracings
	  ■ Identify any potential concerns
	■ Staffing huddles provide situational awareness for patient admissions, unit transfers, and triage care needs
	■ OB provider chart documentation at regular intervals for laboring patients
	  ■ Progress note frequency related to the stage of labor and the fetal heart rate category
		■ Unit-wide buy-in of scheduled huddles
		■ SBAR communication
		■ HRO communication strategies
		■ Chart documentation standards for the unit

Unscheduled	■ Nonurgent clinical concerns brought forward using the RN-OB/CNM chain of communication ■ Urgent clinical concerns brought forward using the RN-OB/CNM Chain of Communication ■ Use of the Unit Chain of Escalation	■ RN-OB/CNM Chain of Communication ■ Obstetric Unit Chain of Escalation

Emergency	■ Team is alerted simultaneously to respond to the type of emergency
	  ■ Fetal cord prolapse
	  ■ Shoulder dystocia
	  ■ Obstetric hemorrhage
	  ■ Obstetric event occurring outside of the obstetric unit
		■ Assess local resources and hospital standards for creating standardized, simple and effective emergency responses
		  ■ Overhead with a call system
		  ■ Smart phone based
		■ Regular simulation
		■ Standardized emergency carts with necessary supplies

Big picture communication	■ Scheduled multidisciplinary newsletter
	■ Scheduled multidisciplinary meeting to discuss unit goals, upcoming or ongoing initiatives
	■ See also: section on supporting infrastructure for additional forms of unit-wide communication
		■ Effective unit leadership
		  ■ Practice Just Culture and HRO behavior
		  ■ Strong verbal and written communication skills
		  ■ Direction of the unit is transparent and known to all team members

is a common theme. High reliability organization tools should be used when developing or modifying communication strategies for the unit. As the infrastructure is planned, layered communication strategies must be integrated into the physical design and patient care goals of the unit. The strategies must be able to accommodate continuous and intermittent communication, timed and unscheduled communication, as well as emergency communication that elicits an immediate response from a team. Additionally, there must be "big-picture," regular, transparent communication to update all team members of the stated goals, direction, and initiatives of the unit, as well as to highlight team members' efforts and successes (Table 13.3).

Unscheduled team communications provide the bedrock of healthcare delivery to the patient but are notoriously unstructured and unclear. There is no singular, established written algorithm that guides nursing and OB provider communication best practices regarding clinical care needs, though team training programs (above) provide core fundamentals to communicating clearly. Commonly, nurses and OB providers rely on innate communication algorithms that are unwritten and evolve over time. Some of these algorithms work well some of the time, but none are reliable every time. Importantly, there is variation in patient care communication from team to team and person to person. This variation may lead to frustration from all sides, including the patient. Importantly, lack of a standard communication format may be associated with critical delays in patient care and increase the risk of a preventable adverse outcome. Thus, formalizing some concepts of communication can improve a unit. Scheduled and structured regular "huddles"—such as at intervals of 4, 6, or 12 hours—to review all of the patients on a unit can provide a routine manner for dissemination of information and review fetal heart tracings. Physicians and midwives performing bedside rounds with nurses—rounding in dyads rather than in silos—allow for communicating a shared mental model of care and in the interpretation of a labor course and tracing management. Multidisciplinary interpretation and management of EFM are critical to creating a safe obstetric environment.

Electronic communication (EHR messaging, email, and texting) is widespread and has been readily adopted into clinical workflows often with little or no forethought. When used appropriately, electronic

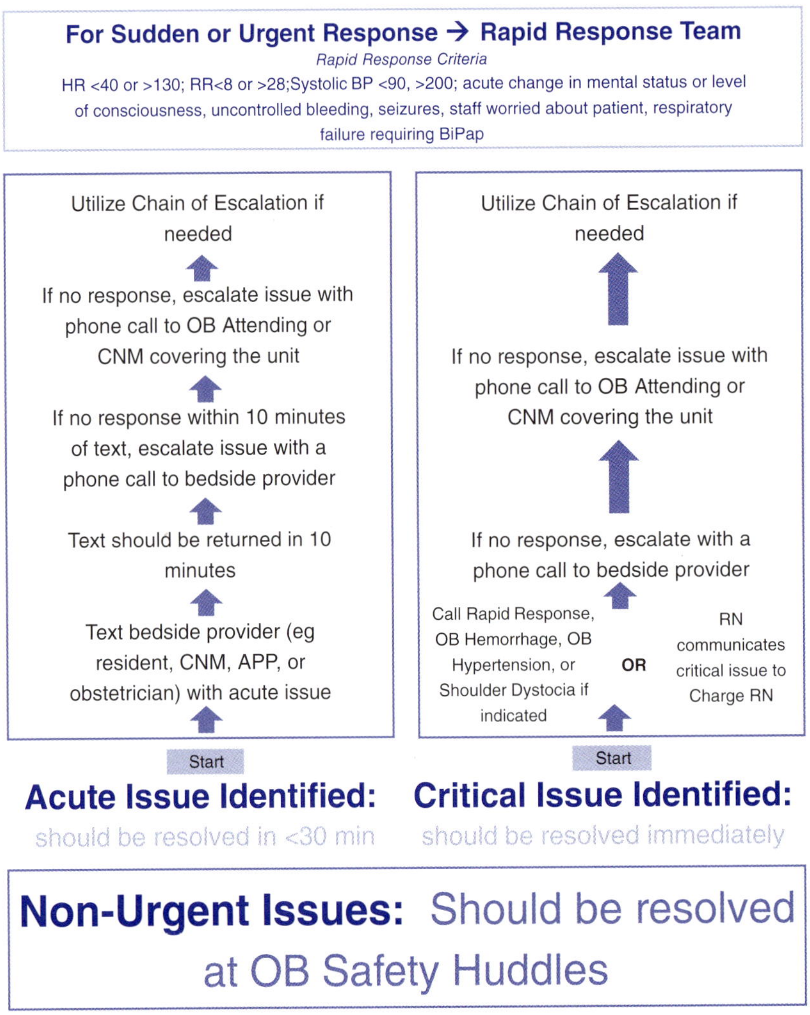

Figure 13.5. Nurse-OB/CNM chain of communication.

communication can provide pertinent information and connect clinical care locations across vast distances. However, there are notable pitfalls with this type of communication, including lack of a timely response to a clinical concern (eg, the message landed in an inbox that is only checked during certain hours) or lack of context (eg, there is no verbal or physical body language in electronic communication). Further, it is sometimes difficult to read the urgency in a text communication, and sometimes nonurgent issues communicated in a text can be misleadingly urgent. Relying on this form of communication at the expense of regular in-person communication has the potential to erode or blunt the development of close working relationships that foster trust, camaraderie, and improved situational awareness. For this reason, a unit can be improved by general standards for how information is communicated in acute, urgent, and nonurgent circumstances. At the very least, obstetric unit leaders should work to encourage verbal and face-to-face communication, in particular for anything beyond the routine.

There is a need for clear, well-developed communication algorithms to promote a work environment that is collaborative and strives to create nurse-obstetrician/midwife communication systems that are easily understood, proactive, and promote teamwork. Importantly, these communication systems should enhance patient safety and the patient experience. The Nurse-OB/CNM chain of communication (Fig. 13.5) is built to model the "chain of escalation." The "chain of escalation" is used to bring clinical and unit concerns up through hospital and medical leadership (Fig. 13.6). This is a critical tool to effectively resolve more complicated unit or clinical scenarios when the right decision is uncertain.

Debriefs and Second Victim Support

Most obstetric providers will experience at least one serious adverse obstetric event during their career. Given this and since even daily clinical care is associated with extraordinary stress, systems for dialog and discussion should be created to support individuals

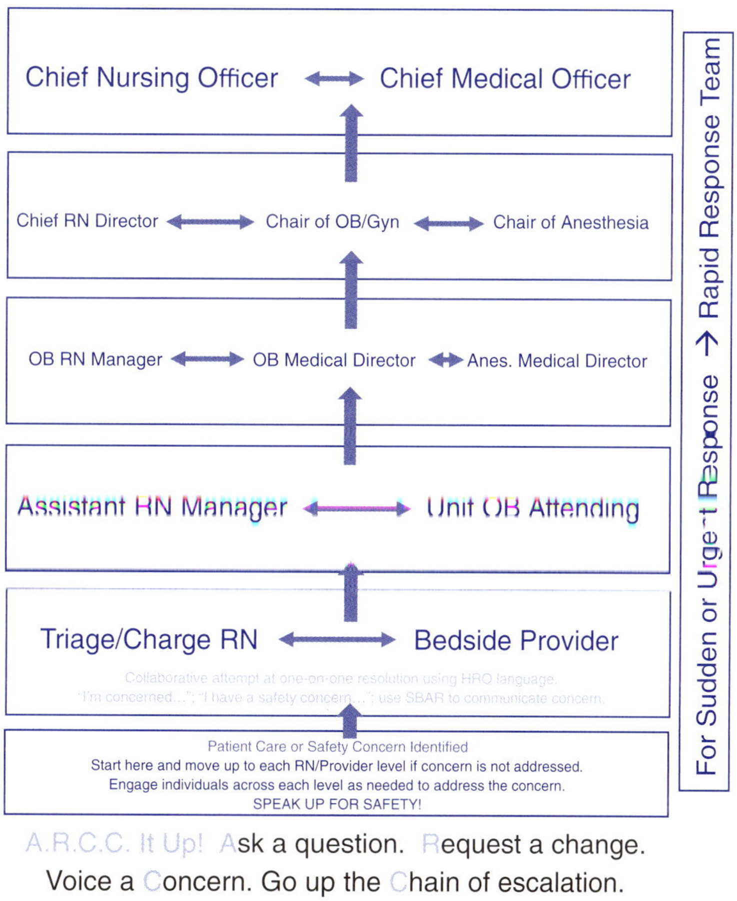

Figure 13.6. Example of obstetric chain of escalation.

and groups. A debrief is the act of reviewing a real or simulated event in which participants explain, analyze, and synthesize information and emotional states to improve performance in similar situations. Incorporation of debriefs into the regular support of our obstetric teams is recognized as a critical component for the development of a safe and high-quality environment for our patients. Debriefs, when done well, are increasingly recognized as a tool to help support HCWs and validate their experiences and feelings when an adverse event occurs.[22-24] Prior to attending a debrief, it is important to recognize the goals of the meeting and establish expectations.

Emotional Debriefs

An emotional debrief provides a time for HCWs to emotionally process and share feelings associated with the course of a specific set of clinical events. All willing team members are invited to be present at and participate in the emotional debrief. The current practice of emotional debriefs on the obstetric unit are based on the infrastructure of Critical Incident Stress Debriefing (CISD). CISD was developed in 1974 and first published in 1983.[25] The primary goal is to provide a supportive, crisis-focused discussion of a traumatic event (critical incident). It is not psychotherapy. It was developed for small groups who have encountered a powerful, traumatic event and aims to reduce the distress and restore group cohesion and unit performance. The objectives are to mitigate the impact of a traumatic event, facilitate the normal recovery, and restore the adaptive functions of healthy people. It serves as a screening opportunity to identify individuals who may benefit from additional support services. The CISD can be adapted to obstetric units to meet the cultural needs and expectations of obstetric HCWs. The emotional debrief is considered a first-line response after an adverse obstetric event and should occur prior to any fact-finding investigation. The debrief can be led by any team member with an expected duration of 20 to 40 minutes. It is not a time to give, have, or seek answers, but it is a time to ask questions and re-state observations or concerns. If time is short because of acuity on the obstetric unit, one may consider reading a "Closing Sacred Moment." It is important to inquire, but to avoid an "inquiry" and provide restoration and not retribution. Judgment and blame are also avoided and there should be sensitivity regarding the potential of the second victim. Figure 13.7 provides an example of a facilitators guide to initiating and leading an emotional debrief.

Operational Debriefs

An operational debrief is an exploratory and fact-finding mission. Information gathered from this debrief will assist in future event review including a root cause analysis (RCA). Application of the known complications test will help determine if the event is a Safety Event: (1) Was the procedure, treatment, or test appropriate and warranted based on nationally recognized standards of care. (2) Was the complication of known risk, was it anticipated before the procedure and was the standard of care applied to mitigate the risk? (3) Was the complication identified in a timely manner (at the time of occurrence)? (4) Was the complication treated according to the standards of care and in a timely manner? If all the four answers are "yes," then this is not a safety event. If the answer to any question is "no"—the event is a safety event.

Second Victim Phenomenon

The term second victim was coined in 2000 and defines a HCW who is involved in an adverse patient event, medical error, or patient-related injury.[26] After an unanticipated adverse patient event, HCWs may experience many of the same emotions/feeling felt by the patient and family members (the first victims) and can lead to a period of intense professional personal anguish.[26-27] Signs and symptoms are similar to acute stress disorder and can include: numbness, detachment, anxiety, anger, grief, fear, frustration, burnout, withdrawal, lack of concentration, and poor memory.[28] Second victims can develop post-traumatic stress disorder. Historically, HCWs (the most critical component of any healthcare system) have received little emotional support from the system. When support is lacking and individuals experience emotional distress from an adverse event, a vicious cycle can ensue with the subsequent development of burnout, depression, and reduced empathy further compromising the HCW's ability to provide safe, high-quality, and compassionate care.[29]

It is critical that the obstetric unit develop a system designed to recognize, responding to, and support HCWs who are exposed to adverse obstetric events. Regular use of the emotional debrief to support team members will provide a foundation for this infrastructure and creates a culture that prioritizes a HCW's mental health and resiliency. Acknowledgment of the second victim and the risk of negative sequelae when team members are exposed to adverse obstetric events validates the need for formal and accessible mental

Emotional Debrief: Facilitator's Guide

Debrief can be led by any team member and can last approx. 20-40 minutes.
If time is not available to debrief, staff can gather in a circle and read the Closing Sacred Moment.

Purpose

"After a difficult event, we often continue to have feelings about what happened and our experience. This is a time to express those feelings, to honor our hard work and the patients/families who were affected, and to care for ourselves and others who we shared the experience with. Thank you for taking this time to be together."

Expectations

"I'd like to set some expectations for our conversation today:"

- Everyone who would like to should get a chance to speak.
- While clinical concerns and questions may come up, this is an opportunity to lean into and process the emotional side of our work rather than problem solve.
- This space is safe and confidential.
- This is an opportunity for participants to offer perspectives of events and create a fuller story of what happened.

Opener

To begin, let us go around and briefly share our experience of this event. You may interpret this simply in terms of your role–e.g., "I was the bedside RN"–or more broadly, in terms of what it was like for you.

Questions to Consider

To facilitator: Conversation may start happening. If so, let it naturally flow. If not, here are some prompts you can pose to the group:

- "What was the hardest thing about this event for you?"
- "What did you appreciate or were grateful for in the work of your colleagues?"
- "What do you think you or we might take with us from this event?"
- Moving to more general reflection: **"What does this event bring up for you in terms of what it's like to do this work? What tends to linger or stay with you after situations like this?"**

Closing Sacred Moment

If there was a death: "Let us take this moment to pause, so that each of us, in silence, according to our faith, philosophy, or beliefs, may recognize the life of _______ and remember his/her parents and all those who love him/her, and to wish for them healing, peace, and loving support." *[pause]*
If there was not a death: "Let us take this moment to pause, so that each of us, in silence, according to our faith, philosophy, or beliefs, may recognize the patient and family members affected by this event, and to wish for them healing, peace, and loving support." *[pause]*

Continued (for all situations): "And let us also take this moment to honor ourselves; our strength, our hard work, and our commitment; and all that has been expressed here today. Let us try to take the time to be kind to ourselves and to be gentle with others. And as we go forth, may we continue to remember the preciousness of life, and all that we do to enable its resilience." *[pause]* "Thank you."

Written by Chaplain Anna Hadfield, in collaboration with YSC Labor & Birth/MSC leadership

Figure 13.7. Facilitators guide to perform an emotional debrief after an unexpected obstetric event.

health care for all HCWs. Mental health resources developed to support second victims should be well advertised and program utilization encouraged. Healthcare worker confidentiality must be ensured. Peer support in the aftermath of an adverse event is shown to be beneficial and formalized programs exist.[22,23] Additional resources include traditional one-on-one support with counseling and consideration of pharmacological therapy; classes and workshops to develop stress management skills and promote resiliency; as well as group sessions for teams or units.

Documentation

Documentation that is contemporaneous, logical, explicit, accurate, and readable is critical for teams to communicate with each other and to provide support for how care was delivered.[30] There are no clear standards for the frequency of documentation on antepartum or intrapartum patients. Nursing documentation is typically guided by hospital policy. Timing of physician and midwife documentation should be based on when clinical assessments are performed, when interventions or management plans are changed, and when there are discussions with patients about plans of care. Some units provide standards for regular intervals of documentation in active labor, while on oxytocin, or in the second stage of labor, though there is no universal professional recommendation at this time.

Specifically related to EFM, documentation language and manner should be standardized. That is to say that a standard and common nomenclature, like that of the 2008 NICHD workshop report, should be adopted and mandated. An electronic health record template that incorporates the components of the standard nomenclature can assist in creating uniformity.

Obstetric Clinician Relationships with Risk Management

The legal and risk management team of a hospital is typically viewed as a black box, if not a point of fear, to an obstetric clinician. This is understandable given the emotional trauma of an adverse event, especially when it may involve possible accusations of substandard performance or litigation. It is also reasonable from the viewpoint that the involvement of risk management can often be considered a stance of defensiveness, when most clinicians are uncomfortable. A successful response to adverse events requires a supportive approach at the onset so that the teams managing and mitigating the response to an event can feel supported by the risk management team. A "just culture" approach recommends that even when an event involves an individual human error or slip, except in cases of reckless or risky behavior, those errors or slips could and should have been mitigated by forces in the system to prevent them from reaching the patient and causing harm. Although unit and hospital executive leadership, with the assistance of the medical staff and human resources departments, drives this just culture approach that supports fallible individuals, ultimately it is the role of the risk management team to provide a safe and stable platform for its use.

OBSTETRIC UNIT SUPPORT INFRASTRUCTURE

The support infrastructure of an obstetric unit facilitates the creation, sustainability, and long-term goals of a high-functioning obstetric unit. The exact support needs of a unit reflect the availability of local resources. Involvement of all types of team members will encourage buy-in and provide diverse points of view as the unit grows, develops, and adapts to new or revised obstetric practices. Once the resources are defined, a thoughtful and deliberate creation of a committee or committees can occur. How, when, and where the committee's work is communicated to the entire obstetric staff must be determined. In addition, if there is more than one committee, intercommittee communication must be determined. Examples of support infrastructure include:

- **Obstetric Patient Safety Committee:** To develop, implement, and sustain OB patient safety initiatives.
- **Obstetric Operations Committee:** To communicate the unit's current projects and long-term goals with the broad obstetric community.
- **Staff Social Committee:** To facilitate a culture of camaraderie and community wellness.
- **Formalized Neonatal Encephalopathy Review** of defined "at risk" neonatal encephalopathy cases: To refine practices that support appropriate use of EFM and promote safe birth.
- **Peer-led EFM Case Review**, also known as "tracing rounds": To provide ongoing EFM education in the clinical space, build team trust, and share the mental model.
- **Multidisciplinary Reviews** and collaboration with other departments across the hospital (eg, regular collaboration with the emergency department): To develop necessary obstetric support in non-OB care areas.
- Participation in larger hospital or system-wide committees that reinforce patient quality and safety: To bring new initiatives to the OB unit and align with hospital safety culture.

EVENT REVIEW AND SYSTEM IMPROVEMENT

Event Reporting System and Event Classification

Proactive risk mitigation to avoid future adverse events depends on a tight system to retroactively assess issues that can be identified as latencies and threats to safety.[31] An event reporting system, supported by a standardized approach for classifying the events relative to the risk to a patient and the level of harm involved, allows for the systematic identification of these latencies and threats. At this time, nearly every hospital with a birthing facility will have an enterprise event reporting system that will include the ability to report events to managers and leaders and that also includes an anonymous option for reporting. Specific to obstetrics, it should be clear to staff what represent triggers to report into the system and, specific to fetal monitoring and birth, those often include 5-minute Apgar <7, arterial cord gases <7.0, shoulder dystocia, intrapartum fetal death, unanticipated NICU admission >36 weeks of gestation. However, these events are just the tip of the iceberg in terms of what can and should be reported on an obstetric unit, as "near miss" events where a latency did not reach or harm a patient are very useful to mitigate risk on a unit, especially if they are seen with frequency or in a pattern. For this reason, unit leadership should foster a healthy reporting culture that rewards event reports, especially for "near misses," rather than considers them punishment, retaliation, or tattling. This is especially true for cases involving potential gaps or deviations in good fetal monitoring practice, where harm can be catastrophic. Near miss events can help a leadership team proactively design interventions to prevent recurrence that may lead to harm; further, these near miss situations can be stimulating educational opportunities for interdisciplinary "tracing rounds" for departmental discussion.

Generally, events reported to leadership should be classified as *known complications, non-safety events, near miss events*, or *serious events*. (Formal classifications systems, such as that of the Healthcare Performance Improvement Group, now a part of Press Ganey, are available.[32]) Using a clear and validated event classification system can allow for data collection and helps guide the leadership team in the next steps needed for review of the event. For instance, a serious event may trigger a formal RCA or apparent cause analysis. A near miss event may initiate a brief and less formal review by an investigatory team, led by a unit director or a patient safety coordinator. In the setting of a series of similar near miss events, it would be appropriate to initiate a higher level and more formal review like an apparent cause analysis. Without a classification system, however, this type of decisions and arrangements would be impossible.

Reporting criteria for outside organizations are dependent on state and accreditation organization regulations. The unanticipated death of a full-term neonate, in any type of pregnancy, is considered a sentinel event for reporting by the Joint Commission (Sentinel Event Policy (SE)).[33] Similarly, death or serious injury of a neonate associated with labor or delivery in a low-risk pregnancy is considered a "Serious Reportable Event" by the National Quality Forum, which is often the basis for state department of health reporting criteria.[34]

Root Cause Analysis

All serious and significant safety events on an obstetric unit require immediate and systematic investigation.[35] As specified by the Joint Commission, an appropriate response to a sentinel event (or other significant safety events) involves:

- A formalized team response that stabilizes the patient, discloses the event to the patient and family, and provides support for the family as well as staff involved in the event
- Notification of organization leadership
- Immediate investigation
- Completion of a comprehensive systematic analysis for identifying the causal and contributory factors
- Strong corrective actions derived from the identified causal and contributing factors that eliminate or control system hazards or vulnerabilities and result in sustainable improvement overtime
- Timeline for the implementation of corrective actions
- Systemic improvement (Sentinel Event Policy)

Root cause analysis is an investigation type designed to determine the direct and indirect causes of an event, accident, or incident that dissects all possible modes and chains of causation, in order to supply the investigation team areas needing improvement. Corrective action plans are designed after the RCA to address each suspected causation. Generally, an RCA should contextualize an individual error within a system. That is to say, individual errors, unless an act of reckless behavior, can generally be attributed to weakness in the system around that individual. An individual can still be held accountable within this just culture framework; however, unless an approach is taken where the individual error can be mitigated in the design of a safe system around them, the same event is likely to recur. It is outside the scope of this chapter to review the key elements of RCA, and there exist definitive and comprehensive primary texts on the subject from the Joint Commission and the Institute for Healthcare Improvement.[36,37]

Formal Disclosure Program

A serious event where a deviation in an accepted practice standard results in harm to a patient is not resolved solely when the investigation is complete, action plans are in place, and even with confirmation that an action plan is sustained. Resolution only occurs when the loop is closed with the patient

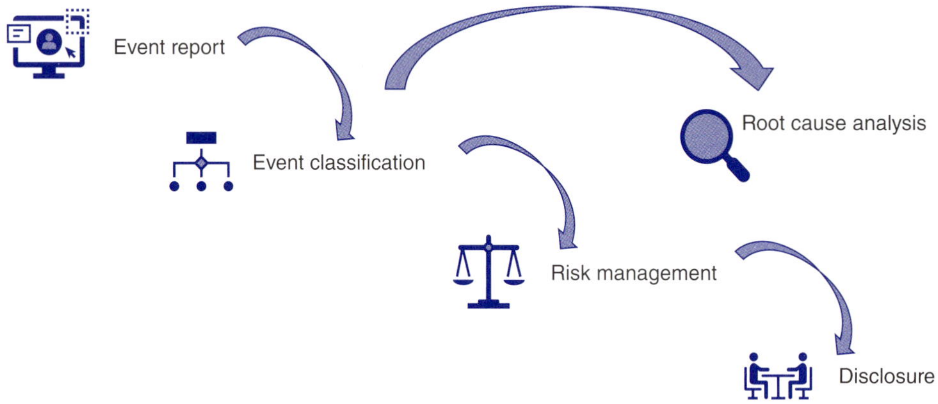

Figure 13.8. Relationship of event reporting, classification, root cause analysis, risk management, and formal patient and family disclosure.

and family. Patient and family disclosure programs involve complete and honest communication with a patient after an unexpected medical event, discussing what happened, linking the error and the outcome, in a way that is meaningful to the patient.[38] Disclosure is important for patients and families as it satisfies their struggle to find meaning in the event that changed their lives. Further, most patients and families are resolved to ensure that an event never affects others, and thus the disclosure of the specific drivers of an event and the steps taken to improve a unit to prevent recurrence. There is evidence that disclosure programs may reduce the malpractice risk of an organization, but this should not be considered a primary driver of a program.[39,40] At the very least it should be comforting to clinicians and administrative members of a hospital that disclosure programs do not increase liability exposure.

Figure 13.8 demonstrates how all of these pieces of a quality assurance and risk management program relate.

SUMMARY

Figures 13.9 to 13.11 reflect the timelines of the hypothetical cases of three patients presented at the beginning of the chapter. Overlying the linear timelines of each case are distinct areas of opportunity representing principles or practices reviewed here. The examples are not meant to explain that any one intervention would entirely prevent what occurred; rather, they represent a bundle of interventions with a good opportunity to prevent failure and an adverse event.

Good practice of EFM interpretation and management requires a robust system built around the clinicians who perform the practice. There is a long-held belief, supported generally in the literature, that EFM in labor has done little to eliminate rare, serious adverse events such as neonatal encephalopathy, cerebral palsy, and infant mortality in otherwise normal pregnancies.[41] Much of the criticism is toward the tool itself and the systems—such as interpretation standards and management

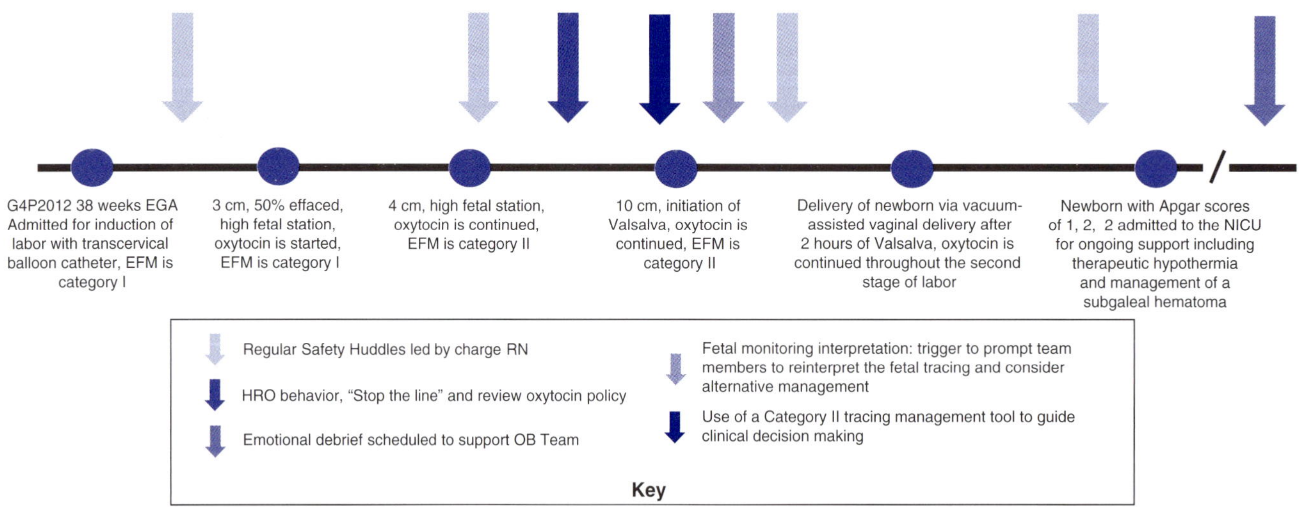

Figure 13.9. Case 1: Areas of opportunity to ensure quality and mitigate risk in fetal monitoring.

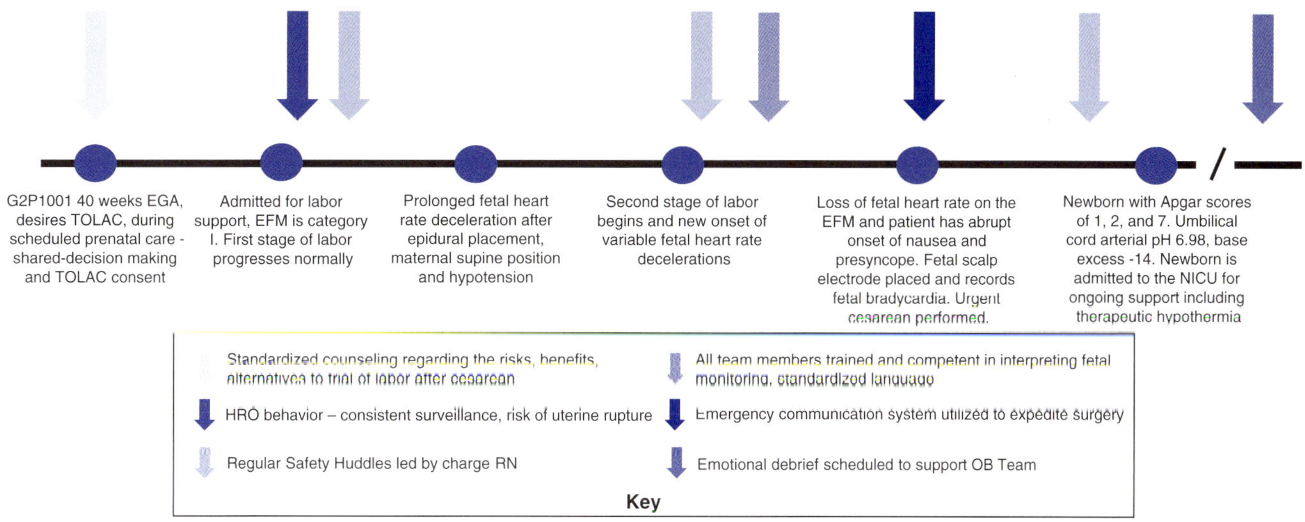

Figure 13.10. Case 2: Areas of opportunity to ensure quality and mitigate risk in fetal monitoring.

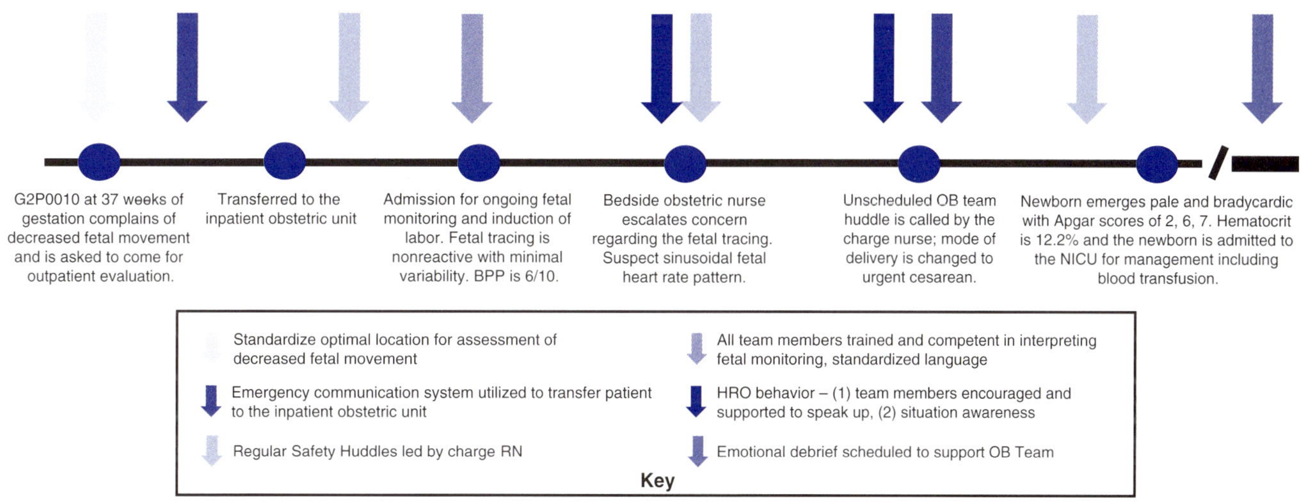

Figure 13.11. Case 3: Areas of opportunity to ensure quality and mitigate risk in fetal monitoring.

guidelines—built to guide clinicians toward good practice. Electronic fetal monitoring may have had a more modest impact than initially envisioned. However, it is probably also fair to say that the impact has probably been muted by a failure, through the first 50 years of use, to apply good safety science and quality assurance practices to the field of obstetrics and the management of labor and delivery. Only in the past 20 years have units organized programs like those discussed in this chapter, which should now be considered the standard best practices to provide strong systems to support individual practice.

REFERENCES

1. Corrigan JM, Donaldson MS, Kohn LT, McKay T, Pine KC. *To Err Is Human: Building a Safer Health System*. National Academy Press; 2000.
2. Dove JT, Brush JE, Jr., Chazal RA, Oetgen WJ. Medical professional liability and health care system reform. *J Am Coll Cardiol*. 2010;55(23):2801-2803.
3. McCaffrey MP, Neumann D, Furniss KK, Lohman SL, Carpenito PM, Johnson VL. The loneliness of the perinatal nurse in litigation. *MCN Am J Matern Child Nurs*. 2008;33(5):281-286.
4. Malpractice Risks in Obstetrics. https://www.candello.com/Insights/Candello-Reports/Obstetrics-Report. Accessed October 14, 2023.
5. Simpson KR, Knox GE. Common areas of litigation related to care during labor and birth: recommendations to promote patient safety and decrease risk exposure. *J Perinat Neonatal Nurs*. 2003;17(2):94-109.
6. Clark SL, Belfort MA, Dildy GA. Reducing obstetric litigation through alterations in practice patterns. *Obstet Gynecol*. 2008;112(6):1279-1283.
7. Pettker CM, Thung SF, Norwitz ER, et al. Impact of a comprehensive patient safety strategy on obstetric adverse events. *Am J Obstet Gynecol*. 2009;200(5):492.e1-e8.

8. Pratt SD, Mann S, Salisbury M, et al. John M. Eisenberg Patient Safety and Quality Awards: impact of CRM-based training on obstetric outcomes and clinicians' patient safety attitudes. *Jt Comm J Qual Patient Saf.* 2007;33(12):720-725.
9. Weick KE, Sutcliffe KM. *Managing the Unexpected: Sustained Performance in a Complex World.* 3rd ed. John Wiley & Sons; 2015.
10. Patient Safety Network (PDNet). High reliability. 2019. https://psnet.ahrq.gov/primer/high-reliability. Accessed October 14, 2023.
11. Chassin MR, Loeb JM. High-reliability health care: getting there from here. Milbank Q. 2013; 91(3):459-490. doi: 10.1111/1468-0009.12023.
12. Agency for Healthcare Research and Quality (AHRQ). TeamSTEPPS. https://www.ahrq.gov/teamstepps-program/index.html. Accessed October 14, 2023.
13. Agency for Healthcare Research and Quality (AHRQ). Hospital survey on patient safety culture. 2004. https://www.ahrq.gov/sops/surveys/hospital/index.html. Accessed October 14, 2023.
14. Setola N, Naldi E, Cocina GG, Eide LB, Iannuzzi L, Daly D. The impact of the physical environment on intrapartum maternity care: identification of eight crucial building spaces. *HERD.* 2019; 12(4):67-98.
15. Ariadne Lab & MASS Design Group. Designing capacity for high value healthcare: the impact of design on clinical care in childbirth. 2017. https://www.ariadnelabs.org/. Accessed October 14, 2023.
16. Berridge EJ, Mackintosh NJ, Freeth DS. Supporting patient safety: examining communication within delivery suite teams through contrasting approaches to research observation. *Midwifery.* 2010;26(5):512-519.
17. Hammond A. A space of possibilities: the importance of birth unit design. *Aust Midwifery News.* 2015;15(3):28-31.
18. Hammond A, Foureur M, Homer CSE. The hardware and software implications of hospital birth room design: a midwifery perspective. *Midwifery.* 2014;30(7):825-830.
19. Pettker CM. Standardization of intrapartum management and impact on adverse outcomes. *Clin Obstet Gynecol.* 2011;54(1):8-15. doi: 10.1097/GRF.0b013e31820a033d.
20. Clark SL, Belfort MA, Byrum SL, Meyers JA, Perlin JB. Improved outcomes, fewer cesarean deliveries, and reduced litigation: results of a new paradigm in patient safety. *Am J Obstet Gynecol.* 2008;199:105.e1-e7.
21. The Joint Commission. Sentinel event data summary. https://www.jointcommission.org/resources/sentinel-event/sentinel-event-data-summary/. Accessed November 2, 2023.
22. Edrees H, Connors C, Paine L, Norvell M, Taylor H, Wu AW. Implementing the RISE second victim support programme at the Johns Hopkins Hospital: a case study. *BMJ Open.* 2016; 6(9):e011708.
23. Schrøder K, Edrees HH, Christensen RD, Jørgensen JS, Lamont RF, Hvidt NC. Second victims in the labor ward: are Danish midwives and obstetricians getting the support they need? *Int J Qual Health Care.* 2019;31(8):583-589.
24. Schrøder K, Jørgensen JS, Lamont RF, Hvidt NC. Blame and guilt: a mixed methods study of obstetricians' and midwives' experiences and existential considerations after involvement in traumatic childbirth. *Acta Obstet Gynecol Scand.* 2016;95(7):735-745.
25. Mitchell JT, Everly GS. *Critical Incident Stress Debriefing: An Operations Manual for CISD, Defusing and Other Group Crisis Intervention Services.* 3rd ed. Chevron Publishing; 2001.
26. Scott SD, Hirschinger LE, Cox KR, McCoig M, Brandt J, Hall L. The natural history of recovery for the health care provider "second victim" after adverse patient events. *Qual Saf Health Care.* 2009;18(5):325-330.
27. Wu AW, Steckelberg RC. Medical error, incident investigation and the second victim: doing better but feeling worse? *BMJ Qual Saf.* 2012;21(4):267-270. doi: 10.1136/bmjqs-2011-000605.
28. Seys D, Wu AW, Van Gerven E, et al. Health care professionals as second victims after adverse events: a systematic review. *Eval Health Prof.* 2013;36(2):135-162.
29. Schwappach DL, Boluarte TA. The emotional impact of medical error involvement on physicians: a call for leadership and organisational accountability. *Swiss Med Wkly.* 2009;139(1-2):9-15.
30. Miller L. Intrapartum fetal monitoring: liability and documentation. *Clin Obstet Gynecol.* 2011;54(1):50-55.
31. Pettker CM. Systematic approaches to adverse events in obstetrics, Part I: event identification and classification. *Semin Perinatol.* 2017;41(3):151-155.
32. PressGaney. The HPI SEC & SSER patient safety measurement guide. 2021. https://info.pressganey.com/e-books-research/the-hpi-sec-sser-patient-safety-measurement-system-for-healthcare. Accessed November 18, 2023.
33. Sentinel Event Policy and Procedures. https://www.jointcommission.org/resources/sentinel-event/sentinel-event-policy-and-procedures/. Accessed August 8, 2024.
34. National Quality Form. List of SREs. https://www.qualityforum.org/Topics/SREs/List_of_SREs.aspx. Accessed November 11, 2023.
35. Pettker CM. Systematic approaches to adverse events in obstetrics, Part II: event analysis and response. *Semin Perinatol.* 2017; 41(3):156-160.
36. RCA2. *Improving Root Cause Analyses and Actions to Prevent Harm.* National Patient Safety Foundation; 2015.
37. The Joint Commission. Framework for Root Cause Analysis and Corrective Actions. 2017. https://www.jcrinc.com/assets/1/7/Appendix_Framework_for_RCA_and_Corrective_Actions.docx. Accessed November 11, 2023.
38. Fein SP, Hilborne LH, Spiritus EM, et al. The many faces of error disclosure: a common set of elements and a definition. *J Gen Intern Med.* 2007;22(6):755-761.
39. Helmchen LA, Richards MR, McDonald TB. How does routine disclosure of medical error affect patients' propensity to sue and their assessment of provider quality? Evidence from survey data. *Med Care.* 2010;48(11):955-961.
40. Kachalia A, Kaufman SR, Boothman R, et al. Liability claims and costs before and after implementation of a medical error disclosure program. *Ann Intern Med.* 2010;153(4):213-221.
41. Alfirevic Z, Gyte GML, Cuthbert A, Devane D. Continuous cardiotocography (CTG) as a form of electronic fetal monitoring (EFM) for fetal assessment during labour. *Cochrane Database Syst Rev.* 2017;2:CD006066.

Index

Page numbers followed by "*f*" indicate figures; those followed by "*t*" indicate tables.